HEALTHCARE
EXECUTIVE
COMPENSATION

A GUIDE *for* LEADERS *and* TRUSTEES

HEALTHCARE EXECUTIVE COMPENSATION

A GUIDE *for* LEADERS *and* TRUSTEES

DAVID A. BJORK

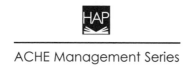

ACHE Management Series

16   15   14   13   12   5   4   3   2   1

Library of Congress Cataloging-in-Publication Data
Bjork, David A. (David Albert), 1947-
   Healthcare executive compensation : a guide for leaders and trustees / David A. Bjork.
      p. cm.
   Includes bibliographical references and index.
   ISBN 978-1-56793-424-3 (alk. paper)
   1. Health services administrators–Salaries, etc.   I. Title.
   RA971.3.B5187 2012
   331.2'81362173–dc23

                              2011046418

The paper used in this publication meets the minimum requirements of American National Standard for Information Sciences—Permanence of Paper for Printed Library Materials, ANSI Z39.48-1984. ♾™

Acquisitions editor: Janet Davis; Project manager: Joyce Dunne; Cover designer: Scott Miller; Layout: Fine Print, Ltd.

Found an error or a typo? We want to know! Please e-mail it to hap1@ache.org, and put "Book Error" in the subject line.

For photocopying and copyright information, please contact Copyright Clearance Center at www.copyright.com or at (978) 750–8400.

Health Administration Press
A division of the Foundation of the American
   College of Healthcare Executives
One North Franklin Street, Suite 1700
Chicago, IL 60606–3529
(312) 424–2800

Brief Contents

Detailed Contents

Foreword

As this foreword is being written, the Occupy Wall Street movement has spread from New York to other major cities throughout the United States. While initially vague in its mission, the movement quickly became a lightning rod for outrage over corporate greed, the growing income disparity between rich and poor, and joblessness, especially among college-educated youth. Coincidentally, union activity began surfacing for some of the same reasons, and labor unrest further contributed to the momentum of this larger movement. Hence, it should be no surprise that executive compensation has drawn the attention of the news media and the unions. With this book, we are fortunate to have a timely and well-researched volume on executive compensation to guide not-for-profit board members and their CEOs in developing and implementing an intelligent, balanced, and defensible executive compensation program.

Unlike other books on executive compensation, this is not a how-to book or technical manual written by attorneys. Rather, it is written by a highly respected and seasoned consultant who has worked in not-for-profit healthcare organizations for 30 years. Dr. David Bjork has heard the debates at board and compensation committee meetings and is intimately knowledgeable about the complexities of the Internal Revenue Service regulations governing not-for-profit, charitable organizations. He also understands how to work with the press regarding stories related to executive pay.

This book will be valuable for compensation committee members as they wrestle with decisions about executive pay and as they explain their decisions to the board, medical staff, press, and public. It will be even more valuable to board members who only have for-profit and public company experience and deal primarily with shareholders.

CEOs will find this book useful as they help their compensation committee balance the public's concerns over the level of executive compensation and the critical need to pay enough to recruit and retain talented leaders who have the skills and leadership traits necessary to successfully lead these enterprises. Much of what we read about executive pay is written by people who do not understand how difficult it is to recruit and retain talented executives and to manage healthcare organizations.

Unlike their for-profit colleagues with equity positions and stock options, most not-for-profit healthcare executives I know do not expect to get rich from their professions, but they do expect to be compensated at a competitive level with their not-for-profit peers. Striking this balance is one of the challenges confronting the compensation committee.

Dr. Bjork has an easy-to-read, conversational way of addressing both sides of an issue—with a balanced, unbiased approach. He shares his wealth of knowledge in reinforcing such truths (and best practices) as the importance of transparency and integrity in the entire process, the independence of the compensation consultant, and the role of the board and the compensation committee in this key governance (not management) function.

I am confident that this book will provide the board and compensation committee members and the CEO the requisite knowledge and insights to undertake their respective responsibilities in a manner that will support their institutions' mission. It will also prepare them for the public scrutiny that will inevitably follow.

Brian E. Keeley
President and CEO
Baptist Health South Florida

Preface

I WAS DELIGHTED to get the opportunity to write this book for Health Administration Press, as I had been wanting to write it for a long time. It was an opportune time to write it, because of all the efforts over the past decade to reform executive pay practices and governance of executive pay, and because of the massive changes facing the healthcare field over the next decade. It is a much different book than it would have been had I written it ten years ago.

One of the best things to come out of governance reform is that trustees are now asking us why executive compensation is structured the way it is, instead of asking us what they should do. They're questioning the validity of traditional assumptions about executive pay, rather than approving whatever consultants or management recommends.

That's why this book is dedicated to two sets of mentors who have taught me to question almost everything I thought I knew about executive compensation: trustees such as George Cadman of Baptist Health South Florida, Steve Broidy and John Law of Cedars Sinai Health System, and Paul McKee and John Dubinsky of BJC HealthCare, who never stopped questioning what I told them, and CEOs such as Don Wegmiller, George Halvorson, and Pat Fry, who always had better ideas than I did and thereby pointed out the folly of believing that the best advice comes from benchmarks, standards, and best practices—or from consultants.

The book is a continuation of the discussions about executive compensation going on in boardrooms across the country. It recognizes that executive pay programs are changing, and what may have been the best way to do something even a few years ago is probably not the best way to do it in the future. It is intended to encourage trustees and CEOs to question past practices and find better ways of structuring pay and benefit programs.

Trustees are doing a remarkably good job wrestling with the issues they need to deal with in governing executive pay. They are striving to ensure that their executive compensation programs are appropriate for their institutions, a good use of resources, and respectful of community values.

CEOs are, by and large, equally intent on seeing that executive pay programs use resources wisely and effectively to promote good performance and support the organization's mission. They know that their organizations can't thrive unless they have a strong team of talented leaders. They understand that any funds spent on executive compensation can't be spent on clinical programs, but they also know that they can't deliver good clinical programs unless they spend enough on executive compensation to have a strong leadership team.

I have intentionally avoided reciting regulations about executive pay and benefits. They change frequently and are complicated enough that no one should rely on my explanation of them. Besides, the unfortunate effect of explicating these regulations has been that too much effort is invested in inventing elegant ways of working around constraints rather than straightforward ways of complying with them. If we all focus instead on simple solutions that executives and trustees can agree are satisfactory, even if not perfect, we can stop talking so much about executive pay and spend time more productively figuring out how to deliver better care at a lower cost.

Introduction

BOOKS ON EXECUTIVE compensation are typically reference manuals or how-to-do-it books. Many of them are technical texts written by consultants or attorneys to show CEOs, human resources executives, and compensation professionals how to design an executive compensation program or how to improve an existing program. Some older books tell CEOs what to ask for and how to get it; some newer books tell trustees how to do a better job governing executive compensation.

This book is not a how-to-do-it manual. It is a dialogue about executive compensation addressed to CEOs and boards of directors' compensation committees. It explores their concerns about compensation philosophy, the structure of the executive compensation program, the balance among its components, the emphasis on pay for performance, the challenges of governing executive compensation, and the challenges of defending executive compensation to the public.

The purpose of this book is to help CEOs and trustees understand why executive compensation programs are structured the way they are, how to make them more effective, how to reach better-informed decisions, and how to explain their decisions to the various stakeholders who are likely to question and challenge their decisions.

Trustees and CEOs of tax-exempt healthcare organizations are expected to explain why they pay their executives as much as they do, why they pay executives more than physicians, why they pay their executives more than public agencies do, why healthcare executives are paid more than their counterparts in privately owned businesses (those owned by the entrepreneur raising the question), and whether the money spent on executive compensation would not be better allocated to a service or product that is more central to the organization's tax-exempt mission.

So why are executives paid as much as they are paid? And why are executive compensation programs structured the way they are structured?

DETERMINANTS OF EXECUTIVE PAY

Four principal factors determine executive pay. The two most important are interrelated: the amount of responsibility inherent in the executive position and the size of the organization in which the executive works. These factors reflect the ideas, respectively, that jobs with more responsibility should be paid more than jobs with less responsibility and that management jobs in a large organization entail more responsibility than the same jobs in a smaller organization.

The third most important factor in determining pay is the organization's compensation philosophy. Few organizations intentionally keep pay below average. Many aim to pay close to average, and just as many intentionally aim to pay well above average.

Performance, the fourth factor, has less impact than the other three. Variable pay or incentive compensation is not a big component of executive pay in tax-exempt organizations. As a result, total compensation does not vary much from year to year, and no convincing evidence indicates that better-performing organizations pay more than others.

PURPOSE OF AN EXECUTIVE COMPENSATION PROGRAM

Organizations commonly explain their executive compensation programs in terms of a threefold purpose:

1. To help recruit and retain the leaders the organization needs for success
2. To motivate executives to meet the organization's most important goals
3. To reward executives for their roles in making the organization successful

The explanation is adequate but does not answer the question "Why so much?" and it obscures the challenges organizations face in finding the appropriate balance between multiple, often conflicting goals. The explanation for a pay program for nurses, for example, or for the workforce as a whole, would include keeping the cost of the program affordable and reasonable—that is, paying no more than necessary to obtain and keep the talent needed.

Because organizations have only one incumbent in each executive role, however, and because these are leadership roles that shape the success of the organization as a whole, CEOs and trustees are more concerned with paying enough to recruit and retain the right people than with controlling the overall cost of the executive payroll. And when they want to control the overall cost of the executive payroll, they generally do so by limiting the number of executive positions, rather than by limiting pay for individual executives.

As hospitals and health systems struggle to find the resources needed to support clinical programs, pay employees competitively, and improve the health of the community they serve, they should aim to explain their executive compensation program in a way that acknowledges constraints and conflicting goals, such as multiple demands on limited resources, expectations that all employees be treated fairly, respect for community values, and regulatory limits on executive pay in tax-exempt charitable organizations. Acknowledging these constraints and conflicting goals can help CEOs and trustees make better decisions about executive compensation and defend the decisions they make.

IMPACT OF TURNOVER AND EXTERNAL RECRUITING ON EXECUTIVE PAY

Considering more than 5,000 hospitals are operating in the United States, executives have ample opportunity for career advancement. Some change jobs every few years. This turnover provides plenty of occasions for employers to decide how much to pay the next incumbent or find out what it costs to hire the right person for the job.

More often than not, employers pay the next incumbent as much as or more than the last incumbent. If they recruit externally, they find out what other organizations are paying experienced executives. If they choose an external candidate, they often find they have to pay significantly more than they paid the last incumbent.

If they promote an internal candidate, they may start her at a lower salary than the last incumbent was paid, but they rarely decrease the salary range and generally bring her up to the middle of the range within a few years.

When a good executive receives an offer from another hospital and the employer wants to retain the executive, the employer often offers a higher salary. When CEOs and trustees know an executive is getting calls from recruiters, they may increase the executive's pay or institute a retention incentive to keep the executive from leaving.

The dynamics of the labor market also drive pay upward. Executives learn that they can increase their pay by moving to another organization. CEOs and trustees learn that they need to keep pay competitive to retain talented executives. They also learn that it can cost more to hire a replacement than to hold onto the current incumbent.

IMPACT OF NOT-FOR-PROFIT STATUS ON EXECUTIVE PAY

Owners of private businesses know how to control costs. If they pay someone more than necessary, it comes out of their profits. If the business is a sole proprietorship, it comes out of the owner's own pocket.

Executives of firms with publicly traded stock know how to control costs, too, as paying more than necessary can reduce their gains on stock options.

Not-for-profit hospitals and health systems need to control costs as well, but neither the trustees nor the CEO lose much if they pay an executive more than necessary. They have little reason to constrain growth in executive pay because they have no ownership stake in the profits of the organization.

IMPACT OF GOVERNANCE ON EXECUTIVE PAY

Executive compensation is shaped by trustees as they set policies, decide whom to hire as CEO, adopt incentive plans and executive benefits, and approve employment agreements. With no ownership stake in the hospital or health system, trustees are often more focused on retaining executives and maintaining morale in the executive suite than on controlling the cost of executive compensation. The trustees are volunteers, after all, and do not want to lose good leaders to better paying jobs if they can retain them by paying them well.

Trustees generally want to keep pay competitive because they want to be able to recruit and retain experienced, high-performing executives. They often set a policy of paying executives well above average to make it easier to recruit and retain talented leaders. Trustees typically defer to recruiters when deciding what to pay a new CEO, and they have little reason to engage in hard-nosed bargaining. They generally defer to consultants in deciding how much to increase salaries or contribute to executive retirement plans to keep them competitive.

More often than not, trustees want an exceptionally good leadership team to make their organization exceptionally good. That desire often leads to decisions to position pay above average to make it easier to recruit and retain first-rate leaders.

Trustees tend to regard CEOs as peers, not employees. CEOs, after all, are also trustees and effectively lead the board in most areas, even though they do not chair the board. Trustees tend to follow the lead of the CEO in most areas because the CEO knows more about running a healthcare organization than trustees do. Trustees socialize with the CEO. They have a hard time maintaining an arms'-length relationship with the CEO when it comes to setting executive compensation because they do not maintain an arms'-length relationship with the CEO on most other matters. As long as trustees are reasonably satisfied with performance, they have a hard time saying no to the CEO.

IMPACT OF INFORMATION ON EXECUTIVE PAY

One of the most important determinants of executive pay is information about how much executives are paid at other institutions. The information is readily accessible in published surveys, magazine articles, IRS Form 990, and the compilation of Form 990s on the Internet at www.guidestar.com. Compensation committees hire consultants to provide the information, then act on it by increasing salaries to keep them at the intended level specified in the board's policy on executive compensation. Executives look at Form 990s from other organizations and expect to be paid as much as their counterparts at those organizations. Human resources staff buy surveys to determine how to keep pay competitive.

Little real arms'-length bargaining on pay in executive compensation takes place, even when hospitals hire new executives. Even then, boards and CEOs depend on recruiters, consultants, or human resources staff to tell them how much they should expect to pay, and that information determines starting pay as much as what the recruit requests.

IMPACT OF REGULATIONS ON EXECUTIVE PAY

Regulations pertaining to executive pay are generally intended to limit pay, or at least discourage pay above a certain level or limit the way pay and benefits can be delivered. Regulations have unanticipated effects, however, and the abundance of professionals who advise boards and executives on compensation, taxation, and financial planning ensures an abundance of creative responses to many of these regulations.

Executive compensation in the tax-exempt environment is subject to the following regulations:

1. Any compensation earned is subject to tax, and tax is due when the compensation is definitively earned and no longer subject to contingencies or risks of forfeiture.
2. Any compensation paid by a tax-exempt organization to a trustee, an officer, or a key employee must be disclosed to the public on the organization's Form 990.
3. A tax-exempt charity may not give any portion of the organization's revenues, income, or charitable assets to a private individual (known as private inurement) and may not pay an insider (anyone in a position to exercise substantial influence over the affairs of the organization) more than fair market value for services rendered.

   Because this regulation was difficult to enforce (the only penalty was revocation of tax-exempt status), Congress added a fourth regulation (see below) that made it possible to punish private inurement with penalties known as intermediate sanctions.
4. Intermediate sanctions regulations (Internal Revenue Code § 4958) allow the Internal Revenue Service (IRS) to require executives (and other "disqualified persons"—trustees, officers, and others in a position to exercise substantial influence over the affairs of the organization) who have been paid more than fair market value to repay the excess benefit, pay a fine of 25 percent of the excess, and pay an additional penalty of 200 percent of the excess amount if they do not repay the excess benefit and the fine within the tax year. It also allows the IRS to impose a smaller fine on anyone (executives or trustees) who knowingly approved the excess benefit.

The first regulation has led to an enormous investment of time and effort to find and promote ways to defer taxation or to deliver compensation or benefits in ways that avoid taxation altogether and to define contingencies and risks of forfeiture that almost ensure payment.

The second, the requirement to disclose compensation on Form 990, has led some organizations to eliminate forms of compensation they would rather not report to the public, such as payment of bonuses to cover executives' taxes on certain benefits or perquisites. But it has also led to a lot of effort to find ways to deliver compensation that would not need to be reported or that could be reported at less than the true cost. It has fed executives' impressions that they are underpaid by giving them access to information on higher-paid jobs; led the public to believe executives are paid more than they are, by requiring that certain elements of compensation be reported twice; and persuaded compensation committees to raise pay more than they otherwise would, by presenting compensation information in a way that is easy to misunderstand and misuse.

The prohibition of private inurement has generally kept tax-exempt organizations from introducing compensation programs similar to stock options and profit-sharing arrangements for executives, but it has also led to designing programs that disguise what would otherwise be gifts or a share of the organization's income as compensation or benefits earned through service.

The fourth regulation, with its threat of intermediate sanctions, has encouraged trustees to keep compensation within the bounds of competitive practice (what other organizations pay executives in comparable positions) and given CEOs and trustees a persuasive reason to say no to requests for higher compensation. However, it has also led to a lot of work finding isolated instances of higher compensation to help justify unusually high pay and developing compelling rationales for paying someone above the high end of the usual range for a job. It has also changed the definition of reasonable pay from appropriate pay for the job or for services rendered to the highest level of pay that can be justified.

The regulations have not been effective constraints on executive compensation. Their biggest impact has been in changing the way pay is structured, delivered, and rationalized.

CHALLENGES OF MANAGING PERFORMANCE IN TAX-EXEMPT HEALTHCARE ORGANIZATIONS

Pay for healthcare executives is as high as it is because the jobs are unusually difficult and few people can handle them well. Most executive jobs in healthcare require specialized knowledge and skills that can be developed only by spending years working in healthcare.

Many critics of executive compensation assume that the jobs of healthcare executives are easy enough that plenty of people could perform them well. Some hospital trustees who run their own businesses assume that they could run the hospital just as well as they could their own businesses.

These critics overlook two facts about hospitals. They are extraordinarily complex organizations, and their margins for error are extraordinarily thin. Operating margins (operating profit as a percentage of revenues) are thinner than in most other businesses, making it difficult to break even and more difficult to earn enough to replace aging facilities and equipment. Hospitals' customers—doctors and patients—want and expect more service than they or anyone else is willing to pay for. The cost of an error is greater in healthcare than in most other businesses—a patient's death, a lifetime disability, or a large malpractice liability.

The hospital has a huge staff and operates 24 hours a day, 365 days a year. It needs to recruit constantly to fill open positions, and it depends more than most organizations on new employees, part-time employees, and temporary workers. Healthcare differs from virtually every other business in that few of its core activities are routine, systematized, or regularly repeated. Almost all patient care activities need to be tailored to the patient: her health, condition, medical history, drug regimen, age, and other factors.

Managing operations in an environment in which the demand for services is totally unpredictable and changes by the minute is harder than running a grocery store, an auto dealership, or an insurance brokerage. Managing a hospital is more difficult than managing a bank or a manufacturing firm or administering a school district, a police force, or the county's operations. Because healthcare administration requires exceptionally good management, interpersonal, and political skills, healthcare executives are paid well.

ORGANIZATION AND CONTENTS OF THE BOOK

Chapter Highlights

Chapter 1: Issues in Executive Compensation. Addressed in this chapter are important issues concerning executive compensation in tax-exempt healthcare organizations: why executive pay is so high, whether it is too high, how to make it more effective, and how to govern it well. Also discussed are pay for performance, causes of inflation in executive pay, and the difficulty of striking the right balance between competitiveness and fairness in an environment of limited resources and narrow margins.

Chapter 2: Compensation Philosophy. Compensation philosophy is the foundation for decisions made about executive compensation. The chapter highlights the importance of the peer group to be used in evaluating the competitiveness and reasonableness of executive compensation and in determining the level of compensation needed to attract and retain talented leaders. In addition, it addresses decisions related to pay for performance; the balance between current and deferred compensation; the role of benefits in a well-rounded compensation package; and the importance of compensation philosophy in explaining the program to stakeholders—executives, trustees, physicians, regulators, the press, and the public.

Chapter 3: Determining the Market Value of Executive Positions. This chapter discusses the methods and techniques compensation professionals use to determine the market value of executive positions. It explores the challenges involved in identifying a reasonable estimate of market value and the need to study the data to determine if it is reliable.

Chapter 4: Getting Base Pay Right: Salary, Salary Structure, and Salary Administration. The principles of salary administration are discussed, as are the issues involved in determining appropriate salaries for executives and explaining the decisions to executives and trustees. The chapter also addresses the challenges involved in shaping and satisfying executives' expectations, maintaining defensible pay relationships, and signaling to employees that executives are paid appropriately.

Chapter 5: Incentive Compensation. The principles of designing and administering incentive compensation plans—both annual and long term—and the challenges involved in making incentive plans effective are the subjects of this chapter. It also explains trustees' role in shaping and controlling incentive compensation plans.

Chapter 6: Benefits. The issues involved in designing, evaluating, and governing executive benefit plans are explored, including the reasons for providing each type of benefit and the relationship between all-employee benefits and supplemental benefits. The chapter also discusses the role of benefits in a well-rounded compensation package, the usefulness of retirement benefits in retaining executives, and the public relations risks inherent in providing large retirement packages to executives. It touches briefly on the regulations that give rise to and limit supplemental benefits for executives.

Chapter 7: Perquisites. This chapter addresses the issues involved in deciding whether or not to provide perquisites to executives—the reasons for providing them, the reasons for avoiding them, the trend to eliminate them, and the difficulty of defending them as an appropriate use of resources.

Chapter 8: Employment Contracts and Severance. In this chapter we discuss the issues involved in structuring employment agreements and severance policies—the advantages and disadvantages of using employment agreements, the relationship between severance and contract duration, terms for contract renewal and extensions, and the connection between employment agreements and contractual arrangements for supplemental benefits. It identifies the typical elements of an executive contract; explains their purpose; and focuses on severance, the principal compensatory element of a contract.

Chapter 9: Governance of Executive Compensation. The board's role in overseeing executive compensation is explored in this chapter. It identifies best practices in governing executive compensation, the rationale for them, and the relationship between the CEO and the board in shaping and administering executive compensation. In addition, it explains why boards are now exerting more control in governing executive compensation, highlights the most widespread weaknesses in governance practices, and identifies steps every board should take to strengthen its process for governing executive compensation.

Chapter 10: Addressing Public Perceptions About Executive Compensation. Tax-exempt organizations, their boards, and their executives face special challenges related to public attitudes toward executive compensation. This chapter helps guide boards and executives in successfully responding to criticism and overcoming skepticism about executive pay.

Best Practices in . . .

Most chapters end with a set of best practices pertaining to the topic covered in the chapter. They are addressed to trustees as advice on governing executive compensation and to CEOs as advice on managing compensation for other executives.

Select Terminology

Throughout the book the following terms are central to understanding the text.

Expected total compensation: Level of total compensation an employer intends or expects to pay, on average, over time and across all executives, for on-plan performance (meeting all or most of the goals set for the year).

Opportunity: Potential to earn compensation at a certain level, such as maximum incentive opportunity of 20 percent of salary, or enough incentive opportunity to reach the 75th percentile of total compensation. Compensation opportunity can be expressed either as maximum opportunity (the most that can be paid when all goals are met or exceeded) or as an expected amount of pay (the average or typical level of compensation paid over a ten-year period for good performance). Often used to describe incentive opportunity; sometimes used to describe total compensation.

Percentage: When referring to incentive opportunity, percentage always refers to salary, as in "He was paid a bonus of 20 percent of salary." When referring to benefits, it usually means percentage of salary but may refer to percentage of pay (meaning salary plus bonus).

Percentile: Position relative to a data set; that is, position above a certain percentage of the other data, as in 90th percentile, meaning above 90 percent of the data points in the data set. For example, if General Hospital positions salaries at the 50th percentile of its peer group and maximum total compensation opportunity at the 75th percentile, its salary range midpoints fall at the middle of all the salaries in its peer group, below the higher half and above the lower half, and its maximum total compensation opportunity is set above the total compensation paid by 75 percent of its peers but below the total paid by the highest-paying 25 percent of its peers.

Positioning/position: Intention to pay at a certain percentile, on average, across all jobs and over time. Positioning salaries at median means the intention to set the midpoint of the salary range for each job at median and to pay salaries that are, on average, approximately at median. It does not mean the intention to pay everyone at median. Individuals can be paid anywhere within the salary range, which for executives typically runs from 80 percent to 120 percent of the salary range midpoint.

CHAPTER 1

Issues in Executive Compensation

CRITICS OF EXECUTIVE compensation raise difficult questions: Why is executive pay so high? *Is* it too high? How can the executive compensation program be made more effective? How can trustees do a better job governing it?

To maintain support for tax exemption and publicly funded health programs such as Medicare and Medicaid, trustees and public relations staff of not-for-profit healthcare organizations need to be prepared to address these questions. Indeed, anyone who is regularly involved with executive compensation—CEOs, consultants, members of the board of directors' compensation committee, heads of human resources—has a responsibility to respond to these questions knowledgeably and thoughtfully.

Organizations approach decisions about executive compensation in their own ways, and the way an organization does so depends on its circumstances, what it can afford, and the values and beliefs that drive its decisions about executive pay. Trustees and CEOs make decisions they think are best for their organizations. We give trustees responsibility for governing executive compensation for precisely this reason—to make sure the decisions are made by wise community leaders who know the organization and its circumstances and values well, and who can be trusted to make informed decisions in the best interests of their organizations.

ARE EXECUTIVES PAID TOO MUCH?

The short answer is no. Executives are not overpaid. If they were, employers would not willingly pay them as much as they do. And when executives change jobs, their new employer would not pay them as much as or more than their previous employer did. There are exceptions, of course, due to special circumstances, but the question is whether executives as a class are overpaid.

But this short answer does not address the emotional intensity associated with the question, which arises from its moral, political, sociological, and economic dimensions. It is not one question, but at least four:

1. Are executives paid more than they should be paid?
2. Why should executives of organizations that are tax exempt and dependent on public funding for Medicare and Medicaid be paid as much as they are?
3. Why should executives be paid so much more than other employees?
4. Are executives paid more than they are worth?

People who are paid a lot less than executives—that is, most people—are likely to think executives are overpaid; they have a hard time imagining that a job or a person can be worth so much. The opinion usually comes with a moral veneer—no one *should* be paid that much. Sometimes the opinion is more explicit—it's wrong or immoral to pay a person so much.

Much of the deep-seated resentment of executive pay in the healthcare field can be attributed to the fact that tax-exempt hospitals are community institutions paid for in large part by taxpayers. It is colored by the opinion that we all have a right to healthcare services—so no one should get rich off them.

In the political sphere, the resentment takes the form of proposed limits on executive pay and other regulations. In some states, for example, no executive of a public hospital can be paid more than the governor. In others, legislators propose limiting executive pay in hospitals to a multiple of average pay for other employees. The US Congress and state legislatures conduct hearings, launch investigations, and express outrage against hospitals for allegedly abusing the public trust. Since 1996, federal law and regulation have threatened to impose fines, or "intermediate sanctions," on executives of tax-exempt hospitals and health systems if they are deemed overpaid, and on trustees if they agree to excessive executive pay.

High compensation for healthcare executives feeds social discontent over the widening disparity in wealth and income in the United States. It also drives boardroom debates about the extent to which executives should be well paid while the hospital is trimming costs everywhere else and asking employees to pay a greater share of the cost of healthcare and retirement benefits.

But labor market forces drive pay for executives, just as they do for other employees. Just as doctors are paid differently than nurses, because their jobs are different and represent a different segment of the labor market, executives are paid differently than doctors and nurses. Hospitals may be tax-exempt charities serving the public good, but they are still big, complicated businesses with narrow profit margins, and they need talented executives to keep them strong. Tax exemption and public funding for Medicare and Medicaid have no bearing on what it costs to recruit and retain executives. Each of the 6,000-plus hospitals in the United States needs a group of executives, creating a dynamic market for executive talent that determines how much executives are paid. There is no rational basis for the view that executives should not be paid as much as they are paid, just a personal attitude, generally held by someone who is paid less.

The intrinsic worth of an individual may be impossible to determine, but the intrinsic value of a job can be quantified. Economists and most workers judge the value of a job by how much it pays. A job is worth what an employer is willing to pay an employee to do it, or what an employee is willing to accept as payment for the job. Virtually no one doubts that principle—except when it comes to executive jobs.

Hospitals and health systems continually look for ways to reduce their costs. When they come across jobs that cost more than they are worth, they eliminate the jobs and either eliminate the work, redistribute it to other employees, or outsource it to cheaper labor. They view executive jobs the same way. When hospitals and health systems find an executive job that seems to cost more than it is worth, they eliminate it if they can and redistribute the work to other managers. The one action they cannot take is outsource the work to a cheaper labor force, because there is no cheaper labor force capable of doing the job well.

Therefore, executives must be worth what they are paid, because employers keep them on the job and willingly continue to pay whatever they are paid. Even when they leave or lose one well-paid job, they can usually find other employers who are willing to pay them just as much as or more than they were paid in their previous jobs.

WHY ARE EXECUTIVES PAID SO MUCH?

Common answers to this question are, "We have to pay that much or they wouldn't work for us," "We just pay the going rate, the same as everyone else," or "That's what it costs to hire someone to do the job." Of course, if the question were that easy to answer, executive pay would not be criticized as often as it is.

But those answers are untrue. Most executives would not quit their job if they were paid a bit less—at least not until they accepted a better paying job. Many hospitals and health systems pay more than the going rate, and those that intentionally position pay above the median cannot claim that they only pay the going rate. Most organizations pay more than they would have to pay to hire someone to do the job; people who could perform the job reasonably well and who would be willing to do so for less than the person chosen are in ample supply.

The dynamics of decision making on executive pay differ from the dynamics of other purchasing decisions, and they often lead organizations to pay more than they need to. Boards and CEOs do not let cost stand in the way when they are recruiting executives. They often decide whom they want to hire before they begin to discuss pay. They sometimes come around to admitting that they cannot afford to hire their first choice, but they just as often end up paying whatever it takes to get their first choice to take the job.

Most discussion of executive pay is based on the assumption that pay is set by labor market dynamics. This ignores the fact that most pay decisions affect what incumbents are paid, not what external recruits are paid. Employers voluntarily give executives raises every year. They voluntarily enhance benefits and perquisites from time to time and sometimes increase incentive opportunities for no compelling reason.

Three principal factors drive executive compensation to today's level:

1. The intent to hire the best talent available for the job
2. The intent to pay competitively enough to retain incumbents
3. The intent to pay above average in expectation of above-average performance

The intentions begin with the board's decision to hire exceptionally talented, highly experienced executives and continue with the board's willingness to pay the salary required to hire and retain them. External recruiting tends to drive pay up. When organizations recruit seasoned executives from other, similarly sized organizations, they generally need to pay well above average, more than they would need to pay to promote an internal candidate.

The intent to pay competitively drives up salary even for internally promoted executives and incumbents, however. Organizations whose policy is to pay at median increase pay faster than the rate of inflation for any executive paid less than median, and organizations whose policy is to pay at the 75th percentile continuously increase executives' pay to stay ahead of the pack.

The intent to pay above average in expectation of above-average performance drives up pay for all executives, whether or not they are performing at an above-average level. Standard salary administration practices call for bringing salaries up to the intended level within a few years, as long as the incumbent performs reasonably well. Furthermore, incentive plans tend to reward institutional performance more than individual performance, so even average performers end up being paid above average.

The reasons executives are paid as much as they are have more to do with logic and belief than necessity:

- Organizations pay supervisors more than they pay their direct reports. They pay managers more than supervisors, department heads more than managers, executives more than department heads, and CEOs more than other executives. Organizations believe that higher-level jobs carry more responsibility than lower-level jobs do and therefore warrant higher pay.

- Following the same logic, bigger organizations tend to pay more than smaller organizations pay. Executives in bigger organizations have more responsibility than their counterparts in smaller organizations and therefore warrant more pay. Most US organizations follow this logic, as do most consultants who advise boards on executive compensation. The results of most executive compensation surveys reflect it as well.

- Hospitals are big organizations—bigger than most other organizations in small and midsize communities—so hospital executives have unusually big responsibilities. In many communities, hospitals are the biggest employer and often the biggest business, as measured by operating expenses. If only for that reason, one should expect hospitals to pay more than the smaller businesses in the same town do.

- Hospital executives' jobs are unusually complex and challenging due to the nature of a hospital's services, the risks entailed in making mistakes, the regulations governing healthcare, and the difficulty of collecting payment for the services provided. So healthcare organizations hire experienced people, who have worked long enough in healthcare to know what needs to be done.

- Boards want highly qualified executives managing their hospitals to mitigate the risks involved in providing clinical care in a heavily regulated and litigious environment. They want to avoid relying on the less experienced executives they would be able to hire if they were to pay less.

- Boards believe they need to pay at median—the 50th percentile—or above to attract high-quality executives, so they intentionally position salary ranges at or above median and offer competitive levels of incentive opportunity and benefits. Almost every organization adopts such a policy and commits to paying more for executive talent than half of its peers—those paying below the 50th percentile—and trying to remain reasonably competitive with those that pay above the median.

- Boards want to maintain good morale on the executive team. They believe they can do so by paying the CEO well, making sure that she is satisfied with her pay, and generally acceding to her requests for raises and bonuses for other executives.

In their book *Pay Without Performance: The Unfulfilled Promise of Executive Compensation*, Bebchuk and Fried (2004, ix) claim that a structural flaw in governance—an imbalance in power—gives CEOs too much influence over their own pay and impedes the effective governance of executive pay. "The absence of effective arm's-length [bargaining with executives over compensation]—not temporary mistakes or lapses of judgment—has been the primary source of problematic compensation arrangements."

While apologists for executive pay have attempted to discredit Bebchuk and Fried's argument (see, e.g., Kay and Van Putten 2007), anyone who has experienced compensation committee meetings appreciates the predicament Bebchuk and Fried's argument represents. Directors are expected to make decisions in the best interests of the corporation, the shareholders, or, in the case of a local not-for-profit organization, the community. When determining executive compensation, however, they often seem to put executives' interests ahead of those of the organization, unless the best interests of the organization are to maintain harmony in the boardroom and morale in the executive suite. Why else would directors agree to pay bonuses to cover executives' tax obligations on benefits and perquisites, eliminate or relax vesting requirements on supplemental retirement benefits, lend the hospital's money to executives to finance deferred compensation in a split-dollar insurance scheme, or adopt countless other approaches to delaying or minimizing tax obligations on deferred compensation?

As long as they are pleased with performance, directors tend to be more generous with CEOs' compensation than CEOs are with the pay of their direct reports. Many committees tend to approve whatever pay or benefits the CEO recommends for other executives because they are accustomed to following the CEO's leads in most areas and regard decisions on pay for other executives as management's turf, not the board's. Directors often regard the CEO as a peer (the CEO is usually a director, too, and due to technical competence, the real leader of the board in most areas), so committees often find it difficult to maintain an arms'-length relationship with the CEO in governing executive compensation.

Executives are paid as much as they are paid because they are in great demand. Hospitals all want to recruit and retain outstanding leaders, and they are willing to pay well to get them and keep them.

DO CONSULTANTS DRIVE UP EXECUTIVE PAY?

Consultants are not responsible for the continuing escalation in executive pay—at least not in tax-exempt healthcare organizations, and at least not now—since boards began to exert more control over executive compensation five to ten years ago. Consultants generally strive to avoid any action that inflates market values or promotes inflation in executive pay. They work for the compensation committee, not for management, and they have an obligation to be as objective as possible in providing data and advice to committees. Nonetheless, the continuing escalation in executive pay is often attributed to consultants.

The reason is that they provide the data that committees use in determining salary increases. Because market values rise every year, analyses invariably show that salaries established the year before are now less competitive than they were when they were set.

But it is the compensation committee, not the consultant, that wants to keep pay competitive. The board has set a policy of positioning pay at median or above, and the committee's role is partly to keep pay at the intended level. The compensation committee asks, "What will it take to keep salaries competitive?" If salaries are already competitive, the consultant replies, "You will need to increase salaries by 3 percent to keep up with the market."

In years past, boards allowed CEOs to choose their own consultants, and consultants knew that the way to maintain the relationship was to keep the CEO satisfied with the results of their work. While consultants understood that their real client was the corporation, the nature of the relationship with the CEO sometimes trumped their adherence to professional standards.

Over the past decade, however, boards and their compensation committees have reclaimed control of the consultant relationship. They now issue requests for proposal periodically and sometimes intentionally change consulting firms every few years to keep consultants from developing a close relationship with management. Many committees now routinely ask their consultants to declare their loyalty to the committee.

Consultants have generally encouraged this change by promoting best practices in governing executive compensation. Most consultants have come to understand that they must demonstrate their objectivity and independence to the committee and guard against being manipulated by management.

Most of a consultant's work is straightforward and technical—collecting and analyzing market data, comparing the client's pay to market data, summarizing the analysis, drawing the obvious conclusions, and offering the obvious recommendations. A typical report amounts to little more than a lot of tables and charts, some observations dressed up as conclusions (e.g., salaries for your executives are, on average, 3 percent below median), and some perfunctory recommendations (e.g., to maintain that market position, you should increase salaries about 3 percent).

Consultants exercise judgment throughout the process, however, in ways that affect their conclusions. They generally know that certain segments of the healthcare industry pay better than others, and that pay levels are higher between Boston and Washington, D.C., and between San Francisco and Los Angeles than elsewhere in the country. They know that large organizations pay more than small ones do, that private institutions generally pay more than public ones do, and that urban hospitals pay more than rural ones do. They know that the more organizations they include in a peer group from a high-paying segment, the less competitive a client will look. Consultants sometimes define peer groups in ways that increase prevailing pay or benefit levels—but so do boards, and it is ultimately the board's responsibility to determine the appropriateness of the peer group.

Admittedly, several techniques that consultants use in gathering data tend to reinforce inflation in executive pay levels or even drive it up inappropriately. One technique assumes that hospitals and systems will continue to increase salaries the next year, as they have in the past, and builds an anticipated inflation factor into estimates of market value. Another compares an organization's size in the current year or the next year with other organizations' size in the past year. (Survey data are always retrospective, so participants' revenues or expenses are almost always last year's dimensions.) The technique with the greatest impact on pay levels, though, is using revenues or expenses, rather than a volume or activity metric, as the measure of organizational size, as charges and costs per unit of service tend to rise a bit every year.

Most economists, financial analysts, and consultants consider revenues and operating expenses good measures of the size of an organization or the scope of an executive position. In the health-care industry, however, the rate of inflation in costs and revenues raises questions about its appropriateness for that purpose. Trustees ask why a 10 percent increase in revenue or a 6 percent increase in operating costs should affect the value of executive jobs when the number of staffed beds, adjusted admissions, and employees has not increased. Why, in other words, should their success in getting better rates from payers mean they should pay their executives more?

Healthcare delivery is far more efficient today than it has been in the past, despite the inflation in costs. Much of the inflation results from the use of increasingly sophisticated equipment and supplies, more intensive interventions, better pharmaceuticals, and sicker patients. The notion that executive jobs in a hospital are worth no more today, on an inflation-adjusted basis, than they were ten years ago is likely wrong, because it assumes that the intensity level per patient is the same as it was ten years ago. Operating expenses may be as good and as appropriate a measure of relative size as we can find, given how weak the alternatives (staffed beds, adjusted admissions, full-time-equivalent employees) are.

On the other hand, two commonly used consulting techniques have the countervailing effect of reducing market value estimates. One uses bonuses or incentive awards earned last year and based on last year's lower salaries in calculating total compensation and in determining whether this year's total compensation opportunity is competitive. Another technique uses market values at the beginning of the year to set next year's salaries. The new salaries may be appropriately competitive on the day they are set but will gradually fall behind the market by the rate of inflation in salaries over the coming year. In the end, consultants have little influence on inflation in executive pay because—in tax-exempt hospitals and health systems, at least—inflation is no higher in executive pay than in pay for other employees.

DO COMPENSATION SURVEYS DRIVE INFLATION IN EXECUTIVE PAY?

Surveys, too, are often blamed for driving inflation in executive pay. But surveys merely convey information. The most important information a new survey conveys is how much salaries have increased over the past year and what the market values are this year, as opposed to what they were last year. The survey information itself has no effect on pay. It is trustees' and executives' commitment to keeping pay competitive, using the information that surveys convey, that drives inflation in executive pay.

Compensation surveys do a good job of showing the range of market pay practices, from the 25th to the 75th percentiles and sometimes from the 10th to the 90th percentiles. The range of market values for a job is so broad that even a salary at the 25th or 40th percentile is competitive, albeit not competitive with the top half of the market. But compensation committees rarely pay attention to the 25th or 40th percentile data. They only want to look at values at or above median. They are not looking for bargains or excuses to hold pay levels down. They are looking for reasons to move ahead with the anticipated regular annual salary increases most large employers deliver every year in the unending effort to keep pay competitive.

DOES EMPIRE BUILDING INCREASE EXECUTIVE PAY?

Some trustees, after watching their organizations expand and seeing the effect that growth has on executive pay, wonder whether executives try to increase the size of their organizations in a gambit to increase their pay. The growth of hospitals and health systems over the past few decades has increased prevailing pay levels for healthcare executives, providing the evidence critics need to make their argument that empire building is partly driven by its effect on executive pay.

Thirty years ago, most hospitals were independent; now, most belong to multihospital systems. In addition, hospitals are generally bigger and more complex than at any time in the past. Many small hospitals have closed and whatever volume they would have had has now been distributed to the hospitals that remain open; some hospitals have merged with others and consolidated their business; and the population is aging, driving hospitals to add capacity, after two decades of reducing capacity in the 1980s and 1990s. Even those hospitals that have not added beds have grown by adding outpatient services and increasing throughput—handling more admissions by shortening length of stay.

The impetus toward growth is less often empire building or executives' desire to increase their pay than a need to respond to external pressures to improve competitive position or economies of scale. Besides, the desire for growth comes as much from trustees as from executives. Trustees who are business executives believe that growth is essential for the health of a business. Businesses are either growing or waning, they believe, and only growing businesses can afford to invest in new programs that will position them for success in the future. By leading this effort to grow, executives have been acting exactly as they have been asked to act by their boards and by society as a whole. Now that they are leading bigger, more complex organizations, their jobs are more difficult, carry more responsibility, and seem to warrant more pay.

Yes, empire building may increase executive pay, but the increase is the result of growth and consolidation in the industry—not a deliberate ploy to increase executive pay.

HOW MUCH OF EXECUTIVE PAY IS RELATED TO PERFORMANCE?

Boards and executives defend executive compensation by pointing out how much of it is based on performance. The reality is that only a small portion of total compensation for executives of tax-exempt hospitals and health systems is tied to performance—except that executives cannot hold onto their jobs long if they do not perform well.

When we talk about pay for performance, we generally mean pay as a reward for current performance, or pay at risk in relation to current performance, not pay as the cumulative result of past performance. In other words, pay for performance essentially means incentive. Incentive compensation is typically about 30 percent of salary for CEOs of independent hospitals and systems and about 15 to 20 percent of salary for vice presidents. It amounts to only 20 percent of total compensation for CEOs and 10 percent to 14 percent of total compensation for most other executives. While not trivial, incentive compensation is not a significant portion of pay, and performance is not a major determinant of executive pay in not-for-profit healthcare organizations.

Furthermore, the portion attributable to incentive compensation is not highly variable—certainly not as variable in healthcare as in other industries. Incentive plans in not-for-profit healthcare organizations are generally designed to moderate the degree of variability in pay. Maximum opportunity is typically only half again as much as the target or expected value. Most incentive compensation plans are not structured as profit sharing, in which the size of a pool reserved for incentive awards varies directly with profits (the most variable and volatile measure of performance in any industry). Instead, most plans use balanced scorecards as their framework, whereby the size of awards is tied to five or more measures of performance. Several measures frequently used, such as patient satisfaction scores, are notably less variable than financial performance metrics. More important, tying awards to multiple performance measures makes awards less variable, as good performance on one measure offsets weaker performance on another.

Most organizations with executive incentive plans pay awards almost every year. Surveys show that in any given year, 80 percent or more of them pay awards, and those that pay awards only once in a rare while are counterbalanced by those that rarely miss paying awards. The consistency of incentive payouts from year to year is a function of the stability seen in volume of activity, operating expenses, reimbursement, patient satisfaction, and clinical quality. This stability is upset only when a serious disruption occurs, such as a strike, a recession, or a defection of a group of specialists.

HOW MUCH PAY SHOULD BE TIED TO PERFORMANCE?

Many trustees would like to see more pay tied to performance. Trustees who favor increasing the amount of pay at risk believe that incentive compensation promotes good performance and assume that increasing the amount of pay at risk will optimize performance. They are generally comfortable with increasing pay at risk because they are accustomed to seeing more pay at risk in their own companies than in the hospitals or health systems they govern. Sometimes they propose increasing pay at risk as an alternative to increasing salaries each year.

Most executives—healthcare and non-healthcare alike—do not favor putting more of their pay at risk, unless it is additional pay. Executives generally reject the idea that they perform better because of incentive compensation, as it implies they would perform poorly without it. They generally admit that they are intrinsically motivated and will perform well whether or not their pay reflects their performance. This does not mean they do not like incentive plans or want to abandon them, just that they view bonuses as appropriate reward and recognition for a job well done, rather than an incentive to perform better than they would otherwise. It also does not mean that they do not want more incentive opportunity—only that they do not want to put any part of their salary at risk.

In addition, they recognize that incentive plans are risky, and that putting too much pay at risk, or putting too much emphasis on one or two measures of performance, could have unfortunate unintended consequences—just as incentive opportunity in financial services can promote excessive risk taking.

Incentive plans engender an unnecessary level of friction and skepticism between trustees and management: Trustees think management sets goals too low and management thinks trustees set goals too high. Increasing the amount of pay at risk, executives suspect, would only increase the friction and skepticism.

Trustees who do not favor increasing the amount of pay at risk recognize that incentive compensation places a burden on them, too. Their approval of such plans means that when the large awards are paid, they must justify them to the public, medical staff, employees, or legislature and explain why total compensation varies dramatically from year to year. They recognize the difficulty in setting appropriate goals and dealing with externalities—events outside the control of management—and the effects of board-approved changes in plans and priorities. Increasing the amount of pay at risk only magnifies the challenges trustees face related to incentive compensation plans.

The utility of incentive compensation is in promoting discipline in planning and goal setting and in focusing attention on a few goals that are more important than the others. Putting no pay at risk, or too little, minimizes the need for management and the board to agree on plans and goals. Placing too much pay at risk raises the stakes to the point that negotiating skills and game-playing strategies can distort planning and goal setting.

The right amount of pay at risk is probably whatever it takes to fill the gap between salary and total cash compensation at the levels specified in the board's compensation philosophy. It is relatively modest if the compensation philosophy calls for positioning both salary and total cash compensation at median (or both at the 60th or 75th percentile). It is significantly more if the compensation philosophy calls for positioning salary at median and total cash compensation at the 65th or 75th percentile. Incentive opportunity is generally modest at tax-exempt healthcare organizations for a good reason—boards and executives have learned through experience how difficult it is to manage pay-at-risk programs.

WHY PAY RETENTION INCENTIVES WHEN EXECUTIVES ARE ALREADY PAID COMPETITIVELY?

Sometimes hospitals and health systems offer executives retention incentives—incentives to stay with the organization for a specified period. This type of incentive amounts to extra pay for staying—nothing else—on top of fully competitive pay for working and performing well.

The purpose of a retention incentive is to ensure management continuity and organizational stability by discouraging turnover at critical times. Occasionally a retention incentive is used in lieu of a signing bonus, a long-term incentive plan, or a supplemental retirement benefit.

The most common uses for retention incentives are to

- retain executives as long as they are needed during a merger and post-merger integration period;
- retain executives when the organization is facing a massive restructuring;
- retain candidates for the CEO position in the years directly preceding the current CEO's retirement;
- retain the leader of a large, expensive project until it is completed;
- persuade an executive to stay after her retirement benefit is fully vested; and
- retain a young, high-profile executive who is looking for promotion opportunity.

Board members generally do not favor retention incentives because they are not contingent on performance. Trustees rarely agree to introduce such incentives unless the board is concerned about losing executives at a time when the organization needs stable leadership or wants the CEO to stay longer than she otherwise might.

Retention incentives work. They are usually effective at retaining executives for a year or two, as long as the plans are rich enough to outweigh any salary increase and hiring bonus another employer might offer.

They may also be unnecessary, as the executives might stay anyway. But waiting until the risk becomes a catastrophe is not a smart approach, as by that time no action can be taken to mitigate the situation. For example, losing an information technology executive in the middle of a $50 million electronic health record implementation project can be a disaster; a retention incentive is a plan for avoiding that disaster. Even situations that may not end in disaster can benefit from having a retention incentive in place. Losing a strong internal candidate to succeed the current CEO, for example, may not be catastrophic, but it imposes risks that the organization might need to get along with no CEO for a while and that it might not be able to find an equally qualified candidate outside the organization.

Retention incentives are problematic, however, because they usually result in overpaying participants for a time. But because retention incentives typically last for only a year or two (no longer than five), the problem is short lived.

Once they have been paid, though, they become problematic in another way, as compensation drops by the value of the retention incentive. Executives may feel underpaid, and boards may encounter pressure to raise salaries, renew the retention incentive, or replace it with a permanent incentive plan.

WHY PAY SPECIAL BONUSES FOR COMPLETING ACQUISITIONS OR PROJECTS WHEN EXECUTIVES ARE ALREADY PAID COMPETITIVELY?

After completion of an acquisition or a major project, organizations may pay a special bonus to the executives who led the effort.

The special bonus serves to thank the executives for the extra work they did to ensure the project's success.

The rationale for paying the special bonus is that no part of the executive compensation program is intended to compensate executives for the extra work involved in the acquisition or special project; in other words, it was additional uncompensated work, not part of the jobs they were paid to do. That rationale presumes, of course, that executives' roles are defined in terms of keeping operations running smoothly, rather than improving operations, finding and making the most of opportunities to strengthen the organization, and leading change. That presumption is wrong, of course—competitive compensation already encompasses pay for these efforts.

The underlying premise of special bonuses is that the executives who led the acquisition or special project added value to the organization, and some of that value should be shared with them. This concept is borrowed from the for-profit sector, where such rewards are fairly common and executive pay programs are designed to share with executives any wealth they create for shareholders.

However, this premise is antithetical to the idea that tax-exempt charities are operated solely for the benefit of society and that no part of their earnings inure to the benefit of private individuals. Sharing with insiders a portion of the value gained from an acquisition could be considered private inurement unless the bonus paid is clearly appropriate for the work done, the work done was not already paid for in some other fashion, total compensation including the bonus is reasonable, and the bonus does not amount to a distribution of charitable assets. An especially damning aspect of special bonuses is that the organization has no obligation to pay them, unlike awards under a formal incentive plan. The deal is done, the project complete; only at this point does the CEO or a trustee suggest giving something away that belongs to the organization.

If the award were structured as a retention incentive tied to completion of the project, or if it were built into a formal annual or long-term incentive plan, the contractual structure would create an obligation to pay and render it a non-gift. The fact that such a bonus is discretionary and retrospective, especially if it is large, and especially if the executives are already well paid, makes it risky, so special bonuses of this type should be used with caution.

WHAT IS THE APPROPRIATE RELATIONSHIP BETWEEN PAY FOR EXECUTIVES AND PAY FOR OTHER EMPLOYEES?

This question is one of social justice, made more compelling by the widening income gap between hourly workers and senior executives. CEO pay has risen to 400 times that of the average worker in big publicly traded firms (Institute for Policy Studies and United for a Fair Economy 2008).[1] In response, people[2] have proposed limiting CEO pay to no more than 20 times the pay of the average worker, citing the much tighter gap in Japan between CEO pay and the pay of the average worker.

Before embracing this populist idea, one ought to consider some of its obvious implications. Organizations that employ many highly skilled technical professionals (e.g., hospitals, software firms, law firms, medical practices) would pay their CEOs far more than would organizations of the same size that rely on many low-skilled, low-wage workers (e.g., retailers, hotels, fast food restaurant companies, firms that outsource most of their work to low-wage foreign countries). Ironically, the firms with higher-paid labor deliver far more of their added value through the intellectual capacity of their workers than the firms with lower-paid labor do, while the firms with lower-paid labor deliver most of their added value through the intellectual capacity of their management team. Using the same ratio across different types of firms seems to deliver the wrong result.

It would mean that CEO pay would be no more in a big firm than in a small firm, if the average workers' pay were the same. Of course, the value of the CEO position is worth more in an organization with 10,000 employees than in an organization with 100 employees, so capping CEO pay to a specific multiple of average worker pay makes little sense. Any appropriate formula would define CEO pay as a factor of organizational size as well as average employee pay.

Most large organizations do have a formula of sorts that ties executive pay to pay for other employees; it is the compensation philosophy. Through that philosophy, the organizations aim for a degree of consistency. If they pay the workforce as a whole at median, for example, they generally pay executives at median, too.

Even better at promoting consistency between executive pay and pay for other employees is a job evaluation system. As long as an organization uses the same compensation philosophy for executives as it uses for other employees and sets pay ranges based on job evaluation points, salary ranges for executive positions will be directly proportional to the scope of job responsibilities.

Some commentators, aiming to move the debate out of political and ethical domains, have tried to redefine it in terms of the relationship between the CEO's pay and pay for other senior executives. That gap, too, may be higher than it should be, but it misses the point of the debate, which is why executive pay keeps rising when pay for the workforce as a whole is flat; why executives should keep their supplemental benefits as companies cut benefits for the workforce as a whole; and why pay for executives of American firms should keep rising even as they eliminate well-paid jobs for American workers by outsourcing work to Mexico, India, or China.

HOW SHOULD WE BALANCE CONCERN FOR PAYING EXECUTIVES COMPETITIVELY WITH OUR NEED TO TRIM COSTS?

For at least the past 30 years, hospitals have been under relentless pressure to reduce operating costs and become more efficient.

Until recently, they have generally not looked at ways to reduce executive compensation, other than by eliminating unnecessary executive positions. While they have looked at every other opportunity to reduce expenses without harming quality, service, or operational effectiveness, they have overlooked opportunities in executive compensation—for fear of alienating executives or losing them to competitors, yes, but mostly because they believe that any cuts would leave their compensation programs less than competitive.

Boards have been perhaps too concerned with making sure executive compensation is competitive. They should instead focus on paying enough compensation to recruit and retain the leadership talent the organization needs to be successful now and in the future. Trustees should consider using voluntary turnover as the test of whether executive compensation is high enough, or too high—but only turnover explicitly linked to accepting higher-paying jobs elsewhere, and only those where the incremental pay is from a lateral move rather than a significant promotion. Too little voluntary turnover is a good indication that pay is higher than necessary, just as too much voluntary turnover is an indication that pay is too low.

Hospitals and health systems should look for ways to trim the cost of executive compensation, just as they look at ways to trim payroll costs for the workforce as a whole. Because they will be increasingly challenged by scarcity of resources in the future, they will need to look at executive compensation as an expense that needs to be managed carefully—more, perhaps, as a matter of being even-handed and thorough than in expectation of reducing costs much.

WHY SHOULD WE GIVE BETTER BENEFITS AND PERQUISITES TO EXECUTIVES THAN TO OTHER EMPLOYEES?

Many hospitals and health systems give better benefits and perquisites to executives than to other employees, presumably because trustees were once told—often by vendors who wanted to sell them insurance—that they needed to give executives generous benefits and perquisites to ensure that their compensation programs were fully competitive.

Some hospitals and health systems, by contrast, give executives less robust benefits than they give other employees, as a result of caps and limits on standard benefits set by regulators and insurance carriers. Capping benefits at incomes of $50,000 or $100,000 or even $250,000 disadvantages executives because the ceiling is too low to allow the promised benefit to cover their full income. A benefit, for example, that promises employees life insurance of two times salary up to a maximum benefit of $100,000 is unfair to employees making more than $50,000 a year. One that promises employees income continuation in the event of a long-term disability of 60 percent of salary up to a maximum benefit of $5,000 per month is unfair to employees with salaries higher than $100,000 a year. Legislative caps on the amount of income that can be counted in determining qualified retirement benefits also intentionally disadvantage higher-paid employees.

It is easy to argue that employers should try to close that gap and cover as much of executives' income as they can at a reasonable cost, to fulfill the implicit promise made to employees in the formula for the basic benefit. It is harder to justify giving executives richer benefits than hospitals give their other employees.[3] Why, for example, should they give executives life insurance of three times salary if they give employees only one times salary? The usual rationale is to meet competitive standards, but that is not a compelling rationale when resources are scarce and hospitals have cut expenses wherever else they can.

Many hospitals and health systems still provide defined-benefit or target-benefit supplemental retirement plans to executives after having eliminated pension plans for other employees on the premise that they are too expensive, and having substituted significantly less generous defined-contribution plans. What is particularly difficult to justify is that hospitals and systems were enriching retirement benefits for executives over the last two decades at the same time they were cutting retirement benefits for other employees.

On the other hand, a strong case can be made for giving executives more vacation time and a larger severance package than are given to other employees. It is difficult to recruit seasoned executives without special executive vacation and severance schedules. Vacation and severance generally start at a low level for new employees and increase with tenure; by moving to a new employer, however, newly recruited executives are giving up whatever tenure they had built up in their last job. Giving executives an enhanced vacation schedule does not cost much because they are not replaced while they are away. Enhanced severance costs more, of course, but the premise of severance is to provide income continuity for the period of time an employee terminated without cause will need to find another job; it takes far longer for executives than for nurses to find their next job after having been laid off. Without offering enhanced severance, though, hospitals would have a hard time recruiting new executives who need to uproot their families and move across country to accept a new position.

By their nature, benefits are paternalistic substitutes for additional compensation. Employers have fallen into the pattern of buying insurance for employees to cover healthcare costs and provide disability and death benefits on the assumption that employees will not buy adequate protection on their own. They provide retirement benefits (in lieu of higher wages) on the assumption that even if they were paid more and given the choice between saving or spending, employees would not generally save enough money to accumulate an adequate retirement nest egg.

But basic benefit packages for the workforce as currently designed encourage employees to take at least partial responsibility for the cost of benefits by making participation in insured benefits voluntary, giving them incentives to forgo health insurance altogether or to choose less expensive high-deductible plans, requiring them to pay a portion of the premiums for insured benefits, or providing all or a portion of the retirement benefit as matched contributions payable only if the employee contributes to the plan.

By contrast, supplemental benefits for executives are usually paid in full by employers. Trustees should consider requiring executives to take on a meaningful level of responsibility for these benefits, as other employees are expected to do. Executives, after all, are in a better position than other employees to make wise choices between cash and benefits; if they are not willing to pay a portion of the premium for supplemental life or disability insurance, or if they would rather take additional cash instead, it is probably not wise for the hospital to pay the entire cost of these benefits. Likewise, if matched savings plans are the best approach to providing retirement benefits to other employees, would they not also be good for executives?

The gradual disappearance of most visible perquisites and certain supplemental benefits for hospital CEOs, such as permanent life insurance and medical expense reimbursement policies, shows that they are not a competitive necessity. Other perquisites and benefits may not be competitive necessities, either.

ISN'T THERE A WAY TO GET EXECUTIVE PAY UNDER CONTROL?

Executive pay is under control. Saying that it is out of control implies that it increases of its own momentum. Executives are paid what trustees want to pay them and in the ways trustees want to pay them. At least they are paid what trustees have agreed to pay them, in ways that trustees have approved at some point in the past, and in ways that trustees continue to authorize.

Executive compensation is controlled by the board's compensation policy and by the actions of the compensation committee. Annual salary increases are typically modest, executive benefits are generally reasonable, and incentive plans reward executives only when and to the extent that their performance meets the board's expectations.

Critics who say executive pay is out control mean that it is too high. What they want to see is pay for executives lowered, and lowered a lot. They may want regulations to limit executive pay, but regulations have not worked in the past and are not likely to work better in the future.

Trustees are not likely to cut pay significantly, at least not enough to satisfy anyone who thinks that executive pay is out of control, and legislators are not likely to limit pay in any meaningful way. There are a few things trustees could do, however, to feel that they are moderating executive pay a bit. They could stop pay from rising faster for executives than for other employees, and they could stop giving executives richer benefits and perquisites than they give other employees. For these measures to be implemented, however, boards would need to change the way they think about executive compensation and adopt some of these best practices:

- Stop placing so much emphasis on paying competitively.
- Stop doing things just because other organizations do them.
- Pay executives as much as necessary to recruit and retain them, but not more. Use the organization's recruitment and retention experience as the litmus test in determining whether pay is competitive.
- Recognize that you cannot pay enough to hold onto an executive whose ambition drives him to look for the next good opportunity for career advancement.
- Avoid customizing benefits, perquisites, or contractual terms for individual executives—even the CEO.
- Address questions about the structure and value of executive compensation with the same rigor used in zero-based budgeting and in making decisions about investments in other programs. In other words, look at resources devoted to executive compensation as resources that cannot be used for anything else.
- Begin and end committee meetings in executive session to give members the opportunity to raise concerns and identify

issues that need discussion without worrying about friction with management.

- Report the compensation committee's decisions to the board in detail. Aim for transparency. If you are not comfortable reporting a decision to the board, it is probably the wrong decision.

NOTES

1. In *CEO Pay and the Great Recession,* the seventeenth annual executive compensation survey, the Institute for Policy Studies (2010) reports that CEO pay declined in 2009 to 263 times average worker pay. In "CEOs Distance Themselves from the Average Worker," the Economic Policy Institute reports that the multiple fell to 185 in 2010, then rose to 243 in 2011 (Bivens 2011). The Heritage Institute (2007) shows an exhibit reporting the multiple as 531 in 2000. Regardless of the year-to-year fluctuation in the multiple, the most commonly cited statistic is the multiple of 400.

2. Including Peter Drucker; see the Drucker Institute (2011).

3. Publicly traded firms are beginning to move away from this practice. The Council of Institutional Investors (2011, 11) and The Conference Board (2009, 9, 20–22) have recommended against giving executives benefits richer than those provided to other employees.

CHAPTER 2

Compensation Philosophy

INTRODUCTION

Compensation philosophy is the foundation for good governance of executive compensation. An explicit compensation philosophy gives the board and the compensation committee a basis for making executive compensation decisions that would otherwise be ad hoc, with no enduring rationale to keep them reasonably consistent over time. It gives the CEO a basis for keeping pay for other executives competitive and fair. And it provides a basis for communicating the compensation program to executives and other stakeholders.

A compensation philosophy makes it easy for the board to delegate oversight of the executive compensation program to the compensation committee, knowing that the committee will act in accordance with the philosophy set by the board. It provides a framework for decision making that helps the committee reach consensus and make decisions quickly.

The more explicit and the more specific the compensation philosophy is, the more it helps guide decision making. But specificity is itself a pitfall. A compensation philosophy that calls for setting pay at a specific level, such as median or average, fuels inflation in executive pay. It reinforces the nearly universal practice of increasing pay every year, by more or less promising to keep pay competitive with a particular benchmark. It implies a greater degree of precision than is warranted by actual pay patterns and the way survey data are used to identify specific benchmarks—and it promotes bigger increases than might otherwise be given. A specific compensation philosophy gives compensation committees and CEOs a reason to increase pay to the benchmark level, even if they would not otherwise be inclined to do so, as it represents a policy to pay executives—experienced ones, at least—at this benchmark level.

When compensation philosophy calls for positioning salaries at a specific level, it gives disgruntled executives whose salaries are lower than what is called for by the philosophy a basis for claiming they are underpaid. Implicit or explicit, specific or not, compensation philosophy represents little more than a commitment to pay as much as other organizations, or to stay ahead of them. A specific compensation philosophy commits the organization to increasing pay whenever prevailing pay levels rise and at the same rate at which pay rises elsewhere. It encourages boards to maintain old compensation and benefit programs as long as they are the competitive norm, even if trustees would not approve the programs today, given current circumstances.

However, sacrificing specificity to avoid the pitfall would deprive compensation philosophy of much of its usefulness in shaping and facilitating decisions. Ideally, compensation philosophy should be expressed as values, beliefs, or general guidelines, not as a policy of paying at a certain level. A policy represents a promise and an obligation. It does not leave trustees much latitude to exercise judgment in making decisions or give the organization much flexibility in dealing with anomalies or unexpected changes in circumstances.

COMPENSATION PHILOSOPHY DEFINED

An organization's philosophy of executive compensation expresses the board's intentions related to paying executives. It represents the views of trustees and the values of the organization.

Sometimes compensation philosophy is a formal written statement. Other times it is expressed only informally and explains how decisions were made in the past or how they are likely to be made in the future. When expressed in a formal written statement, the philosophy outlines the principles the board expects the compensation committee to follow as the committee oversees the executive compensation process. Seldom is the compensation philosophy actually philosophic. It is generally just a set of parameters identifying the intended level of competitiveness for salaries or total compensation—for example, "We set salary ranges at median and total compensation opportunity at the 75th percentile and are willing to pay up to the 90th percentile when performance is extraordinarily good"—more policy than philosophy, with no express rationale for the guidance it provides.

Some rationale usually underlies that policy, however, whether explicit or implicit. The standard rationales include the need to recruit and retain talented leaders and the belief that pay should be tied to performance, either because incentives shape behavior or because superior performance ought to be rewarded.

The underlying rationales that usually go unstated are based on assumptions that have never been proven:

- To recruit first-rate executives, we need to pay above average.
- If we pay above average, we will be able to recruit better executives than if we pay at median or below.
- If we use incentive compensation to motivate executives, we will get better performance from them than if we do not offer incentives.
- Institutional success depends so much on having the right leaders that we need to pay them competitively, even if we do not have the resources to carry out other initiatives we want to support.
- Our executives will leave if we do not pay them competitively.
- Executives know enough about what their peers make elsewhere that they can tell whether or not they are paid competitively.

Criticism of executive pay has encouraged organizations to adopt a more philosophical tone in explaining the rationale for their compensation programs. Some frame their compensation philosophy statements in value-laden phrases expressing the need for talented executives, such as "to lead the organization through challenging times" or "to ensure the organization can continue to meet the community's needs for clinical services." They may add a phrase supporting the belief that pay should be tied to performance.

No matter how it is expressed, an organization's compensation philosophy represents a board policy. If the policy calls for positioning pay at a specific level, it forbids extreme exceptions or at least forces acknowledgment of, and requires some justification of, exceptions. As a directive from the board to the compensation committee and the CEO, it almost requires the CEO to disclose any extreme exceptions to the committee and the committee to disclose any extreme exceptions to the board. If there are only one or two or a few exceptions, they can generally be explained and justified, but if the exceptions are numerous, they are likely to raise questions about whether the CEO and the committee are complying with the board's policy, or whether the policy should be changed to match

---

Structure and Administration Undermine Policy

A healthcare system with an explicit policy of positioning pay no higher than median adopted a standard salary structure with salary ranges stretching from 20 percent below median to 20 percent above. Even though the new structure came with guidelines constraining use of the portion of the range above median, the system continued to follow the same administrative practice it had previously used, which gradually moved all employees to the top of their salary ranges. Soon, most of the system's executives were being paid 20 percent above median, which was at or near the 75th percentile.

---

actual practice. If, for example, an organization pays most of its executives 15 percent above median when the philosophy calls for paying them at median, the philosophy seems like a sham.

Some policies are vague generalities, such as "We pay competitively" or "We pay on par with the other hospitals in town." Others are more specific: "We position salaries at the 60th percentile, offer above average incentive opportunity and average benefits, and position total compensation at the 75th percentile." Sometimes the policy is expressed as a range, as in "We position salaries between median and the 60th percentile" or "We pay between median and the 75th percentile." Some formal philosophy statements are intentionally vague to avoid publicizing the board's intent to position pay above average.

Large organizations often have multiple compensation philosophies for different groups of leaders—one for executives, one for physician leaders; one for senior executives, another for mid-level executives and managers; or one covering senior system-level executives and executives at the largest one or two hospitals, and another for those at the smallest hospitals. On occasion, the compensation philosophy is different for the CEO than for other executives.

Structure Trumps Policy when a New CEO Is Hired

A system had an explicit policy of positioning salaries at the 75th percentile, with the exception of the CEO, whose salary was positioned at median but whose incentive opportunity brought her total compensation to the 75th percentile. When the CEO retired, the board hired a new CEO at a 90th percentile salary without adjusting incentive opportunity and without recognizing and acknowledging the divergence from compensation policy. The expected value of the new CEO's total compensation, if management met its goals, was far above the 90th percentile.

COMPENSATION STRATEGY VERSUS COMPENSATION PHILOSOPHY VERSUS COMPENSATION POLICY

Up to this point we have used *compensation policy* loosely as an alternate term for compensation philosophy. But philosophy differs from policy in practical terms, and both differ from compensation strategy. As stated earlier, *compensation philosophy* is an expression of the organization's beliefs about and intentions in regard to executive compensation.

Compensation policy is a rule or set of rules established by the board that defines what the board intends to pay executives or establishes limits on what the organization can pay without making exceptions to the policy. While compensation philosophy represents permission to pay at a certain level, compensation policy represents a constraint on paying much above or below that level.

Compensation strategy is a process and a plan for implementing compensation philosophy or policy by structuring the executive compensation program. It tends to be more specific and open to change than are compensation philosophy and compensation policy. Compensation strategy addresses the balance among various elements of the compensation program, the emphasis placed on certain aspects of the program, and the reason for designing the program in a particular way to achieve a particular end.

An organization's compensation strategy is a set of decisions about how much emphasis to place on pay for performance (typically a main focus of the strategy), whether to use just annual or both annual and long-term incentives and how to balance them, and how to structure the program to help retain executives. It allocates resources between fixed and variable elements, between current and deferred compensation, and between compensation and benefits to make the best use of resources in recruiting and retaining leaders and aligning them with the institution's mission, strategies, and goals. And it establishes the amount of emphasis the organization will place on security provisions, such as life and disability insurance, retirement benefits, and severance.

WHY DO BOARDS ADOPT A COMPENSATION PHILOSOPHY?

Boards develop a compensation philosophy to provide a framework for making decisions about pay and benefits. With a formal compensation philosophy or policy specifying the level of pay the board deems appropriate, the board may safely delegate to a committee responsibility for overseeing executive compensation, as its existence implies that the committee must inform the board of major exceptions to the policy and ask for approval of any change to the policy.

Additional reasons to adopt a compensation philosophy include the following:

- It helps keep the compensation program consistent over time and as compensation committee members turn over.
- It allows the board to delegate authority to the CEO to manage compensation for executives outside the purview of the compensation committee without giving up its responsibility for ensuring that executive compensation is set at a level the board deems appropriate.
- It helps keep compensation equitable, thereby lowering the risk of litigation on the basis of discrimination against executives in protected classes.
- It tends to limit disparity in pay by identifying a "right rate of pay" for each job. It implicitly calls for bringing low-paid incumbents up to the right rate of pay over time and tends to limit increases for incumbents who are paid significantly more than the right rate of pay for their jobs.
- It communicates the basis for compensation decisions to executives, so they know what to expect and know they will be paid at a reasonably competitive rate.
- It helps the board explain its decisions to stakeholders by expressing the reason for executive compensation levels in terms of paying on par with other organizations or paying what is necessary to attract and retain talented leaders.

- It provides a good reason for rejecting requests for more pay or new programs if the proposed change would move compensation above the benchmark level specified as the right rate of pay.

UNINTENDED CONSEQUENCES

Unfortunately, the specificity that makes a formal compensation philosophy so useful has unintended consequences. One problematic consequence of any compensation philosophy that calls for positioning pay at a specific level is that it promotes inflation in executive pay. Whether the policy calls for positioning pay at median or at the 75th percentile or some other position, it calls for increasing the pay of any executive who is paid less than the intended level.

Most commentators focus their criticism on policies that position pay at the 75th percentile, saying that it raises pay unnecessarily. This assessment overlooks the real problem, which is that most employers intend to pay at median or above. Even if every organization's policy called for paying at median, employers would still raise lower-paid employees to median without reducing pay for employees paid above that level, thus driving up median pay and fueling inflation. In short, it is the commitment to paying competitively that drives inflation, not just a commitment to paying above average.

An effective compensation system ought to pay individuals what they are worth, or what it takes to recruit and retain them, but not more. At any major employer, however, compensation systems focus more on what the job is worth than what the incumbent is worth, and more on consistency and fairness than what it takes to recruit and retain a particular individual. These other unintended consequences of policies that position pay at a specific competitive level show how compensation systems work and how good intentions affect practical decisions about pay.

- A compensation policy reduces flexibility in deciding how much to pay people, as it positions pay opportunity for all jobs at the same competitive level (e.g., all at the 65th percentile) instead of positioning pay for each job where appropriate given its importance to the organization, where appropriate

Standard Approach Eliminates Flexibility and Raises Pay Unnecessarily

A large, diversified healthcare organization that drew its talent from many different segments of the economy had for a long time been using a compensation philosophy of paying between median and the 90th percentile. The intention was to give the CEO the flexibility to pay executives whatever was required to recruit and retain the right incumbent for each executive position without paying any more than necessary. When a new member of the board assumed leadership of the compensation committee, he persuaded the committee to adopt a more conventional approach of positioning pay at the 75th percentile and using standard salary ranges. The organization then began increasing the salary of each executive who was paid below the 75th percentile, and because it no longer had the flexibility to position salaries for the most important leadership positions at the 90th percentile, it began to seek other ways to raise compensation for those jobs.

Several years later, having long forgotten the flexible approach to executive compensation that had worked well in the past, the committee began asking why it took so long to bring newly promoted executives up to the 75th percentile. It should have been wondering instead why it was necessary to pay every executive at the 75th percentile.

for the incumbent given her competencies, or where required for recruiting or retaining the right person for the job.

- A compensation policy tends to augment salary increases by focusing more attention on jobs that are paid less than the specified level than on those that are paid at or above it.
- It promotes an unrealistic sense of precision. Dispersion in executive pay is extraordinarily wide, even within a group of organizations of the same size, with the highest pay for any position more than twice the pay for the lowest. A policy of positioning pay at median or average focuses on a single value, while a policy of paying "competitively" could encompass a band stretching well above and below that single value.
- It implies that pay below median is not competitive, even though half the incumbents in any sample are paid below median, and even though many of those paid below median believe they are paid competitively.
- It encourages paying at least some people more than necessary, because all that is necessary is what it takes to recruit and retain the right person for the job. It leads to big salary increases for newly promoted executives and to paying executives who have no desire to move on to higher-paying jobs elsewhere on par with those who are constantly looking for career advancement opportunities.

ISSUES TO CONSIDER IN DEVELOPING COMPENSATION PHILOSOPHY

Boards and their compensation committees generally set compensation policies in an informal, intuitive manner, focusing primarily on the choice of peer group and the intended competitive position. Even written statements of compensation philosophy rarely include a well-developed rationale because the thought process used in creating the philosophy is heavily influenced by unexamined assumptions and focuses on conclusions rather than reasons for the conclusions.

Trustees might articulate their compensation philosophy differently if they took a more analytical approach to considering the issues discussed below.

- *What do we have to pay to recruit and retain the leadership talent we need to meet our goals and succeed in our marketplace?* This question encompasses a host of issues, but it focuses on the most important factors—what we *need* to pay, not what we *think* we need to pay, and what type of leaders we *need* to succeed in our marketplace. The issue can be addressed by reviewing recruitment and retention patterns and satisfaction with the current management team. A system with very little turnover that relies largely on internal promotions and that performs well with homegrown talent probably does not need to pay as much as one that generally recruits externally to fill open leadership positions.

  Cash compensation, primarily salary, is the currency of recruitment. Benefits do not play much of a role in recruiting executives, except for seasoned, high-level executives who are already comfortably ensconced in a good job, who may demand a good retirement package and generous severance as conditions for moving to a new job.

  Both cash and benefits help to retain executives, but other factors often matter more. People stay in their jobs because they like the work, the organization they work for, and the people they work with, as long as they feel fairly treated and fairly paid. They stay if they have deep roots in the community and would rather not force their families to move.

  Benefits can help retain executives, but the only benefit with much effect on retention is the retirement benefit. It is more effective at retaining older executives than younger ones, of course, and is effective at retaining younger and mid-career executives only if the retirement benefit is generous and would be forfeited on voluntary termination before retirement age.

A hospital that recruits externally for most of its executive positions needs to emphasize cash compensation. One that develops most of its leadership talent internally may not need to, unless it experiences a lot of turnover. A hospital that wants to retain executives until they retire probably needs to emphasize retirement benefits. One that does not expect many of its executives to stay until retirement can probably find a better way to allocate resources.

- *What is the labor market in which we compete for leadership talent?*
  All of the nearly 6,000 US hospitals and the several hundred multihospital systems compete for leadership talent. Each year, 14 to 18 percent choose a new CEO, and a roughly comparable number choose a new chief financial officer (CFO) or chief information officer (CIO).

The size of the executive talent pool is enormous, as each of the 6,000 hospitals has its own set of executives. A significant number of these CEOs, CFOs, and CIOs are looking for new jobs at any given time, and another big group of them is willing to move if the right opportunity comes along.

But the talent pool for any given job is much smaller than the pool of talent because employers and executives both set limits on what factors they will consider. Executives generally look for jobs with more responsibility, more prestige, and more pay than they currently have and rarely move to smaller or less prestigious organizations unless they need the job. They set limits on where they are willing to live. Employers generally look for executives who already hold the job they are recruiting for, albeit at another organization, preferably at an organization just as big and prestigious as the one they are recruiting for. Executives tend to stay within the segment of the industry in which they have already worked. Those in Catholic systems are more likely to move to another Catholic system than to a secular system, especially if the executives are of the Catholic faith. Those from the East or West coasts are more likely to stay in those regions than move to the Midwest, or move all the way across the country rather than take a job in "flyover land." Surprisingly little movement is seen between general industry and healthcare, between for-profit and not-for-profit healthcare, and between urban and rural hospitals. Executives who choose to work in academic hospitals tend to move to other academic hospitals, and those who choose to work in public institutions tend to move to other public institutions.

Similarly, employers tend to prefer candidates who have worked in the same type of institutions and environments. Most hospitals and health systems look for a candidate who fits the values and culture of their organization. That may mean looking for someone from the same region, from the same religion, from the same type of institution, or from a community with values similar to those of the hiring organization.

Executives advance their careers in two ways: by taking on broader roles in their own organizations and by moving to bigger or better-known organizations. Thus, the talent pool for a vacant executive position is made up largely of executives already in the same position in another organization and second-level executives ready to move to a top position. Most candidates who are already employed in the same job are at smaller organizations. The pool of second-level executives ready for promotion includes those working at organizations of the same size, some at bigger organizations, and a lot at smaller organizations. Given the usual path of career progression from smaller to larger organizations, any hospital or system competes for executive talent primarily with smaller organizations when it is recruiting externally and with larger organizations as it tries to retain its leaders. This means that the competitive labor market for leadership talent is broader than we generally think it is when we are recruiting and smaller than we think it is when we are concerned about retaining executives. Because there are many more small hospitals than big ones, the competition is more intense among smaller and midsize hospitals and systems than at larger ones. Once executives gain a leadership job in a big organization, they do not have many more opportunities for career advancement because there are not many bigger organizations, and relatively few that will be willing to pay them more.

• *How much external recruitment is needed? How many positions can be filled by promotion from within?*
Few healthcare organizations, other than large multihospital systems, have enough strong second-level executives to replace senior executives when they leave. Large organizations with strong leadership development programs may be able to fill most executive openings through internal promotions. They may not need to position compensation as high as do smaller organizations that must recruit externally for most leadership positions.

Organizations that position pay at median should recognize a corollary—that they should invest in leadership development programs, as they will have difficulty getting external candidates to fill open positions if they cannot pay more than median.

• *What can we afford?*
Decisions about affordability revolve around allocation of resources. Money spent on executive compensation cannot be spent on clinical programs. Positioning executive compensation at the 75th percentile instead of median can cost even a small organization up to $200,000 extra per year, and a large hospital or midsize system with ten executives an extra $1 million or more per year—enough to pay for several additional positions.

Operating profit margins in healthcare are thin. Hospitals trim payroll costs by eliminating positions, sometimes by reducing benefits, but only rarely by cutting pay. While they try to limit the number of executive positions to control cost, and sometimes eliminate executive positions, they tend to regard executive compensation as a competitive necessity largely exempt from cost cutting. As a result, hospitals often spend more than they need to on executive compensation.

- *How should our compensation philosophy reflect our institution's values? Our community's values?*

In most communities, hospital executives are paid more than almost everyone else in town. As a result, the hospital's executive pay levels seem inappropriately high to most community members—no matter what the compensation philosophy is.

Trustees are supposed to take the organization's mission and values into account whenever they make decisions for the hospital. They are also expected to bring the community's values to bear on decisions. As they make decisions about executive compensation, they should be asking whether average or above-average pay is better aligned with the institution's and the community's values. They should also be asking how well incentive pay, supplemental benefits, and perquisites are aligned with the institution's and the community's values.

Peer Group Chosen to Keep Compensation Low

A large rural hospital in the South Central region of the United States wanted to position executive compensation at median. To avoid paying a median based on a broad national peer group of hospitals its size, it used as its peer group the hospitals in its state, as represented by a survey conducted by the state hospital association. Pay levels were about 10 percent lower in that survey than in national surveys. The board adopted the median identified by the state survey as its compensation position, satisfied that it was using its resources wisely.

For a premier hospital in a large city, an above-average pay policy may fit the image the hospital is trying to portray to attract physicians and patients. The sole provider in a small town or midsize community stressed by the decline of the industrial sector will have difficulty justifying an above-average pay policy—even though it may be harder for these institutions than for a premier urban hospital to attract and retain leadership talent.

Now that IRS Form 990 requires disclosure of certain types of supplemental benefits and perquisites, even boards of large, image-conscious institutions that once happily provided car allowances and country club membership to executives recognize that these perquisites may not be aligned with community values.

Values have changed a lot over the past decade, and many features of executive compensation programs are relics that are less appropriate now than they were when they were introduced. With all the pressure on healthcare providers to be more efficient, boards should take a fresh look at their compensation philosophy and align it with what they expect the institution's values to be in the future, even if that means abandoning traditional programs offered only because they once seemed right.

- *What can we justify to stakeholders?*
  Until recently, compensation for healthcare executives was regarded as confidential. Many compensation committees did not divulge details even to the board as a whole. Now that disclosures of executive compensation on IRS Form 990 are readily accessible on the Internet, the question of what level of compensation the board can justify to stakeholders has become more important than in the past.

  Healthcare economics are getting tougher for most stakeholders—patients, physicians, and employees—but so far have not affected executive pay much. Rising salaries, big incentive awards, and supplemental benefits and perquisites are difficult to rationalize when patients must pay more for healthcare, employees see their benefits being cut, and physicians see their incomes declining or remaining flat.

• *Will paying more get us better talent? Or will we just have an easier time finding good people?*
This question is difficult to answer because there is no good way to measure the caliber of leadership or management talent and no opportunity to conduct controlled experiments or before-and-after tests. There is no way to demonstrate a correlation between better pay and better talent without first reaching agreement on how to measure leadership talent.

No evidence indicates that higher-paid executives are more talented than executives paid at median or average, or that the most talented executives end up at the highest-paying institutions, or that it takes above-average pay to recruit exceptionally talented executives. But there is ample evidence that plenty of talented executives work at institutions that do not pay especially well.

Paying above average does make it easier to recruit, however, and no doubt shortens the time required to fill open positions. It expands the pool of candidates who will consider the position.

What really helps attract better talent is being realistic about where the talent is. There is far more exceptional talent at smaller organizations than at bigger organizations, as there are far more small organizations than big ones. And a hospital is far more likely to be able to recruit an exceptionally talented leader from a smaller organization than from one of the same size. An executive has little reason to move from one hospital or health system to another of the same size, even if the pay is a little better, and an especially talented executive is likely to have better opportunities than a lateral move for marginally better pay.

- *Do we need to pay more to get better performance?*
  Boards sometimes increase incentive opportunity when they want to improve performance, in the hope that if executives are offered bigger rewards, they will deliver better results. Most boards, however, recognize that getting better performance depends on determining *how* to improve performance—not on paying to improve it. Executives are intrinsically highly motivated and will perform well if they know how to improve performance. Low pay is rarely the reason for weak performance, and high pay is rarely the reason for outstanding performance.
- *How much should we emphasize pay for performance?*
  No one has shown that pay-for-performance programs actually improve performance. High expectations probably do more to improve performance than pay for performance does, as executives are highly motivated and want to achieve whatever goals are set for them. What incentive compensation does is focus attention on the goals used to determine awards. It forces managers to define goals clearly; encourages boards and managers to agree on priorities; and increases the level of discipline used in planning, goal setting, and performance measurement. An organization with a strong planning process, good measurement systems, and good communication between the board and management team does not need incentive compensation or merit pay to deliver good results. All that pay for performance does is support the performance management system and reward success at meeting whatever goals are set. Putting more money into rewards for performance is unlikely to improve performance, just as reducing the rewards for performance is unlikely to hurt performance.

Compensation committees often favor increasing pay for performance because trustees are accustomed to much higher incentive opportunity in their own jobs than is typical in not-for-profit hospitals and systems. Some boards are skeptical of incentive compensation, though, stemming from concern that they do not have a good performance measurement system in place or that incentives place too much emphasis on financial performance. The ironic result of this skepticism is that boards are reluctant to tie very much pay to clinical quality, patient satisfaction, and process improvement.

The right level of emphasis on pay for performance is a function of the organization's culture, the intensity of its efforts to improve performance, and the comfort trustees and executives have with the performance management system.

• *Where should we be generous? Where should we skimp?* Compensation philosophy needs to address the balance between fixed and variable pay and between cash and benefits and perquisites. Incentive compensation varies from 10 percent to almost 100 percent of salary, and benefits and perquisites vary from 10 percent to 50 percent of salary. Few organizations can afford to be generous or highly competitive in all areas of compensation, so they must decide what areas to emphasize and what to de-emphasize.

Some organizations decide to be generous with salaries and position them at the 65th or 75th percentiles to help with recruitment; others decide to be generous with incentive opportunity to put more emphasis on pay for performance; some decide to be generous with benefits to help retain executives. It is easy to be generous with one part or another of the executive compensation program, but harder to skimp on something to offset the cost of being generous with something else. Unfortunately, being generous with salaries drives up the cost of incentive awards and benefits, as both are defined largely in relation to base salary.

Few organizations make intentional trade-offs between elements of the compensation program. Those that choose not to use incentive compensation do, because they usually position salaries high to make up for the lack of incentive opportunity. Some that position salaries or incentive opportunity above average leave benefits below average, but that is less often intentional than due to lack of attention.

A thoughtful approach to defining compensation philosophy addresses these trade-offs, even though the trade-offs might not be articulated in any formal statement of compensation philosophy. Organizations make trade-offs such as these in budgeting for everything else. Why not for executive compensation? The compensation committee could start by answering these questions:

—If we are willing to pay a bit above average, should we put the extra money in salaries or incentive opportunity or benefits?

—If we want to save a bit of money on executive compensation, should we cut back on salaries or incentive opportunity or benefits?

—If we would like to shift more money into salaries or incentive opportunity or benefits, would we take it from benefits or incentive opportunity or salaries?

—If we need to increase current compensation, can we pay for it by reducing deferred compensation?

—If we want to put more emphasis on variable pay, can we pay for it by reducing fixed pay?

• *How should we promote fairness? What do we mean by "fair"?* Paying executives fairly is generally taken to mean paying them close to the same competitive level (e.g., keeping most salaries close to median). This approach allows for some variation to account for experience and performance, but not much. Pay systems emphasize fairness now more than in the past to minimize the impact of biases related to gender and race and to reduce the effect of seniority on pay.

Some organizations think it fair to give everyone the same size salary increase. That practice, however, just perpetuates the current dispersion in pay; people paid high relative to market value continue to be paid high, and people paid low relative to market value continue to be paid low.

Bias Embedded in Compensation Structure

A state university medical center used a titling structure for administrators similar to that for professors—administrator, associate administrator, and assistant administrator—and tied pay to rank rather than scope of responsibility. The executives' titles, moreover, bore no relation to scope of responsibility. Two executives—both of them male—in charge of support services (housekeeping, engineering, and food service) and professional services (laboratory, imaging, pharmacy, and rehabilitation) were associate administrators, while the female chief nursing officer (CNO) was an assistant administrator but had significantly more responsibility than the two men did—more employees, a bigger budget, more responsibility for clinical quality and patient satisfaction, and principal responsibility for the core activity of the organization—taking care of patients. The title-based salary structure set the CNO's salary lower than those of her male counterparts. Worse, each of the other female executives at the medical center was an assistant administrator, while most of the male executives were placed in the higher ranks.

ARTICULATING THE RATIONALE FOR THE EXECUTIVE COMPENSATION POLICY

The public expects boards of tax-exempt hospitals and health systems to keep pay for executives modest, and so do legislators and regulators. Knowing that funding for public healthcare programs depends on maintaining broad public support for them, boards should expect to be held accountable for their decisions about executive compensation and be prepared to explain them. A well-articulated statement of compensation philosophy provides the basis for a good explanation.

To be effective, the rationale should explain the reasons health-care executives are paid more than public officials, why big organizations need to pay more than small ones, why hospitals need expert administrators, and why the funds dedicated to executive compensation should not be allocated instead to some other program or service. The rationale could include the following elements:

- A reference to the challenges facing all hospitals and health systems—low margins, difficulty collecting payments, risks and consequences of errors, need to influence decisions made by outsiders (e.g., physicians, third-party payers), expectations for perfect care in a 24/7 operational setting, litigiousness, and difficulty pleasing patients and maintaining employee morale in a stressful environment
- A statement of the board's expectations for superior performance and continuous improvements in quality and service while improving productivity and cost-effectiveness
- An explanation of the need to pay competitively to be able to recruit and retain talented, experienced leaders
- An assertion that the hospital cannot continue to meet its mission to provide care to the community if it is not able to recruit and retain capable leaders (A reference to the number of hospitals that have closed over the past decade could drive this point home, as no one—not even the institution's harshest critics—wants to see the community hospital close.)

MAINTAINING CONSISTENCY OVER TIME

One advantage of having an explicit, specific compensation philosophy is that it helps organizations maintain a consistent approach to setting and governing executive compensation over time.

Challenges from New Board Members

Compensation committee membership changes frequently, as does leadership of that committee. Given the significant role that the chair plays in shaping the committee's process and decisions, guiding the work of the committee's consultant, and advising the CEO on executive compensation, a new chair can bring an entirely new perspective and style to governing executive compensation. An influential new committee member can do the same. New committee members are more likely than continuing members to raise questions about—or even propose changes to—the compensation philosophy, the structure of the executive compensation program, and prior committee decisions.

If the compensation philosophy is informal and explained as "This is what we've done in the past," it is far more open to change—and challenge—than if it has been formally adopted by the board, been in place for a long time, and been repeatedly affirmed by the board over the years. Challenging the appropriateness of the philosophy is more difficult if its rationale is clearly and persuasively articulated than if no explicit rationale is stated. New members of compensation committees do—and should—ask "Why do we do things this way?" A well-articulated compensation philosophy, with a compelling rationale, can answer that question and help keep the compensation program consistent over time.

Challenges from New CEOs

CEOs turn over, too, and new CEOs often bring their own views of compensation philosophy into the discussion, in part on the basis of the compensation policies and programs they worked under elsewhere. A new CEO often tries to modify the compensation philosophy or compensation program, but compensation decisions should reflect the board's views, not necessarily those of the CEO. A board-approved compensation philosophy with a persuasive rationale, especially one that has been repeatedly reaffirmed by the board, helps maintain consistency when a new CEO arrives by making it harder for the new CEO to persuade the board to change its policy.

COMPENSATION PHILOSOPHY'S INFLUENCE ON THE COMPENSATION PROGRAM

The extent to which the compensation philosophy shapes the compensation program depends on the specificity of the philosophy and the level of discipline that management and the board or compensation committee bring to the task of governing and managing the program. The more specific the compensation philosophy, the greater is its influence on the structure of the compensation program and the decisions that determine how executives are actually paid. The more specific the philosophy, the easier it is to determine whether the program and the actual pay practice match the philosophy, and the easier it is to decide how to change the program or the actual pay practice to comport with the philosophy.

If it is specific enough, the compensation philosophy tells the committee and the CEO how competitive salaries, incentive opportunity, benefits, and total compensation should be, and what peer group should be used in determining where to position each element of compensation. It tells the committee's consultant exactly what data, analyses, and recommendations to show the committee and gives the committee and its consultant precise direction on evaluating the competitiveness and reasonableness of total compensation. It helps the committee determine how to refine the structure of the program to keep it aligned with policy.

COMMUNICATING THE COMPENSATION PHILOSOPHY TO STAKEHOLDERS

A well-considered and clearly articulated compensation philosophy simplifies the task of communicating the executive compensation plan to stakeholders. Boards have an obligation to explain the compensation philosophy and its rationale to executives and new board members, of course, but also to other stakeholders— physicians, employees, sponsors, investors, and credit rating agencies, and trustees are coming to recognize that they also ought to explain it to legislators, regulators, and taxpayers (who pay for half of the care delivered to patients)—if they want to maintain the organization's tax-exempt status and persuade legislators and the public that the community should continue paying for public healthcare programs like Medicare and Medicaid.

This obligation to explain the compensation philosophy is not limited to above-average salary agreements. A median- or average-pay policy may seem unnecessary to explain, but it should be explained nonetheless, for a number of reasons:

- A great portion of care is paid for by the public—mostly by people who earn less than healthcare executives do, and for whom even median or average pay seems excessive.
- Hospitals are usually so short of resources that they cannot afford to fund all the systems, equipment, and clinical programs they would like to have; continue providing the same retirement benefit they once offered employees; or keep employees' costs for healthcare benefits constant. And even median or average pay for executives consumes resources that physicians and employees would rather see used in other ways.
- Hospitals' labor costs are so high that leaders are always looking for ways to cut payroll costs—often by trimming employee benefits and eliminating positions. Employees may rightly ask why executive compensation is not equally subject to cost cutting.
- Physicians' income is not rising as quickly as executives' pay is, so physicians may rightly question why executives should get salary increases every year, even if they are paid only at median.

Positioning executive compensation above median or average always calls for explanation because it represents an intention to pay more than necessary and a preferential allocation of resources to executive compensation. There are perfectly good reasons for positioning executive compensation above average, but they should be articulated clearly.

The public expects transparency from tax-exempt charities, just as the investing public does from publicly traded firms. The newest SEC requirements for reporting executive compensation in proxies calls for public firms to disclose their executive compensation philosophy—the peer group used in determining compensation, and the percentiles the compensation committee looks at in evaluating and determining executive pay. No one should be surprised if these requirements are extended to tax-exempt healthcare institutions or become widely accepted, at least, as best practices, brought into tax-exempt healthcare by trustees accustomed to these disclosures in the for-profit sector.

CHOOSING THE RIGHT PEER GROUP

Few hospitals think of themselves as essentially the same as most others; they focus instead on what makes them different from others. Yet few boards and fewer executives insist on obtaining comparability data from hospitals most like theirs, ones that share some specific, special trait. Instead, boards and their consultants typically use a broadly defined national peer group of hospitals and systems similar only in size.

The labor market reflects the fact that hospitals are not all the same. Rural hospitals do not compete with urban hospitals for leadership talent. Nonteaching hospitals do not compete directly with academic medical centers. Children's hospitals do not compete with behavioral or rehabilitation hospitals.

Competition for talent also tends to be limited geographically because of executives' preferences and family ties. Most hospital executives spend their entire careers in the same region, even when they move from one institution to another. This is less the case with specialty hospitals—cancer centers, children's hospitals, academic medical centers—and with the country's largest hospitals and systems, which often recruit nationally for executives.

Pay levels are sometimes higher, sometimes lower in a narrowly defined peer group than in a broad national peer group, but they are often essentially the same. Regional pay levels, for example, are higher in the Northeast and in California than in other parts of the country, especially in major urban areas. But they are essentially the same in the mountain states and the Midwest as they are in the Southeast, for organizations of the same size and complexity. Pay is generally higher in urban areas than in rural areas, especially for small hospitals. But executive pay is generally higher in small rural, subsidiary hospitals than in small, independent rural hospitals. Children's hospitals and private academic health systems tend to pay more than nonteaching institutions. Public hospitals tend to pay less than private tax-exempt hospitals. But pay levels in Ohio, Texas, and Minnesota are essentially the same for hospitals of similar size and with similar services.

A 100-bed independent community hospital in a midsize rural community should be using a peer group of comparably sized independent community hospitals. It should not be setting its pay levels in comparison with children's hospitals, cancer centers, heart hospitals, or rehabilitation or behavioral hospitals. Similarly, a hospital with no teaching program should not use data from academic hospitals to set executive pay levels.

Boards should insist on using a peer group of organizations that are similar in ways other than size—scope of services, geography, and culture, for example—for the following reasons:

1. The board gains comfort in knowing it is indeed paying appropriately and governing executive compensation well.
2. Executives gain comfort in knowing the data used in setting their pay are appropriate.
3. The board can more easily persuade external stakeholders that the data it uses in governing executive pay are appropriate.
4. Executives and the board are protected from unnecessary challenges from the IRS about the appropriateness of data used in governing executive pay.

The last reason may be the most important one, as it is imbedded in intermediate sanctions regulations and, as a result, is widely recognized as a best practice in governing executive compensation.

One requirement for establishing a presumption of reasonableness is that the board or its compensation committee obtain and rely on *appropriate* comparability data on total compensation. The regulations as set forth in IRC §4958-6(c)(2) define *appropriate* as sufficient, given the knowledge and expertise of board or committee members, for them "to determine whether . . . the compensation arrangement in its entirety is reasonable. . . ." Relevant information for determining reasonableness "includes, but is not limited to, compensation levels paid by similarly situated organizations, both taxable and tax-exempt, for functionally comparable positions . . . current compensation surveys compiled by independent firms; and actual written offers from similar institutions competing for the services of" the same person. They also mention local or regional circumstances as one factor to be considered in determining whether pay is reasonable. IRS auditors have been known to ask for regional comparisons where organizations have been using broad national databases for determining executive compensation.

Using a narrowly defined peer group instead of a broad national peer group has a few disadvantages, however. Data from a small peer group are never as reliable or as robust as data from a big peer group. There may not be enough data points from a small peer group to determine the value of nonstandard jobs. Year-to-year changes in

---

Peer Group Chosen to Keep Executive Compensation High

A large hospital in a major midwestern city positioned its executive compensation at median relative to its competitors—all of which were much larger than it was. The resulting compensation plan positioned salaries at the 75th percentile of hospitals its size.

market values are less consistent in a small peer group than in a big peer group because turnover in a few jobs can cause significant changes in market values, especially at the upper and lower ends of the distribution, such as the 75th or 90th percentiles. For this reason, organizations should be wary of using peer groups with less than 15 organizations and should generally compare data from a narrowly defined peer group with data from a broad national peer group to identify whatever statistical anomalies may arise from using a small data set.

DETERMINING HOW COMPETITIVE PAY SHOULD BE

Just as no organization thinks of itself as less than special, none considers itself just average or below average. Most boards and executive teams believe their hospital is above average, and most boards believe their leadership team is above average—at least in some ways, and in ways they value.

This mentality leads to an interesting debate among trustees and between executives and the board. "Because we expect above-average performance, shouldn't we pay above-average compensation?" "Because we consistently perform above average, shouldn't we pay above average?" "Since our executives are some of the best in the country, shouldn't we pay above average?" And at hospitals that routinely perform at the top of the field, the question becomes "Why shouldn't our executives be paid at the 90th percentile?" No hospital or health system intentionally sets pay below average in expectation of below-average performance.

Pay can, and should, reflect performance, but other factors often matter more than performance in shaping philosophy of executive compensation. Small organizations, for example, often set a policy of paying above average to compete for talent with larger organizations. Some set a policy of paying well above average to make sure they can retain executives, in the belief that stability on the management team delivers above-average performance. Prestigious organizations often set a policy of paying well above average, in part to match their image of being the preferred provider in their market.

Boards are beginning to express their compensation policies more in terms of performance relative to the industry. Boards that in the past were comfortable setting pay at the 75th percentile are now adding the contingency "when we perform at the 75th percentile" or the rationale "because we expect performance at the 75th percentile."

The best or right compensation philosophy for an organization can only be determined by the organization itself, or rather by its trustees, in consideration of the organization's values, circumstances, and success in recruiting and retaining executives and trustees' own views of the effectiveness of compensation in recruiting, retaining, and motivating executives. Trustees are charged with this responsibility because they are responsible for seeing that the organization succeeds in achieving its mission, by seeing that the organization has the leaders and the resources it needs to be successful. Trustees, along with the CEO, are in the best position to determine how to obtain, develop, and keep the talent the organization needs to succeed. Some organizations really do have to pay well above average to get the leaders they need, and others have no difficulty recruiting or developing and retaining high-caliber leaders with pay no higher than median. Some organizations really need effective pay-for-performance programs to foster a strong commitment to performance improvement, while others are so strongly committed to performance that they have no need for monetary incentives and rewards. And only someone who knows the organization well, and has known it for a long time, can discern what type of executive compensation program the organization needs.

Almost all hospitals and health systems aim to position executive compensation at median or the 75th percentile or somewhere between the two. Virtually none of them sets a policy of paying below median or below average, and almost none sets a policy of paying above the 90th percentile. While policies on competitiveness of executive compensation vary from one organization to another, four patterns are common:

- Median salaries, median incentive opportunity, median benefits, and median total compensation
- Median salaries, above-average incentive opportunity, median benefits, and 75th percentile total compensation when performance is on budget and otherwise on plan
- Median salaries, median benefits, and enough incentive opportunity to bring total compensation to the 75th percentile only when performance is at the 75th percentile or above
- Seventy-fifth percentile salaries, average incentive opportunity, median benefits, and 75th percentile total compensation

Of course, many compensation programs feature variations on these patterns; for example, some focus on the 60th or 65th percentile rather than the 75th percentile.

Because salaries are the principal determinant of total compensation, a board need only offer average or median incentive opportunity and benefits to maintain the competitive position set by salaries. For example, if salaries are set at the 75th percentile, median incentive opportunity and benefits bring total compensation to the 75th percentile because both are based on 75th percentile salaries.

On the other hand, above-average incentives and benefits have a compounding effect, increasing the competitiveness of total compensation. A policy that sets salaries and incentive opportunity and benefits all at the 75th percentile brings total compensation to the 90th percentile or higher. Many boards do not understand this compounding effect; they assume that they must set each element of the compensation above average to achieve above-average total compensation.

EMPHASIS ON PAY FOR PERFORMANCE

The expression *pay for performance* refers to pay that varies with performance or pay intended to reward performance. At its broadest, it includes merit pay, the salary administration program that ties annual salary increases to performance. In reference to executive pay, though, pay for performance generally means incentive compensation.

For most employees—those who are ineligible for incentive compensation—merit pay is the only method employers use to link pay to performance. For this reason, employers tend to treat it as an important and effective way of linking pay to performance. Because the typical budget for salary increases has been only 3 or 4 percent in recent years, and the reward for outstanding performance is generally a percentage or two higher than the average salary increase for satisfactory performance, the reward for performing better than average is small and pales in comparison with the rewards from an incentive compensation program for executives. The principal determinants of the size of merit salary increases are inflation in prevailing market pay levels and what employers are willing and able to budget for salary increases, not performance.

By contrast, typical incentive awards for executives of tax-exempt hospitals are 15 percent to 30 percent of salary—more for CEOs than for other executives, and more in big hospitals and systems than in small ones. Whatever the opportunity levels, they are generally sufficient to focus participants' attention on the goals they need to meet to earn the awards.

Most observers agree that incentive plans work, insofar as they get people to meet the requirements for earning the awards. Anyone who has seen enough incentive plans and observed the way they work in different settings understands, however, that incentive plans often have unintended consequences. Some trustees and executives are so wary of the consequences that they prefer not to use incentive compensation in executive pay programs.

While some 15 to 20 percent of not-for-profit hospitals and health systems do not use incentive compensation as part of their executive compensation program, most healthcare organizations do. For organizations that have embraced incentive compensation, the question to be answered in developing a compensation philosophy is how much incentive opportunity to offer. The following four factors help frame the answer to this question:

- Whether what motivates executives is the set of goals they are expected to achieve or the money they will receive if they achieve the goals
- The degree to which trustees and executives are comfortable with the performance measures, metrics, measurement systems, and reporting systems used as the framework for incentive compensation

- The gap between the levels of salary and total cash compensation specified in the compensation philosophy
- Whether the organization intends to use just one plan (an annual incentive plan) or two (an annual plan plus a long-term plan)

Most experts argue that the amount of opportunity is less important than the process and structure used in managing incentive compensation—that it is the goals themselves, rather than the potential reward, that motivate executives, and the rigorous discipline incentive plans impose on goal setting, performance measurement, and feedback that improves performance. In other words, above-average incentive opportunity probably has no more impact on performance than below-average opportunity does.

Trustees accustomed to incentive plans in for-profit businesses are often less than completely comfortable with the types of measures typically used in incentive plans by tax-exempt hospitals and health systems. This discomfort tends to lead them to keeping incentive opportunity relatively modest, and significantly lower than typical incentive opportunity in the for-profit sector.

Relatively few tax-exempt hospitals or health systems use both annual and long-term incentives, and most of those that do are large, multibillion-dollar, multihospital systems. Smaller organizations that use both annual and long-term incentives face special challenges in deciding how much incentive opportunity to offer in total and how to balance the opportunity offered in the two plans.

Most boards use one or more of these three methods for determining how much incentive opportunity to offer: mimicking general practice among tax-exempt hospitals and health systems and offering median or average opportunity; deciding to offer more or less than average, whichever the board and CEO believe appropriate for the organization; or calculating the level of incentive opportunity needed to align total compensation with the compensation philosophy.

Some large not-for-profit health systems seem to have used patterns seen in the for-profit sector to determine how much incentive opportunity to offer, but patterns in general industry have not had much influence on incentive opportunity at tax-exempt healthcare organizations. Incentive opportunity is notably higher among for-profit hospitals and health systems than among not-for-profit hospitals and health systems. The one arena in which decisions on incentive opportunity in the not-for-profit sector have been shaped by patterns in the for-profit sector is the health insurance industry, presumably due to intense competition for talent across the boundary between tax-exempt and tax-paying health insurers.

BALANCING FIXED AND VARIABLE PAY

Trustees and executives tend to ignore benefits when deciding how much to emphasize pay for performance. Focusing on the balance between fixed and variable pay can change that decision because it shows how little is variable in most executive compensation packages. When benefits and perquisites are counted, it becomes clear that executive compensation in tax-exempt healthcare organizations is largely fixed, as benefits and perquisites are largely fixed compensation, and benefits and perquisites often outweigh incentive compensation in terms of cost or value. Incentive opportunity of 20 percent of salary for on-plan performance and 30 percent of salary for outstanding performance may seem like an appropriate balance between fixed and variable pay for a $100,000 executive. When one recognizes, however, that the variable component amounts to only 13 percent of total compensation for on-plan performance and only 18 percent of total compensation for outstanding performance, the fixed or guaranteed portion of the compensation package seems to overwhelm the portion tied to performance.

It also leads to the question why benefits are not tied more to performance—especially supplemental retirement benefits for executives. The biggest component of an executive benefits program is often retirement benefits. Retirement benefits—even supplemental executive retirement benefits—are generally fixed, or largely fixed, rather than variable. Some qualified retirement plans count total cash compensation (taxable compensation on IRS Form W-2), but salaries for senior executives, at least, are generally high enough that bonuses or incentive awards do not count. Nonqualified retirement and deferred compensation plans sometimes count incentive awards and bonuses but more often do not. Even when they do count variable pay, they usually guarantee that they will count it, with fixed formulas that count all taxable annual compensation (sometimes even including hiring bonuses and car allowances, sometimes even counting deferred compensation when it vests). Relatively few tax-exempt healthcare organizations make contributions to qualified retirement plans contingent on performance, and almost none make contributions to nonqualified plans contingent on performance—other than making larger contributions when an incentive award is paid and distributing retirement benefits only if the organization remains solvent enough to pay the retirement benefits when they become payable. Retirement benefits—even supplemental retirement benefits and deferred compensation for executives—are designed on the premise that the annual contribution or accrual for retirement is owed to executives for completing a year of service, not that executives have an opportunity to earn a contribution to their supplemental retirement benefit when performance is good.

As long as the focus stays on cash compensation, though, the question of how to balance fixed and variable compensation is the counterpoint to the question of how much emphasis to place on pay for performance. A decision to offer median or average incentive opportunity is a decision to put most weight on fixed compensation and only a small amount of weight on variable compensation. Likewise, a decision to position salaries and total compensation both at median or both at the 60th or 65th or 75th percentiles is a decision to put only a small amount of weight on variable compensation, as there is no room for more than median or average incentive opportunity when salaries and total compensation are both at the same competitive level.

The balance changes significantly with a decision to position total compensation much higher than base pay. When the compensation philosophy calls for positioning salaries at median but total compensation at the 75th percentile, for example, incentive opportunity needs to be twice as much as when salaries and total compensation are at the same competitive level. With a doubling in incentive opportunity, the balance between fixed and variable compensation shifts dramatically. A typical incentive award for an executive increases from 20 to 40 percent of salary, or from 17 to 29 percent of total cash compensation.

Likewise, a decision to use both annual and long-term incentives changes the balance between fixed and variable compensation, because organizations that use both almost always offer a lot more incentive opportunity than those that use only annual incentives—not always twice as much, but usually at least half again as much. Almost never does a board that decides to offer both annual and long-term incentives decide to keep incentive opportunity at median or average levels—in effect, dividing typical annual incentive opportunity in two and leaving so little incentive opportunity in each plan that the administrative burden of managing the plan outweighs whatever advantage the organization gains from using the incentive plans.

INFLUENCE OF PAY MIX ON CULTURE

Few boards or compensation committees spend much time thinking about what the mix of pay implies about the organization's culture and values, or how it contributes to shaping the organization's culture. The mix of pay elements varies from one kind of organization to another, reflecting the organization's culture and values, economic circumstances, or maturity. It varies more in the for-profit sector than in the tax-exempt healthcare sector. Small new entrepreneurial companies tend to skimp on current compensation and emphasize future compensation in the form of stock options. Large mature firms tend to offer fully competitive salaries, incentives, and benefits to help them maintain a stable workforce and executive team. Because most not-for-profit healthcare organizations are big and mature, they generally offer fully competitive pay and benefits. Some organizations are so egalitarian that the executive compensation program consists of nothing more than salaries that are higher than those of other employees; it includes no special benefits, perquisites, or incentive plans for executives (unless an all-employee incentive plan is in place). Others are so generous to executives that every element of the compensation program is notably richer for executives than for the workforce as a whole.

One unintended consequence of a fully competitive executive compensation program is an entitlement mentality. When executive pay is above average, or salary increases are larger for executives than for the workforce as a whole, if executives get richer benefits than other employees, or executives receive visible perquisites like car allowances and club memberships, the board is signaling that executives deserve special treatment, and the executives come to believe that as well.

Boards and executives should realize that executive compensation programs shape stakeholders' perceptions about the values of the organization and that more is at stake in their decisions about executive pay than attracting, retaining, and motivating and rewarding executives. Hospitals' relations with employees and physicians depend on those stakeholders' perceptions of fairness. Hospitals' success at improving clinical quality and satisfying patients' expectations depends on employees' commitment to the hospitals' goals, and nothing undermines their commitment more than their perception that they are being treated unfairly relative to the way executives are treated. Hospitals' tax exemption depends on maintaining support from the public and local, state, and federal authorities, and that becomes more difficult when these stakeholders perceive inappropriate generosity to administrators.

Boards should realize, too, that executive compensation programs shape the way executives make decisions and balance competing priorities. Executives' decisions, in turn, shape the culture of the organization. Compensation programs that are unusually generous to executives encourage executives to believe they deserve special treatment and make it more likely they will look for ways to enhance their compensation than look for ways to control its cost. Incentive plans that put more weight on financial performance than on clinical quality reinforce a focus on cost control and revenue cycle management in ways that make the whole organization cost conscious. Plans that weight clinical quality more heavily than financial performance promote quality improvement efforts and shape an organization-wide commitment to clinical quality and patient safety.

A standard pay mix, one in which salaries, incentives, and benefits and perquisites are all positioned at median or average, may have the least noticeable impact on organizational culture, as it does not emphasize one element more than another and is generally consistent with the way other employees are paid. Even so, it typically shapes culture in four ways:

- Incentive compensation tends to promote a strong performance orientation. It puts a meaningful amount of executives' pay at risk and signals that executives will not be paid fully competitively unless the organization performs well.
- A competitive benefits program indicates that the board values executives enough to be willing to provide supplemental benefits to help retain them. It also shows that the board believes that a strong, stable leadership team is essential to the organization's success and that it is willing to treat executives somewhat better than other employees in order to recruit and retain high-caliber executives.
- A median pay policy sends a strong message to the entire organization that it intends to make the best possible use of limited resources. It supports promotion from within

and, when the board does recruit externally, encourages the organization to choose promising younger executives. It tells executives that the organization is willing to live with a reasonable degree of turnover and does not believe that anyone is irreplaceable.

- A median pay policy represents a conviction that the organization is a good place to work and that executives will choose to work there even if they could make more money elsewhere.

A typical performance-oriented mix of pay, with median salaries and benefits and above-average annual incentive opportunity, has a stronger impact on culture in several ways, including the following:

- It promotes an intense performance orientation and places a significant amount of pay at risk, making clear that managers will not be paid competitively unless they meet the current year's goals.
- It emphasizes operational improvements rather than longer-term initiatives and promotes a high degree of diligence in measuring and monitoring performance and in making midcourse corrections to match changing circumstances.
- It promotes entrepreneurial risk taking by paying big awards for successful initiatives.

A pay program with a special emphasis on long-term performance, featuring median salaries, modest annual incentive opportunity but above-average long-term incentive opportunity, and moderate benefits, has a different effect on culture:

- The emphasis on long-term incentives, more than annual incentives, signals that success in the long run depends on the achievement of major strategic initiatives, at least as much as on effective operational management.

- The emphasis on long-term performance communicates the importance of supporting new initiatives, letting go of the past, and adapting to change as soon as it occurs, and emphasizes the need to keep up with the fast pace of external change.

A pay program with an extremely strong performance orientation, with modest salaries and extremely high incentive opportunity, has the strongest impact on organizational culture. This kind of pay mix is found in for-profit hospital companies and some high-profile not-for-profit systems.

- It communicates that executives' jobs are about making change and achieving goals, not maintaining stability and making incremental improvements.
- It represents impatience for change and a sense of urgency, which often gets communicated to the organization as a whole through higher-than-average incidence of involuntary terminations of people who do not meet expectations or cannot keep pace with change.

A stability-oriented mix of pay, featuring above-average salaries, moderate or no incentives, and above-average retirement benefits, promotes continuity of management and continuity of approach.

- It signals the board's desire to retain executives by promising a comfortable retirement benefit if they stay for the duration of their careers.
- It signals the board's belief that the key to the organization's success is having a stable, first-rate leadership team.
- It promotes a long-term perspective and an incremental approach to making change and discourages unnecessary risk taking.
- It promotes collaboration and encourages people to fit in, increasing the likelihood that they will stay, or be allowed to stay, for the duration of their careers.

Trustees might make the same decisions about executive compensation if they understood how their decisions would affect organizational culture and the way they would be perceived by stakeholders, but they would at least be less surprised by whatever criticism the executive compensation program attracts. They would also have a better basis for making decisions than keeping pay and benefits competitive.

BEST PRACTICES IN COMPENSATION PHILOSOPHY

No doubt some trustees and CEOs would like to know what the best practices are in defining and using executive compensation philosophy well. I do not know of a previous effort to define them, so I offer here a preliminary list:

- Make sure the executive compensation philosophy reflects your organization's mission and values, its leadership needs, and wise use of scarce resources.
- Consider your organization's approach to compensation and benefits for the workforce as a whole, rather than treating executive compensation as an entirely separate matter.
- State the philosophy as a set of general principles or beliefs, rather than as a policy that must be followed; avoid letting a statement of intended competitive position become a promise or an obligation.

Inappropriate Peer Group Positions Pay at 90th Percentile

A small hospital in the South positioned its executive compensation at median relative to its "peers" in the Voluntary Hospital Association, all of which were much larger than it was. The hospital's pay position placed it at the 90th percentile of hospitals its size.

- Choose a carefully tailored peer group of organizations like yours, instead of a generic national peer group, as the source of comparability data to use in setting and evaluating executive compensation data at your organization.
- Set salary and total compensation opportunity at the competitive position that best meets your organization's recruiting and retention needs given the level of competition for talent in your peer group, whatever advantages your institution and community have in attracting and retaining talent, and the type of talent your organization aspires to get and keep.
- Put enough pay at risk to encourage diligence in planning; precision in goal setting; and systematic approaches to tracking, measuring, and reporting results.

Elimination of Incentive Plan Leads to Unintentional Increase in Benefits

A large religious system eliminated its incentive plan but continued to position total compensation at the 75th percentile of its peer group. Executive salaries were positioned at the 90th percentile of the peer group to make up for the lack of incentive opportunity, resulting in an exceptionally rich executive benefits package and a total compensation plan of well above the 75th percentile.

Peer Group Chosen by CEO

A CEO persuaded his board that the peer group for setting his compensation should be for-profit companies larger than his system, as those were the only institutions he would consider leaving the organization for.

- Link any policy of paying above average to a sound rationale (e.g., we will pay total compensation at the 75th percentile when we achieve 75th percentile performance).
- Define the intended competitive position in general rather than precise terms (e.g., "competitive," "middle of the market," "above average," "in the third quartile") to preserve flexibility.
- De-emphasize perquisites and articulate the rationale for providing them, as they attract more attention and criticism than putting the equivalent amount of money into additional compensation or benefits would.
- Review the executive compensation philosophy at least once a year to assess its appropriateness and usefulness in guiding decisions.

CHAPTER 3

Determining the Market Value
of Executive Positions

INTRODUCTION

Debates about executive pay often get mired in the concept of market value. Our society accepts the idea that doctors earn more than nurses and that movie stars earn more than actors in summer stock theater. We understand why plumbers and electricians get paid more than janitors and housekeepers do. People have difficulty, however, accepting the notion that executives deserve what they are paid.

The concept of market value is complex because it must account for multiple labor markets vying for talent, each with its own market values; because the jobs in any occupation vary from one organization to another; and because the best people in most occupations can command pay far above average.

Market value for executive positions varies along several vectors. Large organizations generally pay more than small ones. Independent hospitals generally pay more than subsidiaries. Private not-for-profit hospitals often pay more than public ones. Organizations in large cities tend to pay more than those in small, rural communities. Hospitals in the Northeast region of the United States tend to pay more than hospitals in the Midwest.

The marketplace for talent is not really national—at least not for executives of tax-exempt hospitals and health systems. Hospitals in

New York and Boston rarely recruit in Kansas or Utah, for example. Hospitals in Los Angeles and San Francisco are unlikely to recruit in Maine or Arkansas.

Instead, labor markets are largely regional, and in the country's largest urban areas, they are essentially local. Most positions in New York, Chicago, or Los Angeles can be filled with the talent available within commuting distance of the job.

Labor markets are defined in terms of specialized peer groups and specialized talent. Employers generally aim to hire a candidate who is experienced at doing the work the job requires and at working in an organization similar to the employer's. And candidates typically hope to make the most of their human capital. They can find better jobs, earn more money, and expect more success if they move to jobs similar to those they have performed before and to organizations like those they have worked in before.

Regional Impact on Compensation Philosophy

The board of a premier academic health system with a compensation philosophy of positioning executive compensation at the 75th percentile of the national marketplace began wondering why it was having difficulty recruiting and retaining executives. It discovered that pay levels in the region were 15 percent higher than national norms and that pay levels for premier private academic health systems were 15 percent higher than generic national data from community-based health systems. The health system was offering only median pay for its region and its peer group. The board redefined its peer group for system and flagship executives as a group of 20 leading private academic health systems. The change in the definition raised the 75th percentile by 15 percent and helped solve the system's recruiting and retention problem.

The labor market for any particular executive position, then, is smaller than it might appear to be, and the market value of the position varies according to the labor market from which the employer can draw the kind of talent needed. The fact that executives elsewhere earn considerably more, or less, than average has no bearing on the market value of the position unless these executives are willing to be candidates for the position and are part of the labor market from which the employer recruits. Hospitals and health systems can generally ignore the fact that chief financial officers (CFOs) in publicly traded firms receive stock options and can make much more than CFOs in not-for-profit healthcare organizations, as CFOs of publicly traded firms are generally not part of the labor market from which hospitals and health systems recruit their CFOs. Similarly, hospitals and health systems in the Midwest can generally ignore the higher prevailing pay for healthcare executives in Manhattan, unless they are trying to recruit an executive from Manhattan.

MARKET VALUE DEFINED

The common definition of *market value* for a job is the median or average pay for that job. This definition assumes a crowded labor market—one with an ample supply of labor, a healthy demand for that labor, and plenty of people willing to move from one employer to another.

A more practical definition of market value is the cost of hiring and retaining the talent needed. Because changing jobs entails many costs—loss of seniority, loss of the security and value that come with tenure, maybe the cost of moving and the concomitant disruption of social life and community involvement—people do not move to new jobs without good reason, and the reason is usually higher pay. At the executive level, the cost of changing jobs is substantial, because it often involves relocating and always requires proving one's worth in a new situation. Sometimes it requires giving up substantial amounts of unvested, nonqualified deferred compensation.

So what is the cost of hiring an executive? It is not likely to be median or average pay. If the job can be filled by promoting an internal candidate, it may be considerably less than median. If it can only be filled by recruiting externally and by hiring someone already experienced at doing the same job for an organization of similar size, it will almost certainly cost more than median, as such candidates are generally already earning median pay or more and are unwilling to move without an increase.

And what is the cost of retaining an executive? It may be median or average pay, but it may be more—maybe even a lot more—and it may even be less. If the incumbent likes the job, has ties to the community, and has no particular ambition for a higher-level job, it may be only median or even less. If the incumbent is ambitious and wants a higher-level job, it is likely to take much more to retain her, but retaining her is unlikely, no matter how much you pay, unless she believes she is in line for an internal promotion within a few years.

Understanding market value requires understanding the range of pay for the job, not just the median or average value. At the executive level, the dispersion in pay is enormous, with the high end at least 50 percent more than average and the low end about half the average. Even the standard deviation is wide—at least 30 percent of the central value.

The Concept of Market Value

Market value can be thought of two ways:

- What other, comparable organizations in the region pay the person doing the job (the range of what they pay, from high to low)
- What it will cost to persuade a qualified candidate to take the job (the range of what it will take given what the candidates are making now and other circumstances)

Market value must be thought of as a range of pay to account for the broad dispersion in pay for a job as well as the many reasons executives decide to stay in a job or decide to move to a new position. The range of pay for a job, from high to low or from the 10th to the 90th percentile, shows what executives have been willing to accept as adequate pay and what other hospitals have paid to promote or hire and retain someone to do the job. Given that half the executives in any job are paid less than median, and often substantially less, and given that half are paid more than median, and often substantially

---

How to Determine the Value of a Job

Organizations take one of two approaches to determining the value of a job. The first approach, referred to as market pricing, relies on gathering and analyzing data on pay for the job in question. It is the most common approach to valuing jobs in general and the approach typically used in determining the value of executive positions. The second approach is called job evaluation and relies on evaluating the size and complexity of the job and its responsibilities, then determining its value in relation to other jobs in the same organization. Market pricing emphasizes careful comparisons with what other organizations pay and assumes that what other organizations pay matters more than internal pay relationships. Job evaluation emphasizes internal equity or fairness of pay across the management team and assumes that internal equity matters more than matching what other organizations pay. Both approaches have advantages and disadvantages; as a result, most organizations informally integrate the two approaches. Those that use market pricing try to keep internal pay relationships fair. Those that use job evaluation still aim to keep pay competitive.

---

more, the dispersion in pay for executive jobs makes any notion of market value based only on median or average value too narrow.

That notion is appealing nonetheless because median does represent the central value in the dispersion of actual pay rates, and average does much the same. It seems to imply that median pay is fair pay for the job, or the right rate of pay for the job. But what median pay means depends on one's perspective. A board recruiting a new CEO may regard the median as the least it should expect to pay. A CEO who knows he will be able to fill most executive positions from within may regard it as the most he is willing to pay. A proud organization with a rich bottom line may regard it as the least it would consider fair pay, while a public hospital required to disclose executive pay to the public may regard it as the most it can justify paying.

Salary, Total Cash, Total Compensation

Most people think of market value primarily in terms of salary. It is the usual basis for any discussion of pay with an internal candidate for promotion and for initial negotiations with an external candidate for an executive position. It is also the usual basis for discussion of the relative value of jobs in an organization and for efforts to manage internal equity among members of the executive team.

Trustees serving on compensation committees often think of market value in terms of *total cash compensation*, not just salary, and place more emphasis on the variable portion of pay than it warrants. They often believe, for example, that it should be easy to recruit and retain executives with median salaries, as long as incentive opportunity is high enough. Executives, however, tend to discount the value of incentive opportunity because they cannot count on receiving it.

Focusing only on salaries or total cash compensation ignores the value of benefits and perquisites, and they are often worth 20 to 25 percent of total compensation, as much as or more than incentive opportunity.[1] Any version of market value based only on salary assumes that incentive opportunity and benefits are competitive, just as any version based on total cash compensation assumes that benefits are competitive. Organizations with below-average incentive opportunity often find that they need to pay higher salaries to make up for it, just as those with below-average benefits often need to pay higher salaries to make up for it. Salary may be the starting point for discussions of pay, fair pay, and market value, but the discussion eventually turns to total compensation if there is a shortfall in either incentive opportunity or benefits. Ultimately, an executive's notion of market value encompasses incentive opportunity, benefits, and perquisites as well as salary.

Fair Market Value

Fair market value is defined as the value a willing buyer and a willing seller would agree to in an arms'-length transaction. Fair market value could be more or less than median—more if additional enticement is required to persuade an executive to accept a new position, and less if a candidate, such as an internal applicant, wants a promotion to an executive-level position badly enough that he is willing to accept something less than median pay.

The Internal Revenue Service (IRS) defines *fair market value* in terms of total compensation, not just cash compensation. One requirement for establishing the "rebuttable presumption of reasonableness" to minimize risk of intermediate sanctions (discussed earlier in the book) is that decisions about executive pay must be based on total compensation—not just salary or cash compensation. Consultants and compensation committees now routinely assess the value of total compensation to meet that regulatory requirement.

Fair market value is different from *market value*. Its central idea is the occurrence of an arms'-length transaction—in which neither party has an advantage in determining pay—between a willing buyer and a willing seller. It presumes to represent something like true market value—what any other employer would be willing to pay someone to do the job and what any other executive would be willing to accept as fair pay for the job—but it really represents nothing more than what one employer is willing to pay a particular person and what that person will accept as fair pay. Fair market value can just as well be at the 75th or 90th percentile as at median or average pay, just as an arms'-length transaction can settle on pay at the 10th or 25th percentile.

Arms'-length negotiations for pay take place primarily when an organization recruits external candidates for an open position. In theory, any pay negotiation with an external candidate is an arms'-length transaction. In practice, the compensation levels agreed to in these negotiations are often well above average, especially when they involve a board trying to recruit a new CEO. The concept of fair market value establishes the deal's terms as the market value for the job. Even when a candidate negotiates an unusually rich package—one that is higher than comparability data indicate as appropriate for the job—her compensation can still be considered fair market value because it was negotiated in an arms'-length transaction.

What Other Organizations Would Pay

Because executive pay is generally developed over time, developed one step at a time, and shaped by circumstances that emerge throughout the process, the IRS uses another definition of *fair market value* in situations not involving new hires. According to this definition, *fair market value* constitutes the amount that other similar organizations would pay for the position under similar circumstances. This definition brings the concept of fair market value close to the usual definition of market value and in practice defines fair market value as median or average. Indeed, the IRS does view fair market value for executive positions in tax-exempt organizations as median or average pay and regards any compensation above median or average as potentially excessive.

Going Rate for the Job

Human resources managers, especially compensation managers, think of market value as the "going rate for the job"—the rate they and other employers pay for that job. This notion is similar to median or average but is not necessarily based on a statistical analysis. If used to mean "this is what we pay for the job," the phrase could represent more or less than the average of what other employers pay for the same job. If it means "this is the starting pay for the job," it refers to the lowest rate the organization pays people in the job.

What It Costs to Hire the Right Person

For recruiters, trustees, and CEOs trying to recruit a candidate for an open position, the most important factor is what it costs to hire the right person for the job. This premise has nothing to do with median or average pay because it is arrived at through negotiation with the person they want to hire, who is presumed to be the best candidate of all those who have applied.

Recruiters tend to believe the market value of an open position is generally well above average, as the "right" person will likely require a significant raise to move to the open position. They expect that this person will have an impressive background and a track record of success. While some candidates may be impressive department heads ready for promotion to executive-level responsibility, recruiters have to assume that most impressive candidates are already experienced in executive-level positions and already paid at or above median.

Value of Person Versus Value of Job

Any notion of market pay commingles the value of the job and the value of the person—either the incumbent in the job or candidates for an open job. After all, pay for an incumbent is affected by the incumbent's talent, experience, and ambition as well as by his performance, his ability to negotiate, and any offers he may get from other employers—and by whatever contributions the incumbent makes to the success of the organization besides handling the core requirements of the position. Likewise, the range of pay in the marketplace is affected by the talent, experience, performance, and mobility of the individuals in the job elsewhere as well as by supply and demand and other factors.

When a CEO insists that the market value placed on one of his executive positions is too high or too low, he is often saying it is too high or too low for the way the job is performed by the incumbent. That could mean that the job is different from the norm irrespective of the incumbent, or that it is different from the norm because of the incumbent. Leadership jobs often change a bit from one incumbent to the next, in part because incumbents pursue responsibility for activities they want to lead and avoid responsibility for activities they have no interest in; in part because of the influence leaders wield in the organization as a whole; and in part because of the CEO's decision to assign activities to one executive or another, often for reasons that have more to do with personality or personal capabilities than the logic of organization design. It is not uncommon, for example, for a CEO to say "Our in-house counsel is not really a general counsel" or "My CFO is my second-in-command and much more than a standard CFO."

The standard notion of market value pertains to the job, however, not the incumbent, because market value is considered to be the value other organizations place on the job, or what they pay to get the job done. Considering the variability in job responsibilities and the way the job is performed from organization to organization and incumbent to incumbent, market value is a generalization that cannot adequately reflect relatively small differences in the way a job is structured or handled or in the influence an incumbent wields.

SOURCES OF MARKET DATA

There are two reliable sources of data for determining market value for executive positions. The best is a good survey published by a reputable consulting firm or survey house. The second is the IRS Form 990 reports of tax-exempt hospitals and health systems.

Other, less reliable sources include trade publications (e.g., *Modern Healthcare*) that present a summarized version of data from a reputable survey and anecdotal information gained from search consultants, colleagues, or candidates interviewing for jobs. In the paragraphs that follow, we discuss surveys and Form 990s as data sources.

Surveys

A handful of standard national surveys of executive compensation in the healthcare industry are published by reputable consulting firms, and several dozen more specialized national surveys are published by consulting firms and survey houses. In addition, state hospital associations, consulting firms, and survey houses publish several dozen state and regional surveys; individual healthcare organizations commission custom surveys ("club surveys"); and associations, consulting firms, and survey houses publish surveys of specialty healthcare organizations—home health agencies, long-term care providers, medical groups, cancer centers, independent practice associations, health maintenance organizations (HMOs), and the like.

The best general-purpose surveys for hospitals and health systems are the big national surveys conducted by major consulting firms, because they represent pay practices at hundreds of hospitals and systems of all sizes for thousands of executives. These surveys report enough data to provide reliable statistics on typical pay and range of pay; salary increases; incentive opportunity; the structure of incentive plans; and the types of performance measures used. Some also report reliable statistics on the prevalence, structure, and value of benefits and perquisites for most standard executive positions. They present the data in three to six different size classes and provide charts showing formulas for determining the predicted value of a job at organizations of any size using regression analysis.

The principal weakness of these surveys is that they are broad and national in scope. Furthermore, they generally do not identify the size of the organizations in the survey, so it is difficult to know which organizations are represented in any cut of data; they do not report data in a way that reflects regional differences in pay or differences based on type of organization; and they do not allow the user to analyze pay practices from a custom peer group of organizations most like the hospital or system in question.

For specialized organizations, the best surveys are often specialty surveys of organizations of the same type—academic medical centers, children's hospitals, HMOs, and so on. As long as these surveys have enough participants, they can provide reliable statistics on pay practices for these specialized organizations.

Where pay is higher or lower than the norm because of cost-of-living rates, statewide or regional surveys can provide better data on prevailing pay practices than national surveys can, if enough organizations participate to make the surveys reliable. Surveys conducted by state hospital associations can be adequate sources of data, especially for small and midsize hospitals and systems. The regional, statewide, and local cuts of data in national surveys typically do not calibrate the data according to organization size, making it difficult to determine whether any differences in pay are due to real geographic differentials in pay or only to differences in the size of organizations in the regional samples.

Surveys are only as good as the data submitted to them and the analytical methods used to identify statistics, norms, and patterns. Surveys collect data from human resources staff in hospitals and health systems. These staff may not understand the extent to which the jobs at their organization match the survey's benchmark jobs; they may not have access to all the details of executive compensation, such as the CEO's auto allowance, severance, or club memberships; and their data may not have been entered accurately in the survey database. Furthermore, the survey firm may not test the data for accuracy, follow up on incomplete or inaccurate submissions, or study the computer-generated analyses enough to identify and correct any statistics or conclusions that misrepresent pay practices in the industry.

In the end, any weaknesses in the surveys may not affect the results if there are enough data to overcome the effects of any errors. The big national surveys gather so much data that the medians, averages, and general patterns are almost always reliable. At the extremes of a distribution pattern, however, anomalies and errors in the raw data can distort statistics. Data at the 90th percentile in any survey, for example, are less reliable than data at median, even if the data sample is unusually large.

If the amount of data is insufficient to overcome the effects of errors in the raw data, it is not enough to provide an accurate picture of data dispersion. Any data sample with fewer than a dozen data points is likely to be less than reliable for any statistics other than median and average.

Form 990s

In years past the data in IRS Form 990 had been difficult to interpret, because salaries, incentive awards, and other taxable income were lumped together as a single figure reported as "compensation" and because many organizations found ways to disguise the total value of what they were paying executives. The version of the form introduced for the 2008 tax year makes it easier to understand the data reported, and the instructions make it easier to understand what must be reported. So it is now easier—but still not always easy—to obtain from Form 990s relatively reliable statistics on pay practices at hospitals and health systems. As a result, the data from Form 990s will be more widely used than they have been in the past, and they may come to be relied on as much as published survey data.

The form now reports separate data on salary, bonus and incentive awards, and other cash compensation; deferred compensation; nontaxable benefits; total compensation; and previously reported compensation. It requires description of severance, change-of-control payments, nonqualified deferred compensation and retirement plans, and incentive compensation plans, and indication of the amounts accrued and paid for these purposes must be shown. This makes it relatively easy to assemble a pay database for a custom peer group and use it in determining the market value for a standard senior executive position.

Trustees may be accustomed to using data from proxies of for-profit firms and expect data from the Form 990s to be as reliable as data from proxies. They are not. Any organization using the data from 990 forms to determine market value for executive positions needs to be aware of the various ways in which individual data points may be misleading. Some of these factors are listed in the sidebar titled "Weaknesses in Form 990 Data" and discussed below.

First, the figures report the amount of compensation paid in a calendar year, not the annualized value of compensation for the year or the pay level at the end of the year. If someone worked less than a full year or was paid an award from a multiyear retention incentive or a long-term incentive plan, it is difficult to determine what was earned by working for a full year or what would have been earned if the executive had worked for a full year.

Second, the data are reported by name of the executive (or trustee) with the individual's job title, but the title is often generic rather than specific (e.g., vice president, rather than vice president for patient care). If the individual's job responsibilities cannot be determined, the compensation data reported have little use.

Third, multihospital systems may report compensation for some executives in the Form 990 report for the system and compensation for other executives in separate 990 forms for each hospital or for other separately incorporated businesses, such as home

---

Weaknesses in Form 990 Data

- Titles do not reveal job responsibilities.
- Salary and incentive figures do not include voluntary deferrals.
- Pay data sometimes cover only partial years (for new or terminated employees).
- Total compensation may include hiring bonuses, severance, or distributions of retirement benefits.
- Incentives may include one-time payments, such as hiring bonuses, multiyear retention incentives, or multiyear awards from long-term incentive plans.
- Incentives may include awards for two fiscal years, not just one.
- Deferred compensation may encompass employer-paid contributions to retirement plans, voluntary deferrals of salary, or voluntary or mandatory deferrals of incentive awards.
- Values reported for supplemental defined-benefit retirement plans can distort the value of total annual compensation.
- Some systems split their executives' pay among multiple organizations.
- Some organizations do not report the full value of benefits.
- Some organizations do not disclose deferred compensation subject to risk of forfeiture.

---

health agencies and medical groups. This makes it difficult to get a comprehensive picture of executive compensation at the system as a whole. Some systems apparently continue to divide executives' compensation among multiple entities, masking the total amount of compensation paid, even though this practice is not permissible and has not been for some time.

Fourth, the data obtainable from 990 forms are at least a year old and often older. The Form 990 reports are generally not available until almost a year after the end of the organization's fiscal year, and the compensation data from organizations on a fiscal year ending before December 31 are from the prior calendar year. Sometimes, the most recent data available on the standard reporting site GuideStar (www2.guidestar.org) are two or three years old.

SELECTING DATA TO DETERMINE JOB VALUE

Determining the market value of a job is a matter of finding, selecting, and analyzing the right data. Every decision made in selecting data can affect the estimate of market value determined from it. Using the wrong data can lead to overvaluing or undervaluing the job. Just as important, the wrong decisions make the estimate suspect, because the data will not reflect pay for similar jobs in similar organizations under similar circumstances.

Many separate decisions must be made during the data selection process:

- How to match the job in question with a standard benchmark position
- How to match a job that combines parts of two benchmark positions or is broader or narrower in scope and responsibility than the standard job
- What criteria to use in selecting an appropriate peer group
- How to choose the peer group
- How to find and choose the best sources of data

- How to choose the right cut of data from the survey or database
- How to choose the best analytical technique
- How to validate the data to ensure they are suitable for the job in question

These decisions are discussed in the following paragraphs.

Job Analysis (What Is the Job?)

The first and most important step in determining the value of a job is studying the job and the management structure within which it works to gain a good understanding of the job—to determine the full scope of the job's responsibilities, how much it resembles a standard benchmark position, and how much it differs from the standard. The value of the job cannot be determined without this understanding.

The title of a job does not convey enough information to determine the value of the job. Titles can be misleading because organizations use titles differently; they can be obsolete if the job has changed and the title has not. More important, relying on the title to determine the value of the job presumes that all jobs with the same title have the same responsibilities, and this is definitely not the case. Jobs with the title of chief financial officer vary a lot, as do jobs with the title of chief operating officer (COO). Rank conveys next to no information, other than that an organization with no senior vice presidents or executive vice presidents uses titles conservatively and that one with lots of senior vice presidents or multiple executive vice presidents has decided to use titles as a form of nonmonetary perquisite. Certain executive positions, such as head of managed care or head of business development, vary so much that, without learning about the jobs' responsibilities and how they fit with other jobs in the same organization, one has no idea what the jobs entail.

The structure within which the job operates and the interrelationships among jobs in the organization are both important to understanding the job. A job in a subsidiary hospital often has less latitude in decision making than its counterpart in an independent organization. A job reporting to the CEO generally has more latitude than one reporting to the COO. In many organizations, jobs share responsibility for one activity or another, which makes it difficult to understand either job without understanding how they interact. In most organizations, executives have one set of responsibilities or operations for which they are directly accountable for managing and another set in which they have shared or contributory responsibility for planning.

Organization Analysis (What Is Special About the Organization?)

The second most important step in determining the value of a job (or a set of jobs) is studying the organization in which it operates to identify the organization's defining characteristics— those most important in selecting a group of other organizations similar enough that they can be considered peers. Organization size is always important. Location can be a key factor as well, but the distinction between urban, suburban, and rural may be more important than the city, state, or region in which the hospital is located. Other distinguishing characteristics include geographic dispersion and degree of centralization for multihospital systems, number of employed physicians and degree of integration between hospital and physicians, emphasis on teaching and research and relationship to medical schools and other educational institutions, nature of involvement in managed care, and size and type of subacute care operations. Governance, sponsorship, and control can be important, too, in identifying distinguishing characteristics, as public institutions can differ from private ones, for-profit hospitals from not-for-profits, and religious systems from secular systems.

For that matter, district hospitals differ from city, county, and state university hospitals.

Clinical specializations are distinguishing characteristics when a hospital focuses primarily on one type of care—pediatric care, for example, or cancer, cardiology, behavioral care, or rehabilitation. Children's hospitals are worlds apart from cancer centers and heart hospitals, and psychiatric hospitals have little in common with general hospitals.

Many health systems have become so complex that they have two or three distinguishing characteristics that set them apart from most other systems. Some geographically dispersed, decentralized, religious systems employ a large number of physicians, for example. Some secular systems encompass a large health plan, a large group of employed physicians, and a number of hospitals. And systems like Kaiser, Mayo, and Geisinger are unique.

Choosing the Right Peer Group

The third step in determining the value of a job (or a set of jobs) is choosing the peer group from which comparability data will be drawn. Four factors may affect that choice:

- Cost in time and money (What will it cost?)
- Accessibility of data (How long will it take to get it? How easy will it be?)
- Defensibility (Will observers and the IRS accept this as an appropriate peer group?)
- Persuasiveness (Will executives and the board accept this as an appropriate peer group?)

The right peer group for any organization is presumably a group of organizations just like the one in question. But it is costly and time consuming to identify a group of organizations that have the same characteristics. Organizations that are likely to be challenged on their choice of peer group may find that defensibility is more important than cost and decide to use a custom-tailored peer group to justify the way they pay their executives. Organizations that need to persuade their executives that they are paid competitively may also need to use a custom-tailored peer group that satisfies both the board and the executives that the peer group has been carefully chosen to reflect the distinguishing characteristics the board and executives consider most relevant.

Standard published surveys offer readily accessible data at a modest price, and they are easy to use. For a hospital or health system that is content with generic data, the right peer group may be a national peer group of hospitals or health systems of comparable size. For a hospital or health system with few distinctive characteristics, the right peer group may be a generic national peer group of organizations of comparable size.

Club surveys, too, offer readily accessible, easy-to-use data, and they are generally free, paid for by another party. For an organization lucky enough to be invited to participate in a club survey, the

---

Using the Right Peer Group to Keep Executive Pay Modest

A small integrated delivery system formed by the merger of a large multispecialty clinic and a midsize community hospital wanted to use a peer group of similar highly integrated systems to set its pay levels. Analysis determined that systems in which physicians led the decision making tended to pay less than systems led by lay administrators. This system agreed to use the peer group of physician-led systems, because the executive pay program was modest, the trustees and executives were conservative, and the system preferred to allocate any available resources to clinical programs rather than executive compensation. Because the system had little turnover at the executive level and did not need to recruit executives externally, paying a bit below average did not cause a problem.

---

peer group chosen for that survey may be more or less the right peer group. The peer group was, however, chosen by the survey sponsor and may be more appropriate for the sponsor than for any of the other participants.

Using a custom-tailored peer group is expensive, unless there is a ready-made survey limited to the right type of organizations. It requires commissioning a custom analysis from a consulting firm or a survey house, conducting a special survey to collect data from the peer group, or gathering data from IRS Form 990 reports. The data are never readily accessible, they take time to collect, and someone needs to be paid to collect them. On the other hand, the custom peer group is likely to be more defensible to critics and auditors and more acceptable to trustees and executives.

An organization that decides to use a custom-tailored peer group has enormous flexibility in defining its peer group. It can decide whether to select a specific group of organizations by name, ones executives and trustees all agree are peers; a regional peer group of hospitals or systems of comparable size; or a national or regional peer group of organizations that have similar distinguishing characteristics. A regional peer group can be defined in terms of a single state, a multistate region, a metropolitan area, or part of a state (e.g., Southern California, Upstate New York), or by the distance from a central geographic location. A custom peer group can be as small as ten organizations or bigger than 50. It can be limited to public institutions or private not-for-profit ones, or religious or secular organizations. A peer group for a system with a large physician network can be limited to systems that were formed from multispecialty physician practices or ones that were formed as hospitals acquired small physician practices.

Some organizations decide to define a custom peer group on the basis of performance. But this decision leads to a motley group of organizations of different sizes and distinguishing characteristics, because neither good financial performance nor extremely high patient satisfaction or clinical quality defines a peer group of comparable organizations.

Choosing High-Performing Organizations
Led to Wrong Peer Group

A large not-for-profit multihospital system wanted to set its incentive opportunity and total cash compensation on par with a peer group of "high-performing organizations." It chose a peer group from a survey that reported much higher incentive opportunity and total cash compensation for high-performing organizations than for others. No one told the compensation committee that the high-performing peer group was largely composed of for-profit organizations, which explained why they were identified as high performing (they had high profit margins) and why their incentive opportunity and total cash compensation were so high. Had the committee known the makeup of this peer group, it may have decided that this peer group was not the right one for a high-performing not-for-profit health system to use.

"Aspirational" Peer Group Would Mean Pay
Above the 90th Percentile

An integrated delivery system developed an "aspirational" peer group of organizations it admired and wanted to emulate. It included such internationally recognized names as Johns Hopkins Medicine, Mayo Clinic, Cleveland Clinic, UCLA Medical Center, and Cedars-Sinai, even though the system had only minimal name recognition outside its own region. The system discovered that using this peer group would have positioned its pay practice well over the 90th percentile for systems more like it and decided not to use it.

Choosing the Right Data Source

The fourth step in determining the value of a job (or a set of jobs) is selecting the best sources of data to represent the peer group whose pay practices the hospital or health system wants to use in determining its own pay.

An organization that is content with generic data can choose from a number of national and regional surveys of hospitals and health systems or a survey sponsored by the state hospital association. Some surveys represent hospitals better than systems; others focus only on multihospital systems; and some represent hospitals and systems equally well, by presenting data from hospitals in one section and data from systems in another. Any of the surveys by prominent national consulting firms provide reliable data for most organizations, but some surveys represent small organizations better than large ones, others represent the country's largest health systems better than small and midsize ones, and some represent certain regions of the country better than others. Surveys that provide formulas from regression analysis for determining pay levels for any size organization can be more useful in refining an estimate of market value than those that report pay data only in broad size groupings. A survey that reports data for all systems over $1 billion in net revenue, for example, is only barely adequate for helping a $4 billion system determine the value of its executive positions, as most tax-exempt health systems over $1 billion in net revenue are below $2 billion in size. Likewise, a survey that reports data for all hospitals with less than $100 million in net revenues is hardly adequate for determining the value of executive positions in a $7 million hospital.

An organization that decides to use a custom peer group may be able to use a club survey of organizations like it in sharing some distinctive characteristics other than size. If no ready-made survey adequately represents the custom peer group, the organization will have three choices for obtaining comparability data representing its chosen peer group. One choice is commissioning a special survey to collect comparability data from organizations with the right distinguishing characteristics. Another choice is asking a consulting firm or survey house for a cut of data representing the custom peer group. The third choice is collecting data from the IRS Form 990 report of organizations in the peer group. Most of the major national consulting firms and survey houses have big enough databases that they can deliver cuts of data representing custom peer groups without conducting a special survey. If it is essential to have data from particular organizations, however, or from all the hospitals of comparable size within a 100-mile radius, Form 990 data will need to be used.

Any organization using a custom peer group should consider using a broad national survey for comparison, as the comparison will show how much pay levels in the custom peer group differ from those in the broad national survey. If the difference between the two is significant, the comparison will show trustees the consequences of using the custom peer group. If the difference is minimal, the organization may decide that the cost of using the custom peer group outweighs any benefit gained from using it. Special surveys and cuts of data from a custom peer group often focus on the most common executive positions and do not provide data on less common jobs. The comparison between the custom peer group and a national survey can also provide a factor to use in adjusting data from the broad national survey for jobs that are not adequately represented in the custom peer group.

Choosing the Right Benchmark

The fifth step, and one of the most important, in determining the value of a job is choosing the right benchmark for comparison. The first step—studying the job and the management structure in which it works—should make it easy to decide whether a straightforward match with a standard benchmark position will suffice, whether the job should be matched with several benchmark positions, or whether the job is so different from standard benchmark positions that another approach is needed to determine the value of the job.

Surveys collect and report data on standard positions found in most hospitals and health systems, usually top-level executive positions and heads of operating departments and staff functions. They do not collect or report data on unusual positions because they are too few in number to develop a robust data sample. As a consequence, most organizations will not find good job matches for some of their positions.

Some jobs for which there are no standard benchmark matches can be valued using data representing the labor market from which talent is drawn, rather than representing the job itself. An unusual leadership position that must be staffed by a physician, for example, can be valued by looking at generic data on medical administrators in primary care, and an unusual job requiring a registered nursing background can be valued by looking at generic data for nursing administrators.

Mismatching a Unique Job

A midsize system in the Midwest invests a great deal of money in community development. Its foundation donates money to community organizations and provides seed money to develop new community services. For years, a consultant valued the job of the executive in charge of the foundation as head of development, even though the job had no responsibility for fundraising. It was more like the head of a grant-making foundation or the head of a community development organization than the head of a fundraising organization. Using the wrong benchmark match led the system to pay the job more than it needed to.

Compound jobs combining the responsibilities of two or more standard benchmark positions can generally be handled by matching them with each of the benchmarks they resemble, but the value of the job depends on which responsibility is primary and whether the combination of responsibilities makes the job bigger than the benchmarks. Composite jobs made up of an unusual mixture of responsibilities—such a motley mixture that they cannot be matched with any standard benchmark—are often impossible to match in any way other than in reference to the labor market from which the candidates are likely to be drawn.

Some jobs can be matched to jobs more easily in general industry surveys than in healthcare surveys, whether because the job is more often found in general industry or because the general industry surveys cover certain jobs not covered by healthcare surveys. Second-level executive jobs in information technology, finance, and legal services, for example, can often be matched through surveys dedicated to these jobs in general industry.

Other jobs are best left unmatched rather than using a questionable or inappropriate match. In these cases, the job can be valued by comparison with other executive positions on the basis of internal equity.

Choosing the Right Data Sample

Because size of the organization in which a job works is one of the most significant determinants of the value of an executive position, the most important step in choosing the right data sample or right cut of data from a survey is finding the cut that best represents organizations of the right size. For highly specialized organizations, like academic medical centers, children's hospitals, or comprehensive cancer centers, prestige may matter as much as size, but for most organizations, size is a major determinant of pay because organization size is generally regarded as a good measure of the scope of an executive position.

Most surveys analyze and present data in several ways. The big national surveys typically report system and hospital data separately. They also report several data cuts for organizations of different size—small, medium, and large, at least (see Exhibit 3.1). They sometimes report data for different regions. A few surveys distinguish between public and private hospitals, between teaching and nonteaching institutions, and between religious and secular institutions. Some report regression formulas[2] as well, allowing the user to calculate the predicted value of a job for organizations of any size.

If the median or average size for organizations in a data cut is reasonably close to that of the organization using the data—within, say, 20 percent of its size—the data cut will be fairly reliable for determining the market value of a job. If the cut is too broad, or if the median or average revenue for the cut is much higher or lower than the organization's, the data cut is not likely to provide reliable information on the value of the job. The regression formula may provide a more reliable estimate.

Most surveys also provide a table representing all the comparability data on a particular job, from organizations of all sizes (see Exhibit 3.1). These "all systems" or "all hospitals" cuts may provide a reliable estimate of market value for a job, but only if the median or average size of the organizations in the survey is close to the size of the organization in which the job works. And these "all" cuts will only provide reliable estimates of market value at median—not at the 25th or 75th or 90th percentiles, because those values are likely to represent pay practices at larger or smaller organizations.

National surveys providing regional cuts of data typically present a single cut for each region, representing all the organizations in that region without regard for size. Like a national "all" cut, these regional "all systems" or "all hospitals" cuts will provide a reliable estimate of market value for a job only if the median or average size of the organizations in the region is close to the size of the organization in which the job works.

Exhibit 3.1: Compensation Data for System Chief Operating Officer (pay in $000)

		10th Percentile
Systems < $500 Million Net Revenue	Base salary	$185.6
	Total annual cash	$193.7
	Increase last 12 months (%)	0.0%
	STI award	$2.5
	STI target opportunity (%)	5.0%
	STI maximum opportunity (%)	15.0%
	Total direct cash	$193.7
	LTI award	***
	LTI target opportunity (%)	***
	LTI maximum opportunity (%)	***
	Organization's net revenue (millions)	$127.0
Systems $250 Million to $750 Million Net Revenue	Base salary	$261.0
	Total annual cash	$264.8
	Increase last 12 months (%)	0.0%
	STI award	$12.5
	STI target opportunity (%)	5.0%
	STI maximum opportunity (%)	15.0%
	Total direct cash	$264.8
	LTI award	***
	LTI target opportunity (%)	***
	LTI maximum opportunity (%)	***
	Organization's net revenue (millions)	$314.5

25th Percentile	Median	Average	75th Percentile	90th Percentile	Count
$230.0	$289.5	$281.7	$334.4	$381.7	48
$233.3	$329.2	$313.7	$378.0	$418.2	48
0.0%	2.4%	3.0%	5.8%	7.3%	24
$15.9	$42.6	$51.2	$80.7	$111.1	30
17.5%	20.0%	20.0%	25.0%	30.0%	21
20.0%	30.0%	29.9%	40.0%	50.0%	26
$233.3	$329.2	$314.8	$378.0	$444.0	48
***	***	***	***	***	1
***	***	***	***	***	2
***	***	***	***	***	2
$215.5	$336.5	$317.2	$431.5	$482.0	48
$290.0	$331.5	$335.0	$382.4	$428.8	50
$310.0	$371.8	$379.3	$456.0	$513.4	50
0.0%	1.5%	2.6%	5.6%	7.5%	27
$39.5	$63.0	$67.1	$102.6	$120.2	33
15.3%	23.3%	21.3%	30.0%	30.0%	24
25.0%	30.0%	31.1%	40.0%	45.0%	32
$310.0	$371.8	$380.4	$456.0	$513.4	50
***	***	***	***	***	1
***	***	***	***	***	2
***	***	***	***	***	2
$389.0	$478.8	$484.8	$582.5	$653.5	50

(Continued on next page)

Exhibit 3.1 (Continued)

		10th Percentile
	Base salary	$262.0
	Total annual cash	$262.0
	Increase last 12 months (%)	0.0%
	STI award	$0.0
Systems $500 Million to $1.0 Billion Net Revenue	STI target opportunity (%)	10.0%
	STI maximum opportunity (%)	15.0%
	Total direct cash	$262.0
	LTI award	***
	LTI target opportunity (%)	***
	LTI maximum opportunity (%)	***
	Organization's net revenue (millions)	$568.0
	Base salary	$304.6
	Total annual cash	$324.3
	Increase last 12 months (%)	0.0%
	STI award	$0.0
Systems $750 Million to $2.0 Billion Net Revenue	STI target opportunity (%)	12.5%
	STI maximum opportunity (%)	15.0%
	Total direct cash	$324.3
	LTI award	***
	LTI target opportunity (%)	***
	LTI maximum opportunity (%)	***
	Organization's net revenue (millions)	$810.0

Source: Adapted from Integrated Healthcare Strategies (2010, 110).
Note: STI = short-term incentive; LTI = long-term incentive.

25th Percentile	Median	Average	75th Percentile	90th Percentile	Count
$317.5	$382.4	$372.8	$437.0	$455.0	43
$325.5	$462.5	$430.7	$548.7	$572.0	43
0.0%	1.5%	2.1%	3.0%	6.8%	20
$32.3	$89.1	$80.2	$125.3	$137.8	31
16.5%	25.0%	23.7%	30.0%	40.0%	21
27.5%	35.0%	34.1%	40.0%	50.0%	24
$325.5	$462.5	$430.9	$548.7	$572.0	43
***	***	***	***	***	0
***	***	***	***	***	0
***	***	***	***	***	0
$627.7	$754.0	$752.3	$867.5	$941.0	43
$358.5	$436.2	$442.0	$494.4	$611.2	57
$422.5	$521.0	$536.1	$620.7	$792.1	57
.0%	1.5%	2.4%	4.0%	6.0%	23
$52.2	$106.3	$119.2	$172.0	$239.2	45
20.0%	25.0%	25.5%	31.0%	40.0%	32
30.0%	35.0%	35.7%	45.0%	50.0%	37
$422.5	$521.0	$545.4	$620.7	$792.1	57
$.0	$52.9	$73.6	$89.0	***	7
20.0%	20.0%	24.7%	30.0%	***	7
22.5%	37.5%	44.3%	47.5%	***	8
$890.8	$1,079.3	$1,149.5	$1,300.0	$1,710.0	57

Validating the Data: Getting It Right

The final step in determining the value of a job or set of jobs is validating the data chosen to make sure they are likely to deliver a reliable estimate of market value. If the estimate of market value seems wrong for the job and the organization in which it works, it probably is wrong. Until one is satisfied that the data are right for the job, relative to the other executive positions in the organization, one ought to be skeptical enough to keep looking for a better answer.

Opportunities for mistakes, misinterpretations, and misjudgments abound at every step in the process for determining the value of the job. The data reported in surveys, even the data reported in Form 990s, may be wrong or misleading. The job may have characteristics missed in the initial analysis of its responsibilities, and the benchmark chosen may not be a good match for the job. The organizations in the peer group may differ in significant ways from the organization in question, or it may not have jobs like the one being valued. The surveys chosen may not represent the peer group well, or they may not have enough data on the job to provide reliable information on its value. The data in the survey cut chosen may be misleading for one reason or another. If the answer seems wrong, the analysis may need to be redone.

Published surveys on executive compensation merely summarize the data submitted by participants and report them as a set of statistics. Some data in any database submitted by participants are inevitably inaccurate. More important, some data are anomalous.

The values retrieved from any survey or analysis can be inappropriate even if they are statistically accurate, so it is important to exercise judgment in evaluating the data. The best indication that the values are appropriate is that different sources and different analytical approaches yield consistent values.

One of the best quality controls is comparing data from multiple sources and comparing regression values with median or average values in a cut of data. If the values from several surveys are reasonably consistent, they are more likely to be reliable than if they diverge dramatically, and if the median or average values in a cut of data are reasonably consistent with the value predicted by the regression formula, the values are likely to be reliable.

Another good quality control is internal equity analysis— comparing the values for all the jobs in a management structure to determine if they are appropriate relative to one another, rather than valuing one job at a time. If the values determined for peer jobs, those reporting at the same level, seem to reflect their relative importance, the values are more likely to be accurate than if the value of one job seems significantly higher or lower than it should be. Some surveys include tables showing the typical relationship in job values, often showing the typical value of jobs in terms of a percentage of the value of the CEO's position. When the values retrieved from surveys fall into a pattern similar to the relationships shown in these tables, they are more likely to be accurate than if they diverge significantly from these relative values.

Survey Data Not Right for Relationship Between Two Positions

A midsize system has a large flagship hospital that represents more than half of the system's volume. The president of the flagship hospital reports to a COO for the system as a whole. The market value retrieved from surveys for CEOs of large subsidiary hospitals the size of the flagship hospital is higher than the value reported in the same surveys for COOs of systems the size of the parent, when the system is only a bit bigger than the flagship. The data for both jobs may be completely accurate, but they are inappropriate for this system. The values need to be adjusted to reflect the reporting relationship between the two jobs.

Intuitive evaluation of the relationship between values retrieved from surveys can be another form of internal equity analysis. Some jobs are intrinsically more valuable than others because of the scope or complexity of their responsibilities and their importance to the organization. The position of head of nursing or patient care, for example, is intrinsically more valuable than the position of head of support services (e.g., housekeeping, dietary, engineering, laundry), as long as the head of nursing or patient care has responsibility for all inpatient care in the hospital. If an analysis suggests otherwise, it is probably wrong.

Casual users of compensation data tend to take the data at face value—as definitive information, rather than as a single piece of information. Professionals understand that data must be evaluated, compared with other data, and treated as evidence—not as an answer.

Degree of Dispersion

Median and average values are usually more reliable than 75th and 90th percentile values. Especially in small data sets, the dispersion of data can be abnormal at the upper and lower ends of the set.

Compensation policies that position salaries or total cash compensation at the 75th percentile pose a challenge related to the unpredictability of dispersion. The 75th percentile value for salaries and total cash compensation for most executive positions is generally about 15 to 20 percent higher than median. In some data samples, it is only 5 percent or as much as 50 percent higher. The dispersion in any survey or database is greater for some jobs and less for others. A compensation policy that calls for positioning salaries at median and total cash compensation at the 75th percentile can lead to grossly inequitable levels of incentive opportunity for comparable positions. Values at the 75th percentile can bounce around from year to year, due to change in survey participation or even change in incumbents. An unusually broad or narrow gap between median and the 75th percentile may indicate that the 75th percentile value is not reliable.

Adjusting the Data

Data retrieved from surveys or Form 990 statements usually needs to be adjusted one way or another to determine the market value for a job. They virtually always needs adjusting for inflation in pay levels over time, because compensation data are always old, and one wants to know what the current market value of the job is or what it is likely to be next year. It may also need to be adjusted when the job being evaluated differs significantly from the benchmark position with which it is being compared, to account for the differences in job responsibilities.

Surveys typically ask for data as of a specific date, often a date in the first quarter of the calendar year. By the time the survey is published, many of the salaries reported for the survey will have already been increased. If the new salaries for the calendar year have not been implemented by that date or are not retroactive to the beginning of the year, the salary levels submitted to the survey may be a year old. The request for information on incentive awards typically asks for the most recent award paid, which could be an award granted a year earlier for performance two years ago. Data reported in Form 990s can be even older.

Executive pay has been increasing at the rate of 3 or 4 percent per year in recent years. Any analysis that does not adjust old data for inflation will reflect market pay levels that are six months or sometimes even a year or more old. Most compensation professionals adjust data for inflation, or "market movement," by 3 or 4 percent per year, assuming that market pay levels will continue to rise inexorably.

When a job has significantly more or less responsibility than the benchmark with which it is compared, the value of the benchmark job may need to be adjusted to reflect the size of the job being valued. There are two reasons for making these adjustments. When a job is much bigger or smaller than the benchmark, the employer is likely to recognize the difference and want to pay the executive more or less than the standard market value for the benchmark, to reflect its sense of the importance of the job. When the job is bigger than the benchmark, even if only marginally bigger, the incumbent is likely to recognize the difference and want to be paid extra for the additional responsibility.

Adjustments for job size should be made sparingly, because most executive positions differ from the benchmark job match in one way or another and because differences in job content or job size generally do not have much impact on market pay levels. Most healthcare organizations do not pay a CFO extra, for example, for oversight of medical office buildings and other real estate, of managed care contracting, or even of information technology. Most hospitals and health systems do not pay a chief nursing officer less when many or even most of the nurses report to service line leaders rather than to the chief nursing officer.

Consultants and compensation professionals have developed rules of thumb for making adjustments to account for job size. The following set of statements is one example of these rules of thumb:

- Unless the job is clearly at least one-third bigger (or smaller) than the benchmark, ignore the difference.
- If the job is clearly at least one-third bigger (or smaller) than the benchmark but less than two-thirds bigger (or smaller), adjust the market data by 5 percent.
- If the job is clearly two-thirds bigger (or smaller) than the benchmark but less than twice as big (or small), adjust the market data by 10 percent.

- If the job is clearly twice as big (or small) as the benchmark, adjust the market data by 15 percent.
- If the job is clearly significantly more than twice as big (or small) as the benchmark, the market value of the benchmark is not a good basis for determining the value of the much bigger (or smaller) job.

The most important of these rules of thumb is the first one, because most executive positions vary from the standard benchmark to one degree or another and because jobs change all the time as organizations introduce new initiatives and as they shift responsibilities from one executive to another. Unless adjustments for job size are avoided as much as possible, they will be applied to too many jobs, often without good reason. Organizations are usually far more willing to recognize jobs that are bigger than the benchmark than jobs that are smaller, and they are far more willing to increase the value of jobs as the jobs are growing than to reduce the value of jobs as the jobs lose responsibility.

BEST PRACTICES IN DETERMINING MARKET VALUE OF EXECUTIVE POSITIONS

The following is a list of best practices in determining the market value of an executive position in a tax-exempt hospital or health system.

- Start by studying the job to determine the scope of its responsibilities, its role in the organization, and how it compares with standard benchmark positions. Select the most appropriate benchmark comparison(s) for the job. Decide how to deal with any major differences between your job and the standard benchmark position.
- Determine the most important characteristics of your organization and use them in selecting an appropriate peer group.

Use a custom peer group, if appropriate, rather than a generic one, to get pay data from organizations truly similar to yours, in communities like yours, and in your region.

- If you plan to use a custom peer group, identify specific organizations to include in the peer group or define clear specifications for selecting organizations for the peer group. Order custom cuts of data from one or more surveys, ask a consultant to provide data from the custom peer group, or gather IRS Form 990 reports from organizations in the peer group.

  If you plan to use generic national data, choose several surveys that represent organizations like yours and have enough data to provide a reliable estimate of market value for most of your executive positions. Choose the best cuts of data from each survey to represent your organization's size, and decide whether the regression formula or a cut of data gives a better estimate of the value of the job in your organization.

- Study the relationship between the values drawn from the different sources and identify any anomalies indicating that the values may not be reliable. Check the sources again for a better job match, compare regression values with values from cuts, and look for a better way to extract or interpolate a value that is more consistent with data from the other sources. If the data from one source seem too inconsistent with the data from other sources, consider excluding that source from your analysis.

- Average the values across the different sources.

- Adjust the data as appropriate for (1) inflation over the time that has passed since the data were current and (2) any significant differences between the job at issue and the benchmark job(s) chosen as best matches for the job.

- Assess the overall pattern of market values to determine if it adequately reflects the relative importance of jobs in your organization. If not, decide how to adjust the data to better reflect internal equity.

NOTES

1. Typical benefit costs for executives are about 25 to 32 percent of salary excluding the value of paid time off, and about 36 to 45 percent of salary including the value of paid time off. The costs reportable on Form 990 are often far higher for organizations with defined-benefit supplemental retirement plans.

2. A regression formula is an algebraic formula representing the "line of best fit" from a regression analysis. A regression analysis is a complex statistical evaluation of a large data set that attempts to correlate one value with another. In executive compensation, regression analysis looks for the relationship between pay for a particular job and the size of the organization in which the job works. The line of best fit represents the statistical prediction of the value of the job at any size represented in the data set. The value predicted by the regression formula is similar to median value for an organization of that size, but it is really an estimate of what the median value should be, on the basis of the overall distribution of all the data in the data set.

CHAPTER 4

Getting Base Pay Right: Salary, Salary Structure, and Salary Administration

INTRODUCTION

Salary is the foundation of executive compensation. Incentive opportunity is usually defined as a percentage of salary, many benefits are defined in relation to salary, and total compensation is directly proportional to salary.

That means if salary is "right," or appropriate, total compensation is likely to be about right, and if salary is "wrong," or inappropriate, total compensation is likely to be wrong.

What is the secret to getting base pay right?

- Discovering what other, comparable organizations pay for the same position (job value)
- Deciding what the job is worth relative to pay for other positions in the organization (internal equity)
- Determining what the incumbent or recruit is worth considering her competencies, performance, years of experience in the job, prior experience in other jobs, career potential, and earnings history (personal value)

- Learning (or guessing) how much a candidate is currently paid and determining how big an increase is needed to get him to accept the job (cost of hiring)
- Learning how much another employer has offered an executive and discovering how big an increase is needed to retain her (cost of retaining)
- Deciding what the organization is willing to pay the incumbent or recruit given the value of the job, the personal value of the incumbent or recruit, the organization's compensation philosophy and values, and how much the organization pays other members of the executive team

The most important step in getting salary right is the last one—as once the decision has been made, one is stuck with it, perhaps for a long time. Salaries change slowly, and the relationship among salaries even more slowly.

But salaries do change gradually over time. Most hospitals and health systems, like industrial employers, long ago adopted salary administration programs with annual schedules for reviewing employees' salaries and providing salary increases once a year to keep up with inflation, reward good performance, and recognize acquisition and mastery of job-related capabilities.

Salary administration is the entire process of determining the value of jobs and deciding how much to pay them; reviewing salaries periodically to determine whether they are still competitive and deciding whether to increase (or decrease or freeze) them; deciding whether to recognize changes in job responsibilities with changes in salaries; deciding how much to increase salaries when employees are promoted to jobs with more responsibility; and communicating salaries and salary increases and even the reasons for salary decisions to employees.

Employers invest a lot of time, effort, and money in salary administration. They do so because employers want to keep their pay competitive enough to attract and retain the caliber of employees they need to be successful; because employees expect salary increases every year; because employees want and expect their salaries and salary increases to be fair, relative to salaries of other employees; because employees want to be rewarded for good performance and expect to get salary increases as they demonstrate mastery of new skills; and because organizations worry about losing employees to higher-paying jobs elsewhere.

Insofar as salary administration succeeds at keeping pay competitive and fair, it is well worth doing and worth doing well. It may help retain executives; it may reduce the irritation caused by unfair pay relationships; and it may help satisfy executives that they are paid fairly and competitively. One of its principal purposes, though, is cost control, and one of its goals is spending as little as possible to keep pay competitive and fair. As a result, its principal outcome is constraining payroll costs.

The other outcomes of salary administration are barely noteworthy. As a reward for performance, salary increases are ineffective. The size of salary increases is trivial relative to salary and total compensation opportunity; increases for top performers are barely more than increases for average performers; no employee leaves because his increase was too small, and none stays because his increase was bigger than expected; and few employees believe their salary increase was an appropriate reward for good performance over the past year.

As a retention strategy, salary adjustments are rarely enough to retain someone who is focused on career advancement, although a large enough increase to counter an offer from another employer may be enough to retain someone who would leave only if he could earn a lot more elsewhere. As a system for making pay relationships fairer, salary administration is weak, because there is rarely enough money in the budget to correct inequities.

On the other hand, all those involved in salary administration can take satisfaction from knowing that they are doing the best they can to manage salaries with a limited budget. The CEO believes he has done what he can to see that executives are paid fairly and competitively, and maybe even rewarded for performance. Employees can be satisfied that someone is at least paying attention to their compensation and that they have at least received a token award for working hard for another year. Trustees can be satisfied that they have fulfilled their responsibility for seeing that most executives are paid appropriately, that no one is paid too much, and that the total cost of the executive payroll represents an appropriate allocation of the institution's resources.

SALARY, SALARY RANGE, AND SALARY STRUCTURE DEFINED

Salary (also called *base salary* or *base pay*) is the annual rate of pay for a position. Salary ranges and salary structures are constructs for facilitating decision making and communication about salaries. *Salary ranges* are used to identify an appropriate range for salaries for a job. The salary range is typically centered on the value that is regarded as the right rate of pay for the job; the lower part of the range is regarded as fair pay for someone new to the position who has not yet mastered the job; and the upper part of the range, as fair pay for someone who has consistently performed exceptionally well in the job over many years. Salary ranges are used to give the employer leeway to position salary at the most appropriate position within the range given the incumbent's experience, capabilities, prior salary, performance, and other factors.

Salary structures combine salary ranges in some logical fashion. Rather than maintain separate salary ranges for every job, organizations group together all jobs with similar market value or jobs regarded as peers into grades, classes, or bands and establish a single salary range for each group of jobs.

Many organizations do not maintain salary structures for executive compensation and instead establish a separate salary range for each job. Those that are especially attuned to internal equity or internal pay relationships tend to favor graded salary structures for executives, so we devote a section later in this chapter to discussing them.

OVERVIEW OF SALARY ADMINISTRATION

Salary administration is a systematic process that applies a set of rules and guidelines to determining salaries for an organization's employees. It includes the following components:

- Determining the rate or range of pay for a job
- Determining or refining the pay relationships among different jobs
- Determining annual and promotional salary increases
- Planning and controlling the annual increase in payroll costs

Salary administration allows the CEO and board to delegate to other executives responsibility for determining salaries and salary increases for their subordinates, and it gives the compensation committee a method for determining salary or a salary increase for the CEO that is consistent with the approach used across the organization.

In independent hospitals and health systems, administration of executive salaries is generally controlled by the board or its compensation committee, in conjunction with the CEO. In subsidiary hospitals, it is typically controlled by the system CEO or the executive to whom the subsidiary CEO reports, following whatever policies or guidelines have been established by the board. For sake of simplicity, we discuss trustees' role in governing executive compensation.

Establishing and Approving Salary Ranges

Most large organizations follow a set of rules—implicit or explicit—in establishing salary ranges for a job or assigning jobs to a salary grade. The tasks involved in employee salary administration are carried out by human resources department staff. For executive positions, however, this work is often performed by an external consultant.

Salary administration starts with identifying the right rate of pay for the job, establishing a salary range for the job, and obtaining approval of the range from the compensation committee. Once the initial range has been established for the job, it is generally adjusted once a year to reflect inflation in executive pay, changes in market value, and changes in job responsibilities.

Organizations often have a formal approval process for the salaries of new or restructured positions. The initial range for a position establishes a precedent and a commitment that are hard to overturn later—a commitment to add the position, the precedent of a baseline value for the job, and a commitment to the incumbent to keep salary, incentive opportunity, and benefits competitive with the starting level.

The process for approving annual changes to pay rates or ranges is considered a budgetary issue and this is usually less formal. Most organizations establish a salary budget that controls the rate at which salaries increase. Some compensation committees, however, approve salary ranges for executives every year in addition to or as an alternative to reviewing or approving actual salary increases.[1]

Salary Review Process and Frequency

Most organizations review executive compensation once a year but also have a process for reviewing compensation when positions change or when new executives are hired. The general review entails comparing current salaries (or total compensation) with comparability data drawn from compensation surveys or other sources to determine how competitive they are. Some organizations assess total compensation every year; others do so only once every few years and focus only on salaries in the intervening years.[2]

The purpose of the review is threefold:

- Management wants to determine annual salary increases to keep pay competitive, recognize incumbents' development, and reward performance.

- To fulfill its duty to oversee executive compensation, the compensation committee needs to determine whether executive compensation, including proposed salary increases and incentive awards, is competitive, reasonable, and consistent with the organization's compensation philosophy.

- To establish a presumption of reasonableness for executive compensation, the compensation committee needs to obtain and rely on appropriate comparability data on total compensation before determining any salary increase for the CEO and approving any salary increases for other executives or physician leaders covered by intermediate sanctions regulations.

Determining and Approving Annual Salary Increases

Once a year, the CEO reviews any salary analysis the organization has conducted and determines or recommends salary increases for other executives. Similarly, the compensation committee reviews the analysis and determines a salary increase for the CEO and approves increases for other senior executives. Salary increase decisions typically consider three factors: the relationship of the current salary to the new salary midpoint or market value, the performance of the executive over the past year, and the budget for salary increases.

Guidelines for Determining Salary Increases

The CEO and compensation committee craft executive salary increase guidelines informally in discussions between the two parties, which take place either during the budgeting process or after they have seen the most recent compensation survey or reviewed their consultant's analysis of executive pay. Trustees often start the discussions by asking what the salary increase budget or guidelines are for other employees, then ask the CEO whether there is any reason not to follow the same guidelines for executive salaries.

Determining Promotional Salary Increases

Promotions come in three different types:

1. The executive moves up one level in the hierarchy to another position with significantly more responsibility, as from controller to chief financial officer or from chief operating officer to CEO.
2. The executive gains additional responsibility without moving up a level in the organization.
3. The executive is granted a change in title, which may or may not be accompanied by an increase in responsibility or a move up the hierarchy.

Promotional increases are often bigger than annual salary increases, and they should be, to recognize significant increases in responsibility or significant increases in rank. The size of any promotional increase should depend on how much higher the new salary range is than the old one and on where the executive's old salary fits in the new range. Because the promotion represents a new job for the incumbent, the new salary should ideally be below midpoint, to leave room for increases later as the executive demonstrates mastery of the new responsibilities.

PRINCIPLES OF SALARY ADMINISTRATION

The overarching goal of a salary administration system is to pay people appropriately given the board's compensation philosophy, the competitive rate of pay for the position, a fair relationship with pay for other positions in the organization, the value the incumbent brings to the job, and the amount that the organization can afford to pay. In pursuit of that goal, most organizations articulate six related principles of salary administration:

1. Determine the right salary range for the job.
2. Position the salary appropriately in the range to reflect the competencies, knowledge, experience, and performance of the incumbent.
3. Increase pay to midpoint as the incumbent demonstrates increasing competence in the job.
4. Reward performance by giving bigger-than-average salary increases to the organization's best performers.
5. Keep salaries and increases fair.
6. Control payroll costs by establishing budgets and guidelines limiting the size of salary increases.

These principles are discussed in the following paragraphs.

Determine the Right Salary Range for the Job

The most fundamental principle of salary administration is to start by establishing the right rate and right range of pay for the job. The rate and range of pay should reflect the accountabilities of the position, the knowledge and competencies required to handle the job, and the relationship of the job to other positions in the organization.

The right rate of pay depends on three factors:

- The organization's intended competitive position, as identified in its compensation philosophy and tempered by the amount that the organization can afford to pay
- The market value or going rate of pay for the job
- Internal equity, or the relative value of the job, compared with the value of other jobs

The right rate of pay for the job is independent of the incumbent's or the candidate's capabilities, experience, and performance in the position. It assumes that the job will be done well regardless of who does it and that the incumbent has the requisite skills and experience to handle all the accountabilities and meet all the performance expectations for the position. Most organizations translate the right rate of pay to a salary range to allow some latitude in positioning the salary in the range to reflect the value the incumbent brings to the job.

Set Pay Appropriately Relative to the Value the Incumbent Brings to the Job

The second principle says that the salary should be positioned within the salary range in a way that reflects the incumbent's or candidate's capabilities, experience, and performance, relative to the presumption that the midpoint of the range is the right rate of pay for someone who is fully qualified for the job, who has enough experience in the position to have demonstrated mastery of the job, and who meets all the performance expectations set for the job. It implies that an executive with no prior experience in the job should be paid less than one whose experience has allowed him to master the job and that an incumbent whose performance is merely adequate be paid less than one who demonstrates outstanding performance year after year.

The right pay for a specific incumbent may be higher or lower than the "job rate," or midpoint of the salary range. Thus inexperienced incumbents should be paid in the lower part of the salary range for the job, experienced incumbents who perform well should be paid at or near the midpoint, and truly outstanding incumbents should be paid above the midpoint.

Some hospitals and systems take the notion of the right rate of pay for the job too literally and want to cap pay at midpoint, often based on a belief that rewards for performance should come through incentive compensation, not through salary increases.

Capping salaries at midpoint makes more sense when midpoints are at the 75th percentile than when they are at median, as capping salaries at median raises the risk of losing talented executives to other organizations willing to pay more. The disadvantage of capping pay at midpoint is that it tells executives that once they reach midpoint, they will not be paid more as they gain more experience, no matter how well they perform, unless they move or are promoted to a higher-paying job.

It is easy to understand why an employer would pay a newcomer or a weak performer less than the salary range midpoint that has been established as the right rate of pay for the job. But why would any healthcare organization with scarce resources pay an executive more than the right rate of pay for the job? The usual answer is that the incumbent is exceptionally talented and performs extremely well. The problem with this answer is that pay at the midpoint assumes good performance and complete mastery of the job. Paying more than midpoint implies that the incumbent is capable of doing more than the job is worth (and why pay for that?) or that expectations are set so low that someone who performs the job well is perceived as an outstanding performer.

A better answer has to do with flexibility in pay. The upper part of the salary range serves the same purpose as the lower part of the range. It allows some flexibility in setting a salary where it ought to be set. It allows some flexibility in recruiting experienced outsiders, who may need a salary above midpoint to accept the job; in retaining executives who have received offers from other organizations; or in keeping executives content with their pay. Most executives, after all, believe that they are better than average and want to be paid more than average. Even if salary ranges are positioned well above average, at the 75th percentile or so, executives tend to believe they exceed the expectations set for the job and deserve to be paid more than midpoint. And CEOs and boards are often willing to pay executives above midpoint to reinforce executives' perceptions that they are outstanding performers.

Increase Pay to Midpoint as the Incumbent Demonstrates Increasing Competence in the Job

The third principle is to manage salary increases to keep pay properly positioned in the range to reflect competence, experience, and performance. This principle calls for moving salaries up to midpoint over time as newer executives demonstrate increasing competence in the job. It means giving larger salary increases to people paid low in their ranges than to people who are already paid competitively—as long as they deserve the bigger-than-average increases by demonstrating good performance and growth in the job. The contrapositive of this principle calls for slowing down salary increases for people who are paid high in their salary ranges (unless their performance is so extraordinary that they deserve being paid well above midpoint).

This principle helps normalize over time whatever disparities in pay exist between internally promoted executives, who often start low in the salary range, and those recruited externally, who often start high in the range. It also controls disparities due to tenure, where long-tenured executives are paid high in their ranges and less-tenured executives are paid low in their ranges—even when some of the less experienced executives perform better than those with long tenure.

If a new incumbent with no prior experience in the job should be paid near the bottom of the salary range, how long should it take to get that incumbent's salary up to midpoint? One rule of thumb says that it generally takes three to five years to master a new high-level position, so salary should be brought up to midpoint over a similar period. Following this rule of thumb would require five increases of 5 percent, four increases of 6 percent, or three increases of 7 percent, on top of the rate at which the salary midpoint is moved up during this time frame to keep up with inflation in executive pay.

Most organizations limit the variation in salary increase so much that someone who starts at or near the bottom of a salary range may never reach midpoint. Many increase salaries at about the same rate for all executives, with the result that people maintain the same position within the range year after year. Executives paid low in their range stay in that portion of the range, and those paid high in their range stay there, maintaining long-term disparity in compensation. Unless the disparity is consistently supported by performance or significant differences in capability, it is unfair.

Reward Performance, Not Seniority

The fourth principle of salary administration calls for giving larger-than-average salary increases to employees who perform better than average. This policy helps limit pay above midpoint to those whose performance merits keeping it above midpoint. Giving every employee the same size increase makes the increase no more than a market adjustment to keep up with inflation.

Older executives and some consultants think seniority should be a compensable factor in executive pay, but most other observers believe that competence and performance should be the primary determinants. Experience matters, of course, because it takes time to master a job and demonstrate fully satisfactory performance in it. But once an executive has mastered the job, there is little point in rewarding additional experience. Once an executive's salary has reached the midpoint of the range for the job—the amount the board intends to pay for good performance from a competent, experienced executive—any future salary increases (other than inflationary increases) should reward performance, not experience.

Retention is the one good reason to pay long-tenured executives in the upper part of their salary ranges, especially when the ranges are centered at median. When ranges are centered at the 75th percentile and the organization offers a competitive incentive plan and a competitive retirement benefit, the board has less need to position salaries for long-service executives in the upper part of the range.

Organizations with incentive plans that offer rewards for individual performance should have relatively little need to use the upper part of the range to reward performance. Where there is no incentive plan in place, however, or where incentive awards are largely or entirely based on institutional performance, it is more appropriate to use salary increases to reward performance, even if that policy positions salaries of high-performing, long-service executives in the upper part of the salary range.

Keep Salaries and Salary Increases Fair

The fifth goal of salary administration is fairness. People expect to be treated fairly, and executives are highly attuned to the fairness of salaries and salary increases. The additional disclosures required by Form 990 will only increase their sensitivity to internal equity, as more salaries and salary increases are publicly reported.

People who are not treated fairly, or who think they are not, will likely complain about the situation, which undermines morale. They might even file formal complaints, which could lead to charges of discrimination if the complainant is a member of a protected class of employees. Widely reported findings indicate that female and minority executives are not paid as competitively as their white male counterparts, so employers should be sure that their approach to salary administration is fair. Pay patterns are the evidence on which claims and litigation are won or lost.

In matters of fairness, perception carries as much weight as intent. An environment in which people believe they are paid unfairly, even if they are not, can be just as disruptive as one in which an unfair pay practice actually exists. Explaining the basis for salary administration and salary decisions can diffuse perceptions of unfairness, while secrecy only reinforces them.

Salaries and salary increases both need to be fair and need to be perceived as fair to keep the issue of pay from undermining morale on the executive team. Fairness does not mean that all people are paid the same or that all salary increases should be the same. It does mean, however, that the organization must have a good and persuasive rationale for the differences in salaries and salary increases. A strong, transparent salary administration system based on logical principles that are carefully articulated is an excellent starting point. CEOs and compensation committees should be alert to discrepancies that are or might appear to be unfair. If they are unfair, the CEO and committee should correct them; if they are not, the board should be prepared to explain them.

Control Salary Increases Through Budgets and Guidelines

Much of the focus in salary administration is on determining how much to increase pay. Some of that focus needs to be on controlling the size and cost of salary increases. Managers tend to rate most of their subordinates above average and want to reward them with above-average salary increases. Even with controls, salary increases tend to be larger for executives than for the workforce as a whole. Without controls, salaries would rise even faster.

Organizations control salary increases in three ways. They set salary budgets and expect managers to keep increases within their departmental budgets. They establish salary increase guidelines that strictly limit the size of increases managers can deliver without gaining approval for any exception. And most organizations require approval of proposed salary increases by each manager's superior. Salary increases for senior executives (those reporting to the CEO) generally need approval by the compensation committee, increases for other executives generally need approval by the CEO, and so on.

These controls keep annual salary increases modest, most of the time. Two types of increases, however, fall outside the salary increase budget and salary increase guidelines: promotional increases and market adjustments intended to bring salaries for underpaid individuals up to a more competitive position. Even these increases, though, need one and often two levels of approval.

DESIGNING SALARY RANGES AND SALARY STRUCTURES

Salary ranges and salary structures are tools to facilitate salary administration. Their utility is directly proportional to the number of jobs covered and the number of managers involved in salary administration. They are less essential in dealing with executive compensation because executive jobs are relatively few and the parties involved in salary administration fewer.

Salary ranges are useful, however, in administering salaries and governing executive compensation in larger organizations with 20 or more executives. And salary ranges and structures are essential for a large workforce because they support an orderly system for administering salaries and a logical approach to communicating salary issues to employees and the managers who implement the salary policy. These aspects of salary ranges and structures are expanded on in the following paragraphs.

Designing Salary Ranges

Standard salary ranges establish the limits on acceptable dispersion at 80 percent and 120 percent of midpoint, presuming that pay at the bottom of the range might be fair for someone who has no prior experience in the job and that pay at the top of the range might be fair for a seasoned and exceptionally effective executive who has repeatedly delivered superior results. Some organizations set the outer bounds of salary ranges further apart to allow even more flexibility in positioning salaries.

Some organizations just use markers—such as median and 75th percentile—instead of ranges and tell decision makers to position salaries appropriately between the two points. One reason the use of markers has not become widespread is that the gap between median and 75th percentile varies widely from one job to another. Although the gap between median and 75th percentile is usually about 15 percent to 20 percent, it is less than 10 percent for some jobs and more than 30 percent for others. (Note, however, that some of this variation is anomalous due to small sample size.)

Because the 75th percentile value for a job is typically about 15 to 20 percent above median and the 90th percentile value about 15 to 20 percent above the 75th percentile, the top of a salary range centered at median is often positioned at or a bit above the 75th percentile, and the top of a standard salary range centered at the 75th percentile is often positioned at or above the 90th percentile. For this reason, it is important to use the upper part of the range sparingly, as it represents a significant departure from the board's intent. In fact, some organizations set the limit for ranges centered on the 75th percentile at the 90th percentile to lower the risk that total compensation will be indefensibly high.

Because the 25th percentile is also about 15 to 20 percent below median, a standard salary range centered on median typically runs from about the 25th to the 75th percentiles. Likewise, a standard salary range centered on the 75th percentile typically runs from about median to the 90th percentile.

Designing Salary Structures

Salary structures are designed to put all positions with similar market values or comparable internal worth in a common salary range, or to put all salary ranges into a logical structure made up of a small number of salary ranges. Instead of having separate salary ranges for every job, a salary structure might have 5 or 6 salary ranges for executives, 12 to 15 for managers and non-clinical professionals, and 10 to 12 for nonexempt administrative support staff.

Some salary structures emphasize internal equity. They typically start with a job evaluation, determine grade assignment largely on the basis of that evaluation, and then determine salary ranges for each grade in comparison with market values for the jobs within it. Others emphasize market value. They start with the market value for each job, assign jobs to grades largely on the basis of similarity in market value, and then determine salary ranges for each grade in comparison with market values for the jobs in each grade.

Some salary structures are designed architectonically with ranges that are spaced equidistantly. Others are empirical structures with ranges positioned wherever needed to fit a group of jobs with similar market value. The architectonic approach tends to create more grades than necessary for executive ranks; the empirical approach works better for executive positions because these jobs are relatively few. The architectonic approach is generally better suited to organizations that emphasize internal equity and use job evaluation to determine grade assignments, while the empirical approach is generally better suited to organizations that use market value to determine grade assignments.

Salary structures can have many grades or few, according to how far apart the grades are spaced and how wide the ranges are.

Structures with grade midpoints spaced only 5 to 10 percent apart make it relatively easy to determine which grade best matches the market value for a job and make it easy to move jobs up or down a grade to recognize changes in market value or changes in job design. Those with midpoints spaced 12 to 20 percent apart make it harder to determine which grade best matches the market value for a job when the value is midway between the two; furthermore, the consequence of assigning it to the higher or lower grade is greater when the grades are positioned further apart, so it is harder to move a job up or down a grade to recognize changes in market value or changes in job design.

"Broadbanding" is an approach that uses relatively few grades or bands with very wide salary ranges in order to de-emphasize rank. Some organizations use an approach similar to broadbanding for salary administration at executive levels by putting all vice presidents, for example, in the same salary range, all senior vice presidents in another range, and so on.

Utility of Salary Structures

A formal, graded salary structure seems to simplify salary administration more than it really does. On the surface, a graded structure simplifies communication. A CEO can more easily tell six executives that they are all positioned in grade 14, with a salary midpoint of $100,000 in a range stretching from $80,000 to $120,000, than explain why one job is "worth" more or less than the others—especially when the difference in market value is only a few thousand dollars. But consider how difficult it is to explain why two jobs with similar value end up in different ranges—why a job with a market value of $109,000, for example, has a salary midpoint of $100,000 while a job with a market value of $112,000 has a salary range midpoint of $120,000, or why two jobs with very different market values—say, $89,000 and $109,000—end up in the same range.

A graded salary structure is less flexible than a free-form set of salary ranges developed independently for each executive position. When adjusting salary ranges each year to keep up with inflation, organizations with graded salary structure generally move all salary grades at the same rate rather than adjust each range to match changes in the value of each job. Moving the salary range for a job at a different rate than the structure as a whole is moved requires moving the job up or down a grade, which amounts to reclassifying the job in a hierarchy. So a formal, graded salary structure makes it difficult to keep salary ranges for individual jobs aligned with market value and can make it difficult to recognize changes in job responsibility with a commensurate change in salary opportunity unless the changes are significant enough to move the job up or down an entire grade. If the ranges are only 5 or 6 percent apart, executives can be easily rewarded for a moderate increase in responsibility, while if ranges are 15 or 20 percent apart, it would take an enormous change in job responsibility to justify moving the job up or down a whole grade.

Market values of different jobs change at different rates, so graded salary structures need to be realigned every few years with market values. Some jobs need to be moved from one grade to another to keep salary opportunity reasonably consistent with market value.

Too often, however, grade assignments are taken for granted rather than evaluated regularly and modified when appropriate. Employers are more willing to move jobs up a grade than down a grade. As a result, graded structures tend to lose integrity over time. Some organizations maintain old grade structures long after they have lost their logical relationship to market value.

DETERMINING SALARY INCREASES

Organizations use one of three generic approaches to determining salary increases. The first is the intuitive or discretionary approach. It may be supported by a theoretical model, and it may take any number of factors into account, but it is not shaped or constrained by corporate guidelines or rules. The second is a budgetary approach often referred to as a general increase. Organizations that apply this approach increase all salaries by the same factor or amount (e.g., by 3 percent or by 5 cents an hour), except when a special adjustment is needed to bring the salary to a more competitive position. The third is a sophisticated, disciplined approach that ties the size of increases to performance and often to performance appraisal. This approach is generally referred to as merit pay.

Merit pay typically aims to achieve three separate goals: to reward performance, to keep up with inflation, and to bring salaries up to midpoint of the salary range over time. As merit pay is the approach most widely used in determining salary increases for executives, the discussion in this section focuses on this method, its theoretical underpinnings, and its effectiveness at meeting its own goals. Whether supported by formal merit pay guidelines or influenced only by an abstract model, most CEOs aim to increase salaries for all executives enough to keep up with inflation and give bigger-than-average salary increases to the executives who perform best and to any executives they consider underpaid. Even those who use the intuitive approach probably consider the same three factors as they determine salary increases.

Supporters of merit pay sometimes claim that the entire amount of an annual salary increase is based on performance. It is not. Most of it is a general increase needed to keep salaries even with inflation in pay levels. Construing the increase as nothing but a reward for performance means that the employer has no intent to keep salaries competitive or holds the belief that keeping salaries even with inflation is a reward for performance. This claim overlooks a principal driver of executive compensation: the fear of losing talent if pay is not competitive.

Inflation as Principal Determinant

If there were no inflation, salary administration would focus on giving occasional raises to the 20 percent or so of any group of employees whose performance is so outstanding that they deserve a reward, giving regular increases to new employees as they demonstrate growth in job-related skills and competencies, and giving market adjustments to employees whose salaries were far below competitive levels or far below salaries of their peers. There would be no reason to intentionally increase salaries for all employees every year.

But inflation is significant enough to be the principal driver of salary administration. With inflation as low as it has been for the past two decades, there is little need to increase all employees' salaries every year, but if salaries were increased only once every two or three years, the increases would be much bigger than regular annual increases. Salaries positioned at the 75th percentile would still be competitive (at median, at least) after having been frozen for five to eight years, and salaries positioned at the 60th or 65th percentile would still be competitive after having been frozen for two or three years.

Employers have no obligation to keep up with inflation, whether it be inflation in the cost of living or inflation in market pay levels. They do so voluntarily to keep pay competitive—to minimize the risk of losing employees to higher-paying jobs and to satisfy employees' expectations that they will be paid fairly and competitively.

Inflation in prevailing pay levels is related to but different from and independent of inflation in the cost of living. During times of high inflation in the cost of living, salary increases tend to be lower than the rate of inflation, while during times of low inflation in the cost of living, salary increases tend to outpace the rate of inflation. To avoid confusion between the two, we discuss increases in prevailing pay levels as "market movement," or inflation in pay levels.

Supply and demand drive the rate of pay increases for unskilled jobs and jobs requiring specialized skills, especially hourly jobs with multiple incumbents, such as nurses, pharmacists, and housekeepers. Market movement for executive and management jobs, however, is driven by the expectation of market movement.

A broad, underlying inflation rate affects most jobs more or less equally due to the widespread practice of providing salary increases on an annual basis. Market movement has been so consistent over the past 20 years that observers expect pay levels to continue creeping up 3 percent to 5 percent a year. This expectation in turn fuels inflation in pay because most large organizations intentionally build salary increases into their operating budgets and salary administration systems.

The real drivers of inflation in executive compensation are not supply and demand but executives' expectation of annual salary increases, employers' determination to keep salaries competitive, and employers' fears of disappointing executives. Even sole providers in small and midsize communities that have experienced little turnover for years provide annual salary increases to keep up with anticipated market movement elsewhere in the industry—even though they are not really at risk of losing many executives.

Market Adjustments for Individual Jobs

A market adjustment is a mechanism for delivering a notably bigger increase than normal, often one outside the salary increase guidelines. Labeling the bigger increase as a "market adjustment" implies that the market is driving the increase—that the market value has increased faster for one job than for others or that enhancement of the job's responsibilities raises its market value.

In certain circumstances, an imbalance between supply and demand does drive changes in prevailing executive pay levels. The current emphasis on developing electronic medical records, medical informatics, shared databases, and electronic communication has driven up pay levels for information technology executives and professionals; the industrywide effort to improve clinical quality has driven up prevailing salaries for leaders of that activity; and the trend toward choosing physician CEOs has driven up pay levels for physicians with successful track records as chief executives. Most market adjustments, however, are simply increases so big that they lie outside the organization's salary increase guidelines—increases intended to bring salaries for nominally underpaid executives up to a more competitive level. Once trustees have established a policy of positioning salaries at the 60th percentile (or some other level), once the organization has established a "right rate of pay" for the job and identified a salary range midpoint, the organization tends to think of executives paid low in their salary range as underpaid and decides it needs to provide market adjustments to bring them up closer to the salary midpoint.

Organizations need some way to give bigger-than-normal salary increases to newly promoted executives to recognize their growth in competence. Paying newcomers at or near the bottom of a salary range may be fair for a year or two, but leaving them there long after they have shown that they can handle the job well is not. A properly designed set of salary increase guidelines should allow large enough salary increases for people positioned low in their ranges to bring them up to midpoint in five or six years, or whenever they are fully competent at handling all the accountabilities of the position, as long as they are also performing well in the role. But few guidelines are designed this way, so organizations need to label these increases market adjustments to get salaries up to midpoint.

Salary Increase Guidelines and Budgets

Most large organizations set salary increase guidelines each year. Salary increase budgets and guidelines start with an estimate of the probable rate of market movement for the workforce as a whole. They are often then trimmed in the budgeting process to control cost increases. Salary increase guidelines are designed to keep salary increases within the budget and limit the number of above-average increases. Some salary-increase guidelines call for general increases applied equally to all employees, without regard for position in range or performance. But others call for different rates of increase for different classes of employees—for example, 5 percent for nurses, 3 percent for salaried office employees, and 4 percent for executives—to recognize that market pay changes at different rates for different jobs.

Merit Pay and Merit Increase Guidelines

Merit pay refers to a salary administration system (approach) that considers performance and provides larger-than-average increases to employees who perform better than expected. *Merit increase guidelines* are salary increase parameters that incorporate a factor for performance.

Some organizations use general salary increases to keep up with market movement and handle merit pay rewards independently of inflationary increases. In this circumstance, merit pay is entirely focused on rewarding performance. Given that the intent of merit pay is to provide an additional (or extra-large) increase to people who perform notably above average or above expectations, any special or additional increase for merit should be reserved for a relatively small portion of the workforce, 20 percent or so—even in a relatively small class or group of employees, such as executives.

But the typical approach to merit pay is to bundle the merit component with the inflationary component and the factor that considers position in range. Structured this way, merit pay programs award "merit" increases to the bulk of the workforce and executive team. One reason organizations claim that the entire amount of every annual increase is a reward for performance is to be able to reward all employees for performance after a year of hard work.

Merit pay is often integrated with performance appraisal, so that a salary increase is viewed as a result of performance appraisal. However, this approach can diminish the significance of performance appraisal to a decision about a salary increase. Linking merit pay to performance appraisal reinforces employers' message that all of merit pay is a reward for performance, but executives, having many years' experience conducting performance appraisals and determining merit increases for subordinates, know that salary increases are largely intended to keep up with market movement in salaries and that the portion of any increase tied to above-average performance is small.

When merit pay is structured to encompass an inflationary component, a reward for performance, and a competence-based component to bring salaries up toward salary range midpoint as employees master the job, performance is often weighted the least. The portion devoted to explicitly recognizing above-average performance or performance above expectations is typically limited to 1 or 2 percent of salary. If market movement and the salary increase budget are, say, 4 percent, as they have been over most of the past two decades, the first 4 percent of any salary increase is attributable to inflation and the institutions' intent to keep pay competitive; the incremental 1 or 2 percent meant as a reward for performance is clearly outweighed by the inflationary component.

The portion devoted to bringing salaries in the bottom half of the salary range up toward midpoint is likewise typically limited to 1 or 2 percent of salary—not nearly enough to bring a salary from the bottom of the range to midpoint in a reasonable amount of time.

Exhibit 4.1 shows typical guidelines used by organizations to determine merit increases.

One reason for keeping the performance-based component modest is that most managers want to be able to evaluate most of their subordinates at a level above just meeting expectations. If merit pay formulas link salary increases to performance appraisal and performance ratings, and a sizeable portion of the workforce or the executive team rates above average or above expectations, the merit increase guidelines will break the budget for salary increases unless the increase for above-average performance is at the intended budgetary level.

To bring people up to midpoint over five or six years and provide a meaningful reward for performance to a small portion of the workforce, the budget for salary increases needs to be a percentage or two above the inflationary rate, and merit increase guidelines must keep the increase for average or expected performance at the inflationary rate or lower, as shown in Exhibit 4.2.

Tying salary increases to performance tends to undermine performance appraisal by tempting managers to raise evaluations to justify larger salary increases. Merit pay programs almost inevitably lead to grade inflation and the Lake Wobegon effect of rating too many people above average.

Exhibit 4.1: Typical Merit Increase Guidelines

Performance	Position in Salary Range as Percentage of Midpoint			
	80–89%	90–99%	100–109%	110–120%
Far exceeds expectations	8%	7%	6%	5%
Exceeds expectations	7%	6%	5%	4%
Meets expectations	6%	5%	4%	3%
Meets some expectations	0–4%	0–4%	0%	0%

Exhibit 4.2: More Effective Merit Increase Guidelines

Performance	Position in Salary Range as Percentage of Midpoint			
	80–89%	90–99%	100–109%	110–120%
Far exceeds expectations	9–10%	7–8%	5–6%	4–5%
Exceeds expectations	8–9%	6–7%	3–4%	2–3%
Meets expectations	7–8%	5–6%	2–3%	0%
Meets some expectations	0–4%	0–4%	0%	0%

Rewarding Performance

Most organizations assert that salaries and salary increases reflect performance—meaning individual performance, not institutional performance, and current performance in the job, not past performance in some other job. This assertion encompasses two intentions: to position salary at a level that reflects the incumbent's expected performance and to provide salary increases commensurate with the past year's performance.

The first intention translates to positioning pay above midpoint for an employee who has repeatedly performed at an outstanding level, at midpoint for one who meets all the performance expectations set for the job, and below midpoint for one who is not yet meeting all expectations. The second intention equates to giving bigger-than-average increases to the employees who performed best over the past year, average increases to most, and below-average increases to any whose performance was noticeably less than average or who did not meet all expectations for their jobs.

All discussion of pay based on performance presumes, of course, that whoever is making the decisions can evaluate the incumbents' performance fairly. In reality, different observers rate an employee's performance differently, and performance pay schemes overlook the following facts:

- The evaluation depends on the rater's expectations as much as on the incumbent's performance.
- Each rater has different expectations and different scales for evaluating performance.
- It is often difficult to determine how much of any result is due to the incumbent's performance as opposed to the collective performance of the incumbent's team, the collective performance of the incumbent's colleagues, or external factors beyond the incumbent's control.

Most boards and CEOs often have difficulty delivering distinctive rewards to outstanding performers for three reasons:

- The proportion of executives viewed as being above average or evaluated as exceeding expectations is often close to half.
- Salary increase budgets are too small; not enough money is available to allocate more to the best performers without reducing appropriate increases for good performers.
- Salary increase guidelines rarely allow increases for the best performers to exceed those of average performers by more than one or two percentage points.

How much more is exceptional performance worth than fully satisfactory performance? A "just-noticeable difference" (Weber's law) is often taken to be somewhere between 10 and 20 percent. This notion suggests that people can overlook differences of less than 10 percent in pay but will notice differences of 15 or 20 percent. An executive who believes his performance significantly exceeds expectations and is repeatedly complimented for outstanding achievement is likely to think anything less than a 15 percent premium in salary is insufficient to recognize his stellar performance. Likewise, an experienced, fully competent executive who meets all expectations is likely to think he is worth at least 15 to 20 percent more than a newcomer who is still learning the job.

Salary ranges are typically structured to reflect this just-noticeable difference by setting the minimum salary for a newly promoted executive at 80 percent of the salary range midpoint, the right rate of pay for a fully competent executive who consistently performs well, and setting the maximum salary at 120 percent of the midpoint for an extraordinary performer who has far exceeded expectations year after year.

When merit increase guidelines include an extra 1 or 2 percent for performance, on top of 3 or 4 percent for inflation, the ratio is well above the just-noticeable difference, but the absolute size of the reward for performance seems immaterial because it is only 1 or 2 percent of salary. The problem is that the 1 or 2 percent difference does not come close to a just-noticeable difference in salary until the better performer has received five or ten increases that are significantly larger than average. It would take 15 increases of an extra 1 percent before an executive proud of superior performance is likely to believe he is paid enough above average to adequately recognize that performance.

In other words, merit pay does not effectively reward performance because salary increases are too small to make a notable difference in salary, except over a long time. Recognizing this reality, many organizations de-emphasize the performance aspect of merit pay for executives who participate in incentive plans. Some go so far as to cap salaries at midpoint or even freeze salaries or severely limit increases for executives paid above midpoint on the premise that performance is adequately rewarded through incentive awards.

Bringing Salary Up to Midpoint

Most organizations aim to bring salaries up to the midpoint of a salary range (or some other control point) by the time the incumbent is performing at a fully competent level, or within a few years afterward. Once an organization has defined the right rate of pay for the job and communicates its policy to pay executives at, say, the 65th percentile, it creates an obligation to bring salaries up to that level for incumbents who meet the performance expectations set for their positions.

Salary administration systems generally do not achieve this target in a reasonable amount of time, so organizations resort to periodic special adjustments to do so. Their struggle starts with a statistical problem. The bottom of a typical salary range for executives and salaried employees is typically 80 percent of midpoint. It takes a 25 percent increase to bring a salary at the bottom of such a range up to midpoint. Getting to midpoint in, say, five years, requires annual salary increases 5 percent above the inflationary rate. The biggest increases should accrue during the first few years on the job, however, because that is when most learning and growth occur. The first several incremental increases should be 6 or 7 percent above the rate at which salary ranges are moved, or above the general rate of inflation in executive salaries. But if inflation is increasing salary range midpoints by 4 percent a year, attaining midpoint in that time frame would require increases of 10 or 11 percent a year for people at the bottom of the range, which would be hard to justify when seasoned executives performing equally well are getting increases of 4 percent a year. As a result, it often takes much longer than five years for people to reach midpoint. Some executives never reach it, even though they may be fully competent and performing well in the job.

Delivering salary increases big enough to bring salaries up to midpoint from the lower part of the range over a few years would require explaining why the salary increase guidelines favor people who are nominally underpaid rather than the organization's best performers. Instead, most organizations resort to periodic special adjustments to get salaries up to midpoint. This approach allows them to keep merit increases for nominally underpaid executives on par with those for others while delivering separate special adjustments, and it eliminates the need to explain why someone who is growing in competence but is still not fully proficient should get a bigger salary increase than a seasoned executive who is fully proficient and performing well.

Paying to Retain

Most CEOs and trustees believe that high salaries help retain executives. That is one reason so many hospitals and health systems intentionally position salaries at the 65th or 75th percentile, one reason they intentionally bring lower salaries up to midpoint, and one reason they like to position salaries high in the range for executives considered critical to the success of the organization. High salaries may help retain executives, by satisfying them with their pay, but salaries are not very effective at retaining executives. High salaries make it more expensive for another employer to recruit executives, but there are always plenty of employers who are willing to pay more to get the candidate they want to hire.

There is no evidence that turnover is lower where salaries are positioned at median than where they are positioned at the 75th percentile, and there is no evidence that turnover among executives paid low in their range is higher than among executives paid high in their range.

Neither a high salary nor a big salary increase has much bearing on most executives' decisions whether to stay or move on. For executives focused on career advancement, the first opportunities and the best opportunities are almost always somewhere else, unless their supervisor is close to retirement. For executives who have deep ties to the community and the hospital, few opportunities elsewhere will be attractive enough to disrupt these ties enough to get them to move. For someone who wants to move, the incremental pay is not enough to retain him, and for someone who would stay anyway, the incremental pay is a waste of scarce resources.

Matching an offer from another employer may be enough to retain an executive, but it often is not because factors other than pay weigh at least as heavily in decisions to change jobs. Paying extra to retain executives may be necessary under certain circumstances, as when the organization is in transition, facing unusual challenges, or undertaking a major project. But retention is better accomplished with a retention incentive or a generous retirement benefit than a salary increase.

RECOGNIZING COMPETENCIES AND EXPERIENCE

Just as salary administration systems tend to exaggerate the emphasis they place on pay for performance, they tend to overvalue experience and undervalue competence and competencies. Performance in hospitals and health systems is the result of the interaction of leadership, teamwork, collaboration, and employee engagement in pursuit of clear goals, following a methodical process, and supported by good information and real-time feedback. Performance at the executive level is less a matter of individual output than of effectiveness in setting appropriate goals, promoting collaboration, shaping processes, and encouraging continuous improvement.

Competencies are those capabilities that represent the difference between merely satisfactory performance and superlative performance. Competence, by contrast, implies knowledge, skills, and adequacy. Several examples of executive competencies include:

- the innate drive to improve institutional performance,
- the ability to inspire widespread commitment to institutional goals, and
- an intuitive understanding of the way changes in systems and processes affect other systems and processes.

Salary administration for executives can be construed as tying pay to competence and competencies rather than performance. Salaries should presumably be low in the salary range when people are learning the job, but they should be increased steadily as executives demonstrate that their competence in their role is increasing. Once executives achieve full competence in their role, they should presumably be paid at midpoint, or the right rate of pay for the job.

The bottom half of the range, in particular, is a scale for tying pay to competence. Salary increases for people paid low in their range should reflect growth in the job so that they are paid at a competitive level when they show that they are fully competent in all aspects of the job.

The top half of the range is usually considered a scale for recognizing superb performance above what is expected from the job, but it could be viewed instead as pay for competencies. Pay for performance should be a reward for recent performance, not past performance, and thus should ideally be paid as a lump sum (a bonus or an incentive award), not as an annuity (salary). Paying for competencies, however, is paying for current leadership and anticipated results—those that can be expected from leaders who are able to inspire organization-wide commitment to continuous improvement and engage the workforce as a whole in making the hospital the best it can be.

Competence in an executive position requires strong leadership competencies. Unlike job-related skills and knowledge, leadership competencies cannot be developed in a few years. Leadership competencies are developed over a career through extensive experience and failures in supervising, managing, leading, and guiding others. Someone without strong leadership competencies should never be promoted to a leadership position, as it is unlikely that anyone could develop these competencies quickly enough to become effective in a job that requires leadership competencies more than any other abilities.

Even the bottom half of the salary range, then, presumes that incumbents have strong leadership competencies. The midpoint of the range should be an appropriate salary for an executive with strong leadership competencies of the kind that deliver good performance year after year. Only exceptionally strong competencies that make executives far more influential and effective than expected should require recognition with a salary in the upper part of the range.

Why should an organization pay for capabilities beyond those required to perform the job? Some excess capabilities—such as being exceptionally smart—bring little value to a hospital or health system. Leadership competencies, however, deliver high value to the organization, as these are the capabilities and qualities that lead an organization to superb performance.

Organizations with sophisticated leadership development programs focus on developing leadership competencies. They often use competencies, rather than performance, as the basis for determining salaries and salary increases. Competencies are not easy to measure or evaluate, but they do represent the most important value an executive brings to the organization—unlike performance, which can be measured easily but tends to represent the results of many people working together.

RELATIONSHIP BETWEEN PERFORMANCE APPRAISAL AND PAY

Most organizations that use merit pay link the size of salary increases to performance appraisal scores, with the summary score from the annual performance evaluation determining the performance-related component of the annual salary increase. This approach undermines performance appraisal, as supervisors and subordinates focus on the overall score rather than the feedback, coaching, and guidance performance appraisal is intended to deliver.

Knowing that the score determines the size of a salary increase, supervisors tend to rate their subordinates where they need to in order to generate the salary increase they want to deliver. Managers and even human resources staff come to view performance appraisal as little more than a method for determining salary increases. Linking salary increases to performance appraisal tends to drive up performance ratings to the point that a sizeable portion of the work force is rated as exceeding expectations.

Salary increases can be based on performance without tying them formulaically to performance appraisal scores. Some organizations use an informal approach to linking salary increases to performance, which allows the appraisal to stand on its own and serve effectively as an opportunity to provide an honest evaluation of performance, coach subordinates on developing their capabilities, and find ways to improve both individual and organizational performance.

If performance appraisal is worthwhile—if it improves institutional performance by improving individual performance—it is worth doing well, which means conducting appraisals independently of salary administration. If, on the other hand, performance appraisal is nothing more than a method of determining or justifying salary increases, it should either be eliminated or streamlined to make salary administration less burdensome.

COMMUNICATING PAY TO EXECUTIVES

Most large organizations invest a lot of effort in communicating compensation to employees; sometimes they invest even more effort in communicating compensation to executives. In the interest of transparency, they tell employees what their salary range is, where their salary sits in the range relative to midpoint, and how salary increases are determined. In order to motivate employees, they communicate the goals they need to achieve to earn an incentive award. To help employees understand the value and cost of benefits, they explain how the benefits work and give employees tables showing a tally of the total cost of their compensation and benefits package.

Because executives, managers, and supervisors administer salaries for subordinates, employers explain the guidelines and rules to be followed in determining salaries and salary increases. They explain the structure and administrative rules for incentive plans to all participants in incentive plans, and if the plans include measures of individual performance, they tell executives how to set appropriate goals for subordinates and how to determine awards for individual performance. As a result, executives generally know a lot about the organization's compensation and benefits programs.

But communicating about compensation is difficult. It may seem straightforward, but it is not, because people tend to hear what they want to hear and focus on what they want to be paid, more than on what is said. And much of what is said is bound to be misunderstood.

Commitment to transparency may lead employers to communicate more than they need to about salaries and salary administration. Some authorities would argue that the less said, the better. The only message about salary that needs to be communicated to an employee is what next year's salary will be. Telling the employee what the salary range midpoint or the value of the job is opens the door to questions from any employee paid less than midpoint. Telling employees what the salary increase guidelines are opens the door to questions from anyone whose increase was below average. Telling employees that their salary increase was on par with increases for most other employees opens the door to questions from anyone whose performance evaluation was above average as well as from anyone who has been getting other positive feedback on performance. If salaries for seasoned employees lag midpoint, communicating this much detail about salary administration may engender dissatisfaction with pay rather than gratitude for the transparency. If increases for best performers or those who are rated above average are not large enough to matter, communicating salary increase guidelines or average increases for other employees may only engender cynicism about the employer's commitment to rewarding performance.

Nonetheless, most hospitals and health systems want to explain how the salary administration system works. Executives know how the system works, of course, as they need to administer it, so they expect transparency and will ask for explanations if they do not get it. In communicating salary to executives, the following are the points an organization committed to transparency is likely to want to make.

Communicate the value of the job. Present the salary range midpoint as the right rate of pay for the job, given the compensation philosophy set by the board. Be sure to explain that this is what the organization is willing to pay a seasoned, fully competent incumbent to get the job done, to meet all performance expectations set for the job, and to otherwise perform well as a member of the organization's leadership team.

Communicate the salary range. Present the salary range, explain that a salary anywhere within the range can be fair pay for the job, show where the executive's salary falls in the range, and explain the basis for that positioning.

Communicate the basis for future salary increases. Explain how annual salary increases are determined, show executives the salary increase guidelines, and tell them that salary increases are largely limited to keeping up with inflation once salaries reach midpoint. Sharing the parameters for future increases lets the executive know what type of increases to expect, how long it may take to get to midpoint, and how unlikely it is that they will ever reach the maximum of the salary range.

The downside to communicating the salary range and its midpoint is that it may lead anyone whose salary is below midpoint to feel underpaid and may lead those who are paid above midpoint to wonder why the midpoint is so low. After all, being paid below midpoint implies that the employer does not think the employee is worth a salary at midpoint, and being paid above midpoint could imply that one is overpaid and lead to constraints on future increases.

The downside to communicating salary administration guidelines is that no matter how clear the explanation or how many contingencies are mentioned, some people will hear a promise of future salary increases and look at the top of the range as their rightful pay opportunity when, in truth, few people ever reach the top of the range. Remember that most executives believe they are above average and exceed expectations set for their job, rather than just meet them. They expect an above-average score on performance appraisal and an above-average salary increase, and they expect, eventually, to be paid in the upper half of the salary range.

Organizations committed to transparency should communicate more, rather than less. Remember, however, that salary administration is just a set of administrative concepts and tools, not a set of rules. Salary administration systems exist to simplify the task of managing pay—not to communicate intent to pay in a particular way.

With that caution in mind, the systems and tools used in salary administration should be labeled as guidelines, rather than policies or procedures, to preserve flexibility. Telling managers how to determine salary increases for subordinates calls for emphasizing the need to control costs and the importance of internal equity and consistency. Communicating directly with employees about their compensation, however, calls for emphasizing process ("This is the way we go about making decisions"), concepts ("Anything within this range can be considered fair pay for the job") and contingencies ("Assuming we can afford it, you perform well, and we don't change our approach to salary administration"). Communicating salary administration as policies or standard practices conveys a suggestion of a contractual promise and could even invite litigation.

BEST PRACTICES IN GETTING SALARIES RIGHT

Following is a list of best practices in getting salaries right:

- Start by setting pay for the job right, in relation to market value for the job, pay for other positions in the organization, your organization's compensation philosophy, and what your organization can afford to pay.
- Set pay for the incumbent relative to the value the incumbent brings to the job, considering the person's competencies, experience, and performance.
- Set pay for a new recruit relative to the person's experience, previous pay, and what it takes to get him to take the position, as long as that is reasonable considering the value of the job and pay for other members of the executive team.
- Increase salary over time to bring it to the salary range midpoint (if you use salary ranges, or to the value of the job, if you do not) as the incumbent demonstrates increasing competence in the position and consistently performs well.

- Recognize competence and competencies, not seniority, as seniority by itself is not worth much.
- Reward performance by giving better performers larger salary increases, but recognize that incentive awards and promotions, not salary increases, are the real reward for superior performance.
- Aim to keep salaries fair, relative to one another, but recognize that your best performers should be paid more competitively than the others.
- Use your salary increase budget well. Do not waste scarce resources by treating everyone the same or let rules or merit pay guidelines keep you from doing what you need to do.

NOTES

1. Some organizations, consultants, and attorneys believe that approving salary ranges, rather than actual salary, meets the requirements for the rebuttable presumption of reasonableness in Internal Revenue Code §4958, as long as the compensation committee has determined that total compensation opportunity is reasonable even if executives' salaries were at the top of the salary range and incentive awards were paid at maximum value.

2. Although the best practice is to review total compensation every year, especially for senior executives who might be exposed to intermediate sanctions, annual review is probably unnecessary when total compensation opportunity is moderate, so that even with maximum incentive awards it is still well within the usual bounds of competitive practice.

CHAPTER 5

Incentive Compensation

INTRODUCTION

Incentive compensation is the most interesting element of executive compensation, and probably the most important, because of its relationship to performance. The board and its compensation committee focus on incentive compensation more than on other elements of the compensation program, and so do executives.

Incentive plans are performance management systems that offer pay contingent on performance. This contingency requires an elaborate apparatus of goal setting, performance measurement, and award determination as well as a strong governance process to keep the plan from being controlled by management.

Incentive plans lie at the intersection of management's responsibility for planning, goal setting, and achieving success and the board's responsibility for setting direction, providing guidance, and evaluating management's performance. Because they link goals to pay, incentives intensify the negotiations between management and the board over plans, budgets, and goals.

At the beginning of the year, when trustees need to approve goals, negotiation over goals can generate tension. No executive wants to have goals set so high that they cannot be achieved, or so high that they seem unreachable. They want goals set at a level that seems reasonable, so it is reasonably likely that the goals can be met and awards will be paid. Trustees want good performance, and while they may be perfectly willing to pay awards, their role in the process is to set goals high enough that the organization needs to perform well before awards will be paid. This difference between trustees' and management's points of view often generates tension and sometimes even skepticism, distrust, and resentment.

At the end of the year, when trustees need to evaluate performance and determine or approve awards, tension may arise again as trustees and management discuss why goals were met or missed or how unforeseen circumstances may have affected results. If performance far exceeded the goals set for the year, executives tend to think it was due to their own efforts, while the board may think the goals were too easy. If performance fell short of the goals, the board may think it was due to poor management, while executives may think the goals were set too high.

As long as the negotiation over goals and awards avoids acrimony, distrust, and resentment, this dynamic is healthy. Trustees and management both do what they are supposed to do. Trustees make sure the goals are not too easy, and management gets the opportunity to keep the goals realistic enough that it can meet them consistently, year after year.

Management has the advantage in this tug-of-war because it controls most of the information used in the debate. Trustees determine the outcome, however; trustees must approve the goals, evaluate the results, and authorize the awards. Trustees who compare their institution's performance with benchmarks in the industry and norms in the right peer group can effectively counterbalance whatever advantage management has in deciding what represents a good level of performance.

OVERVIEW OF INCENTIVE COMPENSATION

Most hospitals and health systems use annual incentive compensation as part of their executive compensation programs. Some use both annual and long-term incentives.

Incentives are now generally viewed by boards and management as an essential part of the pay package—as pay-at-risk, variable pay, or pay for performance—rather than as bonuses, which convey the notion of extra pay for performance above and beyond expectations. Some boards and executives still view incentive compensation as something to be paid only when performance is exceptionally good, even though that view is obsolete.

Annual incentive plans are designed to reinforce the annual operating plan in that their goals are generally drawn from the operating plan, they coincide with the fiscal year, and the awards reflect performance over that fiscal year.

Lack of Rewards Leads to Turnover

A large healthcare system introduced its first executive incentive plan as it began recruiting new executives for many of its leadership positions. The compensation committee maintained the mind-set, however, that salaries were sufficient pay for meeting expectations and that incentives should be paid only for outstanding performance far above expectations.

The newcomers all joined the system from organizations that had been paying incentives on a regular basis and that held the contemporary view of incentives as an integral and essential part of the compensation package. For the first few years after introducing the incentive plan, the compensation committee set goals so high that they were virtually unattainable. As a result, no awards were paid for the first few years, even though the new executives improved the system's performance enough to please the board. The newly recruited executives could not persuade the board to set goals at a more realistic level and eventually realized they had taken a pay cut to join the system. Over the next few years, most of those executives moved on to positions elsewhere.

Long-term incentive plans are designed to promote sustained performance or to reinforce longer-term plans or goals that do not fit a 12-month performance period. They typically cover a three-year period, although performance periods may overlap, with a new three-year cycle starting every year or every other year. As there is no natural three-year business cycle, long-term incentives are not necessarily designed to support three-year strategic plans, the way annual incentives support the annual operating plan and budget. The goals are often developed for the long-term incentive plan itself, when there is no three-year strategic plan to draw goals from.

Annual plans generally cover the entire executive team. Long-term plans are generally reserved for senior-level executives.

Utility of Incentive Plans

The principal utility of incentive compensation is in the discipline it imposes on the organization—discipline in planning, goal setting, performance management, performance measurement, and governance. Organizations that do not use incentive compensation often have vague plans, imprecise goals, and weak governance processes. Few hospitals or health systems invest the requisite time and effort in goal setting and performance measurement if the effort has no consequences for executive pay. But because incentive plans require precision in setting goals, evaluating performance, and determining awards, and probably because of their consequences for executive pay, trustees seem more engaged when debating and refining goals for the incentive plan than when reviewing and approving budgets and operating plans.

Organizations reap one signal advantage from using executive incentive compensation: trustees and executives need to reach agreement on which goals are most important and which ones represent priorities for the year. Incentive plans focus executives' attention and effort on accomplishing what is most important. Hospitals' strategic and operating plans inevitably encompass many goals, while incentive plans generally limit goals to a few. If organizations also reap an advantage from improved performance, it is due to this focus on a small number of goals and the discipline required in planning how to meet the goals.

Pros and Cons

Most executives and trustees believe that incentives help improve institutional performance. Others, however, are wary of incentives and, believing that the disadvantages of using them outweigh the advantages, avoid using them altogether, keep them totally discretionary, or keep incentive opportunity modest.

Exhibit 5.1 lists the principal advantages and disadvantages of offering incentive compensation.

But it is not incentives themselves that are effective or ineffective—it is the way they are used. Incentives can lead to positive results when they are well designed to fit the organization and its circumstances, when the goals are appropriate and the measurement systems effective, and when management and the compensation committee manage the plan well.

PURPOSE OF INCENTIVE COMPENSATION

The ultimate purpose of executive incentive plans is to promote the success of the organization by focusing participants' attention on the organization's most important goals and priorities. Incentive plans are systems to support the most important duties of the board—to guide management in achieving the organization's mission, to establish clear performance expectations and evaluate the CEO's performance, and to support the CEO's efforts to make the organization as successful as possible.

We often ascribe other purposes to incentive plans—motivating executives, tying pay to performance, rewarding good performance, reinforcing business plans, and so on. These are all attributes of incentive plans, but they are not purposes.

The reason for focusing singularly on this purpose is that Internal Revenue Service (IRS) private letter rulings make it clear that incentive plans are a legitimate use of a tax-exempt charity's resources only if the plans support the organization's tax-exempt mission. If they do not, any awards disbursed through them may amount to private inurement and misuse of charitable resources.

Executive incentives, then, meet their purpose only if they focus on the right kinds of performance, and only if they reward institutional success or individual performance that supports institutional success. A plan that focuses exclusively on financial performance does not meet the test because financial success is not the mission of a tax-exempt organization. A plan that focuses exclusively on individual performance may not meet the test, either, unless the goals are defined to support institutional success.

Exhibit 5.1: Advantages and Disadvantages of Using Incentives

Advantages

- Leaving a portion of pay at risk keeps pay opportunity competitive without guaranteeing that it will all be paid every year.
- Incentive compensation gives the board the opportunity to clarify its expectations and priorities.
- Incentives provide the CEO a system to help manage performance of other participants.
- Incentives can promote teamwork across functions and departments.
- Incentives focus participants' attention on the goals set for the plan.
- Incentives motivate participants to perform better, at least on the goals set for the plan.
- Variable pay rewards participants in proportion to performance and allows employers to pay especially big rewards when performance is especially good.
- Pay at risk helps control the cost of executive compensation and allows trustees to trim compensation when performance is poor or when the hospital cannot afford to pay it.
- Incentives increase discipline in goal setting and performance measurement by emphasizing the importance of precise goals and accurate reports.

Rewarding Inappropriate Goals Led to Private Inurement

A hospital in a small midwestern community used an incentive plan borrowed from a trustee's business, which emphasized individual performance. Without good guidelines, participants set goals for losing weight, improving their golf scores, and reading the Bible more often. Paying awards for achieving these goals amounted to private inurement and misuse of charitable resources—rewarding executives for achievements totally unrelated to the hospital's mission and giving executives more than the value they contributed to the organization by achieving these goals.

Exhibit 5.1 (Continued)

Disadvantages

- Incentive compensation interferes with budgeting, planning, and goal setting, because it gives executives a vested interest in setting goals that are easy to achieve.
- Maintaining an incentive program requires extra work, especially if individual goals are set for each participant.
- Incentives tend to oversimplify the challenge of managing the organization well by focusing on just a few goals.
- Goals are difficult to define in a way that does not overemphasize one metric at the expense of others.
- Most incentive plans overemphasize financial performance, setting them at odds with the mission of tax-exempt healthcare organizations.
- So much of performance is the result of extraneous events or circumstances that awards do not accurately reflect the efforts of participants.
- Plans often put so much emphasis on individual performance that they reinforce a silo orientation.
- Incentive awards, especially long-term awards, are based more on how well a participant anticipates change than on how well she actually performs. In other words, if you guess right, you win; if you guess wrong, you lose.
- Incentives reward the wrong people—those who make decisions, not those who have the often harder job of implementing those decisions.

INCENTIVE PLAN DESIGN PRINCIPLES

From all the published advice on designing incentive plans, one can cull a few universal principles, shown in the list below, but none of them explain how to design an incentive plan. Instead they warn against copying another organization's plan and trying to reward every important outcome.

- Keep it simple.
- Reward what is important, not just what is easy to measure.
- Customize the structure and measures to match the way the organization plans and manages.

The two best tests of an incentive plan's effectiveness are whether the plan encourages participants to focus on the organization's highest priorities and whether it pays the right amount of money to the right people for doing the right thing. Blindly following preconceived notions of "best practices" can limit a plan's effectiveness. (For example, many trustees and CEOs consider it totally inappropriate to pay awards when financial performance is below budget, which implies that the incentive plan is just a profit-sharing plan only incidentally focused on rewarding other measures of success. Some see no reason to reward significant improvements when the outcome is below average, even if the significant improvement represents remarkably good performance for the year.)

Incentive plans are flexible structures that can and should be modified over time to keep them as effective as possible. Plans that stay the same for years tend to lose their effectiveness in achieving the organization's most important goals. Just as there is no best design for every hospital, there is no best design for all times, only one that is best for current circumstances and priorities.

The structure is only a framework for an incentive plan. What makes a plan effective are the measures, the discipline with which the measures and goals are chosen and defined, and the frequency with which participants are reminded of the goals and how to reach them.

Trustees and CEOs must actively manage an incentive plan to keep it effective. If the measures stay the same year after year, the plan can become stale and lose its motivational impact. If the CEO does not regularly remind participants of the goals and focus their attention on what needs to be done to earn an award, it will not achieve the desired results.

Incentive plans need to have internal champions, and the best internal champion is the CEO. A CEO who does not support incentive compensation cannot be a strong advocate for the incentive plan. Trustees sometimes insist on introducing an incentive plan or structuring it in a particular way without the CEO's complete support, which dooms it, unless the board wants to take on responsibility for actively managing it.

Regardless of the structure, incentive plans never work perfectly, and they rarely treat participants entirely fairly. They cannot encompass every measure of performance, they are not sensitive to the trade-offs managers make between one measure and another to optimize overall performance, and they are not designed to fairly reward differences in participants' efforts or contributions to organizational success. Efforts to improve their structure often lead to other flaws. Recognizing that incentive plans cannot get everything right makes it easier to keep them simple and straightforward—which, in the end, is more likely to make them effective than any effort to engineer the perfect structure.

PERFORMANCE MANAGEMENT

More than anything else, incentive plans are systems for boards and CEOs to manage performance of the institution as a whole. For this purpose, they are more effective than performance appraisal and merit pay, because these focus on individual rather than institutional performance and because the stakes are higher with incentive compensation than with merit pay. With so much money involved, boards and CEOs put more effort into managing incentive plans than they put into performance appraisal and salary administration. If only by default, incentive plans become the primary system for managing executives' performance.

Hospitals and health systems have been using a balanced scorecard approach (Kaplan and Norton 1996) to setting goals for their incentive plans since well before the concept became a fad in the for-profit sector. By setting goals representing financial performance, clinical quality, patient service, and operating efficiency—the main components of a balanced scorecard—they capture the most important aspects of operational performance. Some organizations add or substitute measures of employee engagement, physician satisfaction, or volume of activity; in long-term incentive plans, they often substitute measures of growth or market share, and creditworthiness.

Performance management at the top of an organization tends to focus on organizational success, not individual performance. Incentive plans are ideally suited to supporting organization-wide performance because their structure allows them to focus all participants' attention on measures of institutional success.

Team Goals Versus Individual Goals

Every organization must decide whether to focus its incentive plan on organization-wide performance, departmental performance, or some combination of the two. At the executive level, most plans emphasize organization-wide performance. The emphasis changes at middle management levels, where most organizations place as much or more weight on departmental performance as on organization-wide success.

The usual distinction between organization-wide and individual goals is misleading and involves a misnomer. The distinction is between team goals and individual goals or between organization-wide and departmental goals. Individual goals are really job-related goals, as opposed to organization-wide or team goals. Job-related goals for a chief nursing officer would pertain to the entire nursing division; for a chief financial officer, to organization-wide financial measures such as days in accounts receivable; for the head of a home health agency, service line, or any other business unit, to the success of the business unit.

Many organizations find that incentive plans are not a particularly good way to manage job-related performance, because institutional success requires a high degree of teamwork, coordination, collaboration, and integration. Budgetary goals set at the department level, for example, tend to discourage collaboration and cross-departmental teamwork; indeed, many departmental goals reinforce a silo orientation, as they ask the department head to focus resolutely on optimizing the success of the department and pay next to nothing for collaboration, cooperation, or teamwork.

The usual reason for tying a portion of incentive opportunity to individual performance is to create a "line of sight" between participants' daily job activities and what they personally need to do to earn an award. To create this line of sight, most organizations set customized goals for each participant related to her responsibilities and tie a portion of incentive opportunity to these awards.

The other reason for tying a portion of incentive opportunity to individual performance is to deal with the "free-rider problem." Boards may worry that if incentive awards are entirely based on institutional performance, some participants receive a larger award than they deserve. But the free-rider problem is an issue of performance more than pay, so the problem cannot be solved by making some portion of incentive opportunity, or even all of it, contingent on individual performance. Instead, the organization should determine why the participant is underperforming, then either help him perform better or replace him.

The better reason for tying a portion of incentive opportunity to job-related goals is to explain clearly what each participant needs to accomplish to make the organization as a whole successful. Organizations can define goals and performance expectations without tying them to incentive opportunity, of course, but the employees tend to take it more seriously and do a better job when the goals are tied to pay.

While an executive incentive plan should ideally reward participants in proportion to their contributions to institutional success, every effort to customize the plan to reflect individual performance increases the risk that the plan will treat individual participants unfairly, as job-specific goals cannot be calibrated to represent the same degree of difficulty for all participants. At the same time, placing emphasis on individual performance dilutes emphasis on institutional performance and promotes a silo orientation that can undermine institutional success.

Keeping all the goals focused on organization-wide performance is often the best solution for hospitals with small management teams and for incentive plans with just a few participants. Multihospital systems sometimes find an ideal balance by limiting goals to one set for the system as a whole and another set for each hospital and other major business unit. Performance expectations and goals still need to be set for every division, department, service line, and function, but they do not need to be incorporated into the incentive plan.

Where department heads and middle managers participate in incentive plans, organizations generally decide to tie a major portion of their incentive opportunity to departmental performance. Recognizing that putting too much emphasis on departmental goals can undermine teamwork and collaboration, hospitals and health systems often find an ideal balance by emphasizing institutional performance more than departmental performance.

REGULATIONS PERTAINING TO INCENTIVE COMPENSATION IN TAX-EXEMPT ORGANIZATIONS

Two closely related sets of regulations pertain to incentive compensation in the tax-exempt sector: intermediate sanctions regulations and the Internal Revenue Code's (IRC) prohibition of private inurement and private benefit. They are supported by IRS advisory interpretations on intermediate sanctions and the use of incentive compensation by tax-exempt charities.

The IRC states that no part of the net earnings of an organization may inure to the benefit of a private shareholder or individual. Precedent broadens the rule to forbid giving anyone a right to a share of the organization's revenues or giving any organizational assets to an insider (*insider* is defined in the introduction to this book). Given that incentive plans started out as profit-sharing mechanisms in the for-profit sector, use of incentive plans by tax-exempt charities has always entailed a risk that they violate this prohibition. Over time, however, tax-exempt healthcare organizations have learned how to structure incentive plans so that the risk is largely related to overpaying someone in proportion to the value of services delivered, not to the question of whether the plan shares a portion of net earnings with participants.

Private Inurement and Private Benefit

The premise for granting tax-exempt status to hospitals and health systems is that these organizations exist and are managed for the benefit of the communities they serve, not for the benefit of insiders or other individuals. Arising from this premise is the prohibition against private benefit and private inurement.[1]

An incentive plan at a tax-exempt charity should be structured carefully to avoid the risk as well as the appearance of private inurement and private benefit. Any talk of "having skin in the game," "having a stake in our success," or "phantom equity" elevates this risk, so trustees should avoid it, as it implies they do not understand the prohibition, it could lead to plan designs that clearly flout the prohibition, and it could even be used as evidence that they are intentionally engaging in private inurement. Plans based on models from the for-profit sector can expose tax-exempt organizations to private inurement, as can plans that overpay executives. Any indication that the incentive plan is designed, managed, or manipulated by executives for their own benefit suggests private inurement.

Over the years, consultants and attorneys have identified ways to minimize the risk of violating these prohibitions. Among the most important are the following:

- Setting limits on the size of incentive awards
- Tying awards to goals rather than defining awards as a percentage of earnings or revenues
- Avoiding plans structured as profit-sharing pools or phantom equity
- Making sure that plans emphasize measures such as clinical quality, patient satisfaction, and community benefit as much as financial success

IRS Guidance

The IRS has articulated a three-part test for determining whether an incentive plan (or any other compensation or benefit plan) used by a tax-exempt organization avoids private inurement (IRS 1969, 1987a, 1987b; McDowell 2007, 17–27):

1. The plan must be designed to support the tax-exempt mission of the organization.
2. The plan must be controlled by a disinterested third party (generally the board or its compensation committee).
3. The compensation delivered through the plan and the resulting total compensation must be reasonable compared with incentive awards and total compensation paid by comparable organizations.

In addition, the IRS considers the following factors in determining whether a particular plan amounts to private inurement (IRS 1990, 1987a, 1987b, 2006; Brauer and Kaiser 2000):

- Whether the amount of compensation available under the plan is capped
- Whether the plan has a real and discernible business purpose demonstrating that the plan furthers the organization's charitable mission
- Whether the compensation depends on the participant's performance and not just the revenues or profits of the organization
- Whether the plan appropriately balances measures of clinical quality and patient service with measures of financial success
- Whether the plan is a device to distribute a portion of the profits to persons in control of the organization
- Whether the plan has the potential to reduce the charitable service or benefits the organization would otherwise provide

Intermediate Sanctions

The Taxpayer Bill of Rights 2 gives the IRS the authority to impose penalties ("intermediate sanctions") on insiders who are beneficiaries of private inurement ("excess benefit transactions") and on any executive or trustee who knowingly approves the excess benefit transaction. Intermediate sanctions regulations in IRC § 4958 can be imposed if incentive awards bring total compensation above fair market value for the services provided. The regulations provide a safe harbor (known as "rebuttable presumption of reasonableness") for minimizing the risk of intermediate sanctions if (1) the compensation arrangement and the resulting total compensation are approved in advance by an authorized, disinterested third party; (2) the authorized party has, in approving the arrangement, obtained and relied on appropriate comparability data on total compensation; and (3) the terms of the decision, the process followed in making it, the vote of the individuals approving the transaction, and the source of the data are adequately documented in timely minutes.

Intermediate sanctions regulations say little about the structure of an incentive plan, who participates in it, or how it is administered. They pertain to incentive compensation in four ways: (1) if incentive awards push total compensation up so high as to be unreasonable, they allow the IRS to impose intermediate sanctions; (2) they allow the reasonableness of total compensation to be determined only at the time awards are being considered for approval by the committee; (3) they establish a safe harbor for a new employee whose compensation is fixed in a contract, which would be invalidated by participation in an incentive compensation plan that allows any discretionary judgment in determining the size of an incentive award or the goals on which awards are based; and (4) they allow the compensation committee to establish the presumption of reasonableness by citing superior performance as a rationale for paying an executive above the usual range of the comparability data.

THE ROLE OF THE COMPENSATION COMMITTEE IN OVERSEEING INCENTIVE PLANS

Any incentive plan in which the CEO participates must be administered by the board or its compensation committee, serving as the disinterested third party mandated by the IRS. (If the CEO does not participate in the plan, he is allowed to administer it.)

In principle, trustees exercise control of an incentive plan every time they make significant decisions about it. They control the design of the incentive plan at the outset when they authorize its introduction, approve its structure, determine who participates in the plan, and set or ratify incentive opportunity. At the beginning of every year, they exercise control when they approve the performance measures and the goals for the incentive plan and as they either implicitly reauthorize the plan and agree to continue offering incentive opportunity at the same level to the same participants or explicitly authorize changes to the plan or the list of participants. Then, at the end of the year, they control the plan when they authorize payment of incentive awards after evaluating performance relative to the goals set at the beginning of the year.

In practice, however, trustees' role in controlling and administering the plan is constrained by their dependence on management for leading the planning and goal-setting process, proposing performance measures and goals, proposing participants, tracking performance, analyzing and reporting data on performance, evaluating performance on nonquantitative measures, identifying externalities that should not affect award size, and calculating the size of proposed awards.

Incentive plans take on a life of their own whereby participants and trustees alike assume they will be renewed each year in their current form as long as no one objects to them. In most organizations, trustees' role is limited to reviewing, refining, modifying, and approving goals proposed by management and reviewing and authorizing payment of awards proposed by management. If all or a portion of the CEO's award is discretionary, however, the committee may exercise more control in determining that award.

What should the committee do, then, to meet the IRS's standards for avoiding private inurement with an incentive compensation plan? Once the plan has been approved by the board as a whole (and it should be, because an incentive plan is a contractual obligation), the committee should formally make the following decisions before reauthorizing the plan for another year:

- Who should participate (rather than permanently authorizing all executives to participate in perpetuity)
- How much incentive opportunity is appropriate for each participant or class of participants (rather than assuming it should stay the same year after year)
- What goals should be set to support the organization's tax-exempt mission

At the end of each year, after determining awards, it should evaluate the plan and determine the following:

- Whether awards and the resulting total compensation are reasonable and appropriate
- Whether the plan supports the organization's tax-exempt mission
- Whether the structure of the plan or any of its features should be modified for the coming year

Even if the evaluation is perfunctory, it is worth undertaking to remind the committee of its responsibility to exercise control of the plan.

Another way a committee can demonstrate that it controls an incentive plan is to adopt a formal plan document and a set of administrative guidelines that assign certain responsibilities to the committee. The principal value of these documents is to establish and record the rules the committee should follow when it needs to decide how to deal with unusual circumstances, when a dispute arises, or when it encounters a problem it needs to solve. But they also remind the committee that it has an obligation to exercise control and that it has complete discretion to administer the plan as it sees fit.

Formal Plan Documents

A formal incentive plan document is a legal document that acknowledges the board's approval of the plan, describes the plan in detail, identifies who will administer the plan and who has authority to make decisions about it, and delineates the rules for modifying the plan. It usually assigns responsibility for administering the plan to the compensation committee and generally preserves as much flexibility for the committee as possible by allowing it to exercise discretion in determining whether to pay awards and how big they should be.

Even though any significant change in participation, incentive opportunity, or structure should probably be brought to the board for approval, a typical formal incentive plan document gives the compensation committee full authority to administer the plan and establish the rules by which it will be administered and encompasses these other elements:

- It charges the committee with making a number of decisions each year—selecting participants, setting incentive opportunity, selecting performance measures, setting goals and weighting them, evaluating performance, and determining awards.
- It defines eligibility for the plan and establishes a process for selecting participants.
- It sets limits on awards, such as a maximum size and a hurdle rate for financial performance below which no award can be paid.
- It establishes rules on the effect of death, disability, termination, and retirement on a participant's right to an award.
- It specifies that the plan is no guarantee of employment, that awards payable cannot be pledged or encumbered in any way, and that the employer has the right to deduct withholding taxes due on awards.

Most formal plan documents also give the committee the right to exercise discretion in determining award size, to take into account the effect of externalities on performance, and to avoid having to pay awards under circumstances in which doing so could harm the institution's reputation (e.g., if it has been publicly embarrassed by a serious lapse in quality). Some plan documents charge the committee with periodically reviewing the plan to determine whether it continues to meet the criteria the IRS has spelled out in private letter rulings for avoiding private inurement—deciding whether the plan continues to support the tax-exempt mission of the organization and ensuring that the awards paid and the resulting total compensation continue to be reasonable.

Specific details, such as a list of participants, incentive opportunity levels, performance measures and goals for the year, and the like are often documented separately, sometimes in appendices to the formal plan document, rather than incorporated in the body of the document itself, as many of these details change from year to year.

Administrative Guidelines

The administrative guidelines for an incentive plan prescribe the process and the rules the compensation committee intends to follow in administering the plan. Administrative guidelines tend to be more specific than the formal plan document, as their purpose is to spell out the rules the formal plan document gives the committee the authority to establish.

The guidelines typically deal with practical matters that help the committee maintain consistency from year to year:

- Can awards be paid before or only after receipt of the annual audit report?

- If participants leave the organization before the end of the year, are they eligible for a pro rata award?
- If participants leave after the end of the year but before awards are paid, are they entitled to an award?
- Do incentive awards count as part of the basis for determining benefits?
- How do midyear salary increases affect award size?
- Can new participants be added to the plan during the year?
- How long does a newcomer or a newly promoted executive have to work to earn a pro rata award?

Incentive opportunity, performance measures, goals and weights, and lists of participants or participant categories are often documented separately in an illustration attached to the administrative guidelines.

Too often incentive plans have no formal documentation—nothing more than a set of recommendations from a consultant or an illustration of the performance measures, goals, and weights set for the year and a record of the incentive opportunity levels that have been applied in the past. With no formal documentation of the plan, precedent takes over and trustees and executives assume that the plan will continue from year to year with the same structure, the same participants, and the same opportunity levels.

How can the committee claim to exercise administrative control of the plan when there is no document indicating that the committee has full authority to make all decisions regarding the plan? Absent such a document, the committee may not even know what it has a right to do.

PREVALENCE OF INCENTIVE COMPENSATION

Annual Incentives

About 75 percent of all hospitals and 80 percent of all health systems use annual incentives as part of their executive compensation programs. Some that have no formal annual incentive plan pay discretionary awards often enough that it makes sense to say they have a discretionary plan. Others pay awards occasionally, but probably not often enough to claim they have a practice of doing so.

Most executives consider an annual incentive plan such an integral part of their pay packages that organizations without an incentive plan may find it difficult to recruit. To do so, they generally need to pay salaries high enough to make up for the lack of an incentive plan.

Long-Term Incentives

Long-term incentives are far less prevalent than annual incentives, especially in smaller hospitals and systems, but they are fairly common among the country's largest health systems. Almost a third of secular health systems with more than $1 billion in operating expenses have a long-term incentive plan in addition to an annual incentive plan. Prevalence is somewhat lower among large Catholic systems.

These statistics understate the true prevalence of long-term incentives, as some organizations use special-purpose plans like long-term incentive plans and annual plans with deferral features as substitutes for long-term plans:

- Some systems and hospitals use multiyear retention incentives to retain executives over a period of change, reorganization, executive succession, or post-merger integration.
- Other organizations establish special-purpose incentive plans for certain executives, such as special multiyear incentives related to developing a new hospital or a new health plan, completing a major new system, or completing a proposed merger.
- Several systems and hospitals use a hybrid short-term/long-term incentive plan, which provides significantly more incen-

tive opportunity than a typical annual incentive plan would by itself.

- Others couple unusually rich annual incentives with mandatory deferral of some portion of the awards, rather than introduce separate long-term incentives.

The prevalence of long-term incentive plans is increasing slowly over time. A few tax-exempt healthcare organizations introduce new long-term incentive plans every year.

At the same time, some organizations abandon long-term incentive plans every year. Sometimes boards or management decide their long-term incentive plan involves more work than it is worth.

ELIGIBILITY AND PARTICIPATION

Annual Incentives

Most annual incentive plans cover all executives. A few plans are limited in scope of coverage and include only the top layer of senior executives.

Eligibility is usually determined by title (e.g., vice president or above) or reporting level (e.g., all executives reporting to the CEO, COO, and/or CFO). Sometimes it is determined by membership in a group (e.g., members of the management council).

Participation in management incentive plans drops off below the executive level, especially in smaller and midsize organizations. In larger hospitals and systems, though, it is more common than not for department heads to be included in an incentive plan. In more than half of these organizations, directors are eligible for incentive compensation, either through a separate incentive plan for department leaders—and sometimes all managers as well—or as participants in the executive incentive plan. In smaller independent hospitals and systems, the prevalence of incentives for department heads is lower; about a third of these organizations offer incentive compensation to leaders at this level.

A relatively small percentage of hospitals, just 15 to 20 percent, use all-employee incentive plans. Sometimes middle managers participate in this type of plan instead of the executive incentive plan. A few hospitals and systems have only an all-employee plan, in which executives participate, sometimes at the same opportunity level as all other employees and sometimes at a higher opportunity level.

Long-Term Incentives

Eligibility is defined much more narrowly for long-term incentive than for annual incentive plans. Typically, eligibility is limited to senior executives responsible for developing and leading the implementation of the organization's long-term business plans. A very few organizations let all executives participate in the long-term plan. Whereas annual incentive plans may have as many as 30 or even more than 100 participants, long-term plans typically have 5 to 12 participants. In multihospital systems, eligibility typically includes senior system executives and the president of each hospital. With the exception of hospital presidents, executives in subsidiary operating units are seldom included in long-term incentive plans.

Eligibility is typically defined by officer status or level (e.g., corporate senior vice presidents and affiliate presidents) or by membership in a core group of senior executives (e.g., the president's council). The intent is to limit eligibility to executives who are deeply involved in shaping, planning, and executing major corporate strategies.

INCENTIVE OPPORTUNITY

Incentive opportunity is usually defined as a percentage of salary (e.g., "Her incentive opportunity is 25 percent of her salary"). It is sometimes defined only as maximum opportunity (e.g., "Her maximum opportunity is 25 percent of salary") but often as a range or a three-point scale centered on the target or expected value and anchored at maximum and threshold values above and below the expected value (e.g., "Her incentive opportunity is 20 percent at target, 30 percent at maximum, and 10 percent at threshold").

Opportunity is occasionally defined as a dollar amount (e.g., "If you meet this goal, we will pay you $10,000").

Executives often focus on maximum opportunity as what they hope to earn. In evaluating incentive opportunity and its effect on total compensation, however, trustees and their consultants generally focus on the expected value of an incentive plan as what they expect will be paid, on average over time, when performance is reasonably good.

Annual incentive plans define opportunity only at maximum value about as often as they use the three-point scale. Long-term incentive plans usually utilize the three-point scale.

Organizations that define incentive opportunity only at maximum generally expect to pay awards close to maximum value—not necessarily every year, but as often as the organization meets its goals. On average, awards under these plans tend to be about 80 percent of maximum, and sometimes higher.

Organizations that define incentive opportunity at threshold, target, and maximum generally expect to pay awards at or near target level. Threshold opportunity is typically set at one-third of maximum; target, at two-thirds of maximum. On average, awards under these plans tend to be about two-thirds of maximum.

This difference between the two approaches makes it difficult to compare incentive opportunity at organizations that define opportunity only at maximum with incentive opportunity at organizations using the three-point scale. Where incentive opportunity is defined only at maximum level, the maximum tends to be lower than where opportunity is defined at three levels—but incentive awards and the expected value of awards are not necessarily lower.

A plan in which opportunity is defined only at maximum, with maximum opportunity at 30 percent of salary and with awards generally about 80 percent of maximum, is on par with a plan that defines threshold, target, and maximum opportunity at 12 percent, 24 percent, and 36 percent of salary, respectively.

When incentive opportunity is set only at maximum, goals are likewise defined at just one level, whereas goals are generally set at three levels when incentive opportunity is defined by three levels. This difference has significant implications for the way organizations think about goals and incentive opportunity. Organizations that set goals and incentive opportunity at just one level tend to expect most goals to be achieved and set goals so that they can probably be achieved. Organizations that use the three-point scale for incentive opportunity and goal-setting tend to expect performance at the target level but acknowledge that actual performance might be well above or well below the target level. Use of the three-point scale tends to promote more variability in award size—both above and below the expected size—than plans with opportunity defined only at maximum. Plans with opportunity defined only at maximum tend to pay awards at or close to maximum, or nothing at all, whereas plan with the three-point scale can pay awards near threshold or maximum as often as near target value.

Annual Incentive Opportunity

Exhibit 5.2 shows the typical levels of target and maximum annual incentive opportunities at not-for-profit healthcare systems and hospitals, where opportunity is defined at both target and maximum levels as a percentage of salary.

Where opportunity is defined only at maximum, maximum opportunity is typically on par with or slightly higher than the target opportunity levels shown in Exhibit 5.2.

Discretionary bonus plans tend to pay very small awards, often in the vicinity of 10 percent of salary or less. Discretionary plans tend to be conservative because there is no clear basis for deciding how much to pay. Boards tend to be more comfortable paying large awards when the incentive plan has a well-defined structure, set of measures, and set of rules to follow.

Incentive opportunity even in tightly structured plans can be low. Small independent hospitals and government hospitals sometimes set target or maximum incentive opportunity as low as 10 percent of salary, even for the CEO.

Exhibit 5.2: Typical Annual Incentive Opportunity as a Percentage of Salary, by Type and Size of Organization

Systems and Large Independent Hospitals

Position	Target Opportunity	Maximum Opportunity
CEO	30–35%	45–52%
Senior executives (e.g., COO, CFO)	25–30%	37–45%
Vice presidents	20–25%	30–37%
Directors	10–15%	15–22%

Large System-Affiliated Hospitals

Position	Target Opportunity	Maximum Opportunity
CEO	25–30%	37–45%
Senior executives (e.g., COO, CFO)	20–25%	30–37%
Vice presidents	15–20%	22–30%
Directors	5–10%	7–15%

Small System-Affiliated Hospitals

Position	Target Opportunity	Maximum Opportunity
CEO	20–25%	30–38%
Executives	15–20%	22–30%
Directors	5–10%	7–15%

Long-Term Incentive Opportunity

Because long-term incentive plans typically last three years, it is important to think of long-term incentive opportunity in terms of its annualized value. A plan with target opportunity of 30 percent of salary paid at the end of the third year is worth only 10 percent of salary on an annualized basis if the plan allows for a payout only once every three years. If the plan starts a new three-year performance cycle every year, however, the annualized value of the plan will be 30 percent of salary, as an award can be paid every year once the first cycle is completed. If the plan calls for starting a new performance cycle every other year, the annualized value of the plan is 15 percent of salary, as an award of 30 percent of salary can be paid every other year.

Long-term incentive opportunity is somewhat lower on an annualized basis than annual incentive opportunity. Emphasis on long-term incentives has been increasing, however. Typical opportunity has been rising over the last decade in the not-for-profit sector, just as in the for-profit sector, where long-term incentive opportunity has grown to several (or, for CEOs, many) times as much as annual incentive opportunity.

Exhibit 5.3 shows median annualized incentive opportunity as a percentage of salary in long-term incentive plans in the country's largest and most prestigious not-for-profit health systems.

Long-term incentive plans usually use the three-point scale in defining incentive opportunity. As with annual incentive plans,

---

Exhibit 5.3: Long-Term Incentive Opportunity in Leading Systems

Position Level	Median Annualized Target Opportunity	Median Annualized Maximum Opportunity
President and CEO	27.5%	45%
Executive vice presidents	20%	35%
Senior vice presidents	20%	30%

threshold is generally set at one-third of maximum opportunity and target at two-thirds of maximum.

Total Incentive Opportunity

Long-term incentive opportunity is almost always additive. In organizations that use both annual and long-term incentive plans, annual opportunity is usually just as high as typical opportunity at organizations that only use annual incentives. In organizations that use both annual and long-term incentive plans, total incentive opportunity is about 55 percent at target and 80 percent at maximum for CEOs, and about 35 to 45 percent at target and 50 to 60 percent at maximum for other system executives.

Relation of Incentive Opportunity to Compensation Philosophy

Much of the variation in incentive opportunity is based on compensation philosophy. Organizations that position total compensation opportunity at median or average tend to have lower incentive opportunity than those that position total compensation opportunity at the 75th percentile. Where the intended competitive position is higher for total compensation than for salaries, incentive opportunity needs to be high enough to fill the gap. Where salaries and total compensation are both positioned at the same competitive level (e.g., both at median or both at the 75th percentile), there is less room for incentive opportunity.

STRUCTURE OF INCENTIVE PLANS

Some incentive plans are tightly structured, with interlocking gears that determine the precise value of awards once performance has been measured. Others are loosely structured and leave room for discretion in determining award size. Most incentive plans are based on one or another of a few models. Even so, their structures vary in many ways.

The structure of an incentive plan can be described in terms of these elements:

- Duration of performance period
- An element that controls funding of the incentive plan
- Balance between team goals and individual goals
- Interaction among different performance measures
- Scale for setting goals and determining awards
- Provision for discretionary adjustment in award size
- Deferral of awards

Each element is discussed in the paragraphs that follow.

Duration of Performance Period

Annual plans are structured to coincide with the organization's fiscal year. Some all-employee plans that are otherwise structured on an annual basis pay awards on a quarterly basis.

Long-term plans are usually structured to last three years. Trustees accustomed to stock options with a ten-year life think of three-year plans as midterm incentives, but few organizations are willing to structure plans with longer periods because the external environment changes so rapidly.

Overlapping long-term cycles. Most long-term plans are structured with overlapping cycles, so that a new cycle begins every year or every other year. Those with nonoverlapping cycles begin a new cycle only once every three years.

An Element That Controls Funding of the Incentive Plan

Boards should ensure that incentive awards are funded by current operating earnings, not reserves or investment income, and do not

> ### Complexities of Overlapping Cycles
>
> Overlapping cycles complicate the roles of trustees and
> executives with responsibility for administering incen-
> tive plans, especially if a new long-term cycle begins each
> year. Near the beginning of each year, management must
> propose and the compensation committee must establish
> a new set of goals for both the annual and the long-term
> plans. At about the same time of year, management must
> report on performance and the committee must evaluate
> and determine awards for both the annual plan and the
> just-completed three-year cycle of the long-term plan.
>
> Difficult and time consuming as this effort may be for the
> committee, consider how difficult it must be for participants
> to grasp how the plans fit together—or to remember how
> they differ. At any one time, after all, four incentive plans—
> the annual plan and the three cycles of long-term plans—are
> running. Participants are supposed to pay attention to all
> four sets of goals—which may all be different from one
> another.

absorb too large a share of operating income. They usually control
funding for incentive plans in one of two ways. The first is to use
a hurdle or circuit breaker that must be surpassed before the plan
can be funded, regardless of how good performance was on other
measures. The second is to use a profit pool that determines how
much money is available for paying awards. A variation combines
the circuit breaker with the concept of a profit pool; it uses a three-
or four-step scale that reduces awards when operating margin is
below budget and increases awards when it is above budget.

In tax-exempt healthcare organizations, few plans are structured as profit pools, with the pool defined as a percentage of operating earnings or net income, as this structure seems to violate the

prohibition against private inurement. Some plans are structured this way, nonetheless, either explicitly or implicitly:

- A formula that limits incentive awards to one-half of operating earnings, for example, is a profit-sharing pool defined as a constraint rather than a funding mechanism.
- A formula that adjusts the size of awards downward when operating earnings are below budget and upward when budget is exceeded is a profit-sharing pool in disguise.

Instead, most plans have a hurdle that must be surpassed before awards are paid. These hurdles or circuit breakers are generally defined in terms of the current year's budgeted operating margin or an absolute level of return. They may also be defined in terms of patient satisfaction, clinical quality, accreditation, or charitable care. Some structures feature multiple circuit breakers, each controlling a portion of the incentive plan funding—say, one-third apiece for surpassing hurdles for operating income, patient satisfaction, and clinical quality.

Funding mechanisms for long-term incentive plans. Most long-term incentive plans use a hurdle or circuit breaker defined in terms of financial performance, after accounting for annual incentive awards. The hurdle typically measures financial performance over the entire three-year period as cumulative operating profit, average operating margin, or maintenance of a good credit rating.

Balance Between Team Goals and Individual Goals

A typical annual incentive plan uses a combination of institutional (or team) goals and individual (job-related) goals. But many incentive plans in independent hospitals, single hospital systems, or even highly integrated organizations use only institutional goals. Very few executive incentive plans use just individual or job-related goals and no team goals, as indicated by the following statistics:

- About 40 percent of annual incentive plans are based entirely on team performance.
- About 60 percent of annual incentive plans use a combination of team and individual goals. On average, the balance between team and individual performance tilts toward team performance and allocates 60 percent of incentive opportunity to team performance and 40 percent to individual performance. However, team performance may be weighted as high as 80 to 90 percent for senior executives and 100 percent for CEOs.

Exhibit 5.4 shows a typical allocation of opportunity to team and individual measures.

Most boards and CEOs want to use incentives to drive institutional success, not to reward individual performance. They view incentives as a management system to build commitment to institutional goals and find other ways to manage and reward or recognize individual performance. Organizations that keep the incentive plan largely or entirely focused on institutional success still use performance appraisal and merit pay to focus, motivate, recognize, and reward individual performance.

Most multihospital system incentive plans use a combination of systemwide, entity (hospital or other business unit), and individual

---

Exhibit 5.4: Typical Balance Between Team and Individual Goals in Annual Incentive Plans

Position	Team	Individual
CEO	100%	0%
COO, CFO	80%	20%
Staff vice presidents	70%	30%
Operations vice presidents	60%	40%
Directors	40%	60%

or job-related goals. Thus, their executives are often measured on two sets of team goals: one at the system level and one at the business unit level. Some use only these two sets of team goals and no individual or job-related goals.

Plans that cover department heads in addition to executives tend to put more weight on individual performance for the department heads than for the executives. Many of these plans use only systemwide goals for the CEO; a combination of systemwide, entity, and individual goals for most other participants; and entity and individual goals (in hospitals) or systemwide and individual goals (in the system's central office) for department heads.

Decentralized systems tend to allocate most of the weight for hospital executives to hospital performance. Those that are fairly centralized tend to balance the weight between system and hospital goals to promote integration across the system. Weighting typically varies by the level of participant, as shown in Exhibit 5.5.

This approach leads to allocating incentive opportunity among systemwide goals, entity goals, and individual goals in the manner shown in Exhibit 5.6.

Awards Based Solely on Individual Performance

In a twist on the usual pattern, a two-hospital system on the East Coast has an incentive plan that bases awards entirely on individual performance. Performance appraisal and merit pay, by contrast, are based largely on institutional success and performance on team goals. As a result, salary increases are the same size for all members of the executive team, while incentive awards can vary substantially from one executive to another. Institutional success, then, generates small rewards, while individual performance generates larger rewards. Trustees and executives alike seem content with this odd inversion.

Exhibit 5.5: Typical Balance Between System and Hospital Goals in Annual Incentive Plans in Moderately Centralized Multihospital Systems

Position	System	Hospital
System CEO	100%	0%
System executives	100%	0%
System directors, managers, and supervisors	100%	0%
Hospital presidents and vice presidents	30–40%	60–70%
Hospital directors, managers, and supervisors	10–20%	80–90%

Exhibit 5.6: Typical Allocation of Opportunity Among System, Entity, and Individual Goals in Annual Incentive Plans in Moderately Centralized Multihospital Systems

Position	System	Hospital	Individual
CEO	100%	0%	0%
Broad system executives (e.g., COO, CAO)	80%	0%	20%
System executives	60%	0%	40%
System directors, managers, and supervisors	40–50%	0%	50–60%
Hospital presidents	30%	50%	20%
Hospital vice presidents	30%	40%	30%
Hospital directors, managers, and supervisors	10%	30%	60%

Balance between team and individual goals in long-term incentive plans. Long-term plans are with rare exception entirely team oriented. In independent hospitals and centralized systems, long-term plans generally use the same goals for all participants. In decentralized and moderately centralized multihospital systems, long-term plans may include both system and entity goals. They virtually never use individual goals.

Interaction Among Different Performance Measures

Performance is evaluated independently on each performance measure, and awards are often calculated separately on each performance measure. Some incentive plans, however, are structured so that performance on one measure affects the value of performance on the other measures. Annual incentive plans structured as profit-sharing pools in the for-profit sector are two-dimensional, with the pool of funds available for awards determined by financial performance and the size of awards earned for performance on nonfinancial goals modified by the size of the pool. Some hurdles and circuit breakers are defined in a way that makes the plans two-dimensional; instead of eliminating awards altogether if the hurdle is not surpassed, the plans use a scale that adjusts award size in proportion to operating income.

Interaction among measures in long-term incentive plans. A common structure for long-term incentive plans is a two-dimensional matrix that sets up interaction among the measures used. Performance on one dimension (e.g., financial performance) determines the value of each unit, and performance on the other dimension (e.g., growth) determines how many units are earned. This structure is similar to a performance unit or performance share plan used in for-profit companies as a long-term incentive.

Scale for Setting Goals and Determining Awards

Every incentive plan that bases incentive awards on performance in relation to goals uses two sets of metrics and two scales—one of each related to performance, the others related to award size. Linking the scale for award size to the scale for performance, however, makes the two scales look like one, albeit with two sets of labels.

In setting a goal one usually thinks of one number or one result to be achieved. In setting a goal for an incentive plan, however, one needs to decide whether exceeding the goal is worth more than achieving the goal, and whether getting close to the goal is good enough to warrant paying something, even if only a modest award.

In a game, one either wins or loses; getting close doesn't count, and beating one's opponent by a long shot doesn't count more than just squeaking by. In healthcare, as in any business, however, exceeding a goal is better than just meeting it, and getting close to the goal is often good enough. Setting a goal for a business or healthcare organization entails making assumptions about the future—what the competition will do, how the economy will fare, and what regulators may change—so business planners tend to think in terms of a range of possible outcomes, not just a single number.

Goals for incentive plans are often defined as a range of potential outcomes—a goal, to be sure, representing expected or hoped-for performance but also a point that represents satisfactory performance, somewhat below the real goal but still good enough to warrant paying an award, and a range above the goal that represents superb performance that may be worth a bigger award than what is promised for meeting the goal itself.

Some scales have only one point, representing the goal itself. These are pass/fail goals. Beating the goal counts no more than reaching the goal, and finishing short of the goal, even by an eyelash, counts not at all.

Other scales have multiple points, often one representing the goal itself, one representing the lowest level of performance that merits an award, and one representing the level that merits a maximum award. Some have only two points, one representing the goal itself, the other representing the lowest level of performance for which a goal will be paid.

Three-point scale. Many incentive plans used by tax-exempt hospitals and health systems set goals at three levels: expected or on-plan performance, outstanding performance, and satisfactory performance somewhat below plan. The same scale represents the expected or target-level award for on-plan performance, a maximum award for outstanding performance, and a small award for satisfactory performance.

Exhibit 5.7 demonstrates the three-point scale.

Many three-point scales allow interpolation between the bottom and the top of the scale, so every incremental increase in performance generates an increase in award size. Others represent a set of steps, with no interpolation between them, so awards have only three possible values—minimum, target, and maximum.

This approach works best with relatively few performance measures and with goals that are quantitative, as setting standards at three different levels requires careful, time-consuming work. Choosing the point below which no award will be paid is just as important as choosing the point at which a target-level award will be paid, and choosing the point at which a maximum award will be paid is almost as important.

One variation on the three-point scale uses pass/fail goals but counts the number of goals met to determine award size (e.g., three of five goals achieved equals threshold; four of five goals

---

Exhibit 5.7: Three-Point Scale

Performance Measure	Performance Standards		
	Satisfactory	On-Plan	Outstanding
Cost per adjusted admission	$16,500	$16,300	$16,100

	Incentive Opportunity		
	Threshold	Target	Maximum
	3%	6%	9%

equals target; five of five goals equals maximum). This method works well for an organization that uses many measures or whose goals are not quantitative.

Another defines a three-point scale for incentive opportunity but sets goals at only one level—on-plan performance. Performance is evaluated subjectively, and an employee who meets plan earns a target-level award, one who far exceeds plan earns a maximum award, and one whose performance is satisfactory but slightly below plan receives a threshold-level award.

Consultants generally recommend using a three-point scale, as it represents a realistic approach to goal-setting in a business context and a reasonable approach to defining the relationship between performance and pay. It assumes that goals are directional in nature, rather than an end point; it assumes that most of the time, results will be somewhat above or below the goal itself; and it assumes that an organization should be willing to pay something, at least, for performance a little bit below the goal and something extra for performance above the goal.

Two-point scale anchored at maximum opportunity. Some plans set goals at only one level—on-plan performance—or two levels— on-plan performance and satisfactory performance somewhat below plan. The scale for incentive opportunity promises a maximum award for on-plan performance, and the scale descends from there. Performance is sometimes measured as percentage of goal achieved and the awards calculated as a percentage of maximum, on a scale that goes all the way down to 0 percent. When the scale uses two points, the lower one may be set to generate a threshold-level award at half or one-third of maximum, with a sliding scale between the two points, or nothing at all. A scale that pays nothing for performance at, say, 80 percent of goal would generate an incremental award of 5 percent of salary for every 1 percentage point increase in performance.

Using a two-point scale seems simpler than using a three-point scale, but a two-point scale still requires thoughtful calibration of the linkage between performance and award size. A two-point scale in an incentive plan is a conundrum. It acknowledges that reasonably good performance a bit below plan is good enough to deserve an award but does not admit that performance far above plan is worth more than performance at plan. A two-point scale with the lower end anchored at zero is absurd, as it pays a modest award even for reaching just 10 percent of the goal and pays an award of 90 percent of maximum for performance 10 percent below the goal. The lower end of a two-point scale for performance should generally be set no lower than 80 percent of the goal because performance further below the goal is seldom considered satisfactory.

Scales in long-term incentive plans. Long-term incentive plans typically feature a scale that defines goals at three different levels: satisfactory (threshold opportunity), on-plan (target opportunity), and outstanding (maximum opportunity) performance. Long-term plans are usually tightly structured and rarely discretionary. Most use a sliding scale, with awards determined by interpolation between levels.

Provision for Discretionary Adjustment in Award Size

One fundamental principle of governing executive compensation is that boards and their compensation committee should use good judgment in deciding how much to pay people. This principle has become embedded in incentive plans as rules that allow compensation committees to exercise discretion in determining award size.

Most plans allow boards to exercise judgment in deciding how to deal with externalities, unusual and nonrecurring events, changes in strategy, and unforeseen changes in circumstances. Many explicitly give the board the latitude to adjust the size of awards otherwise earned by a set amount, say, an increase or decrease of as much as 25 percent of the size of the award before adjustment. Others give the board the latitude to determine awards on a discretionary basis by evaluating performance relative to goals, rather than measuring it, and deciding how big the awards should be, rather than calculating award size according to a formula.

Other plans explicitly allocate a portion of incentive opportunity to a discretionary element. This lets the committee and the CEO take into account elements of performance that are not explicitly incorporated as goals. The discretionary component may consider all aspects of performance, as performance appraisal does, or it may consider only special achievements or failures, as in these examples: "Not only did she meet all her goals but she also did a very good job on this project," or "He did meet all his goals, but at the expense of letting other responsibilities slide."

A surprising number of incentive plans are entirely discretionary. Some have the infrastructure of tightly designed plans but explicitly allow the board total discretion in deciding whether to make awards and determining how big they should be. Some have well-defined opportunity levels but charge the board with determining awards on a discretionary basis by evaluating overall performance on the business plan for the year.

Discretionary elements of long-term incentive plans. Most long-term incentive plans have a rule that allows the board or its compensation committee to exercise discretion in determining the size of awards, especially in the event of unusual externalities and unforeseen changes in circumstances. Virtually none of them explicitly allocate a portion of incentive opportunity to discretionary evaluation of performance, however.

Deferral of Awards

Incentive awards are generally paid soon after the end of the performance period, but many employers allow executives to defer incentive awards if they choose, using either qualified savings plans or nonqualified deferral plans.

Some employers mandate deferral of some portion of executives' incentive awards. Few do so with annual incentive awards, but more do with long-term awards, particularly when long-term cycles end every other year or every third year, in order to smooth out income.

Long-term awards are often paid in two or three partial payments according to the number of years between the ends of performance cycles. That way, an amount can be paid each year, assuming an award is earned at the end of each cycle. If the cycles are three years long and do not overlap, the award is often paid in three equal parts, one per year, until the end of the next cycle. If the cycles overlap by one year, the award is often paid in two equal parts. The portion that is deferred is generally subject to a cliff vest, meaning participants forfeit the deferred portion if they leave the organization before the day the incentive is paid.

PERFORMANCE MEASURES AND GOALS

Performance measures are the core of an incentive plan. Choosing the right performance measures and the right way to measure performance are the key to making the plan effective. Choosing the right performance measures and setting the goals right matters far more than the structure of the incentive plan.

The right measures and the best way of measuring performance vary from organization to organization and from year to year in accordance with circumstances, values, plans, and priorities. Most advice about choosing performance measures starts with limiting the measures to a few, say three to five, and to those that are quantitative. Better advice is to choose what is important to achieving the organization's mission, not what is easy to measure; to choose measures that best represent overall organizational performance; to choose measures already embedded in the operating plan, rather than metrics developed just for the incentive plan; and to choose measures that reflect the way the CEO manages the organization, rather than ones used primarily for the incentive plan.

The more the metrics for the plan—the performance measures, the scales used for measuring performance, and the goals or performance standards set for the year—are aligned with the metrics used in managing the organization on a daily, weekly, and monthly basis, the better the plan is likely to work. If they are tightly integrated with the organization's planning, management, and reporting systems, they will be part of the fabric of management, rather than a separate performance management system run primarily to determine the size of incentive awards.

The performance measures and goals an organization uses in an incentive plan should be developed in the planning and budgeting process and then embedded in the operating plan. Goals drawn directly from the operating plan are more likely to receive sustained attention all year long than goals developed independently just for the incentive plan.

As the compensation committee determines the performance measures, goals, and weights for the coming year, debates often crop up about what to measure and how to measure performance for the incentive plan. That the debates crop up in compensation committee meetings rather than in the planning and budgeting process may seem odd, but deciding how much to pay for performance seems to demand more diligence from trustees than reviewing and approving the annual operating plan (or the quality plans). This suggests that the organizations have not yet decided how to manage their business, as measuring performance is such an essential part of managing a business and deciding how to improve its performance. The question of whether financial performance should be measured for the incentive plan in terms of net operating margin, net income, cash flow, or cost per discharge is really asking how the organization should be managed, and how performance should be monitored and reported to the board.

A typical plan uses a handful of measures covering financial performance, productivity or cost-effectiveness, clinical quality, and service quality. Some plans also use measures of growth or volume, and some use measures of employee satisfaction or engagement.

Many hospitals and systems organize the performance measures for their incentive plan around a construct such as a balanced scorecard or a set of pillars representing the most important categories of performance. Some, for example, use a four-quadrant balanced scorecard with measures focused on patients, employees, clinical quality, and financial results. Others use a set of five or six pillars to organize strategies, plans, and goals.

Performance Measures in Annual Plans

Most annual incentive plans used by tax-exempt hospitals and health systems measure performance in the following three areas:

1. Virtually all annual incentive plans include a financial measure.
   - Eighty percent use net operating income or net operating margin.
   - Some measure cash flow (earnings before interest, depreciation, and amortization, or EBIDA), cost-effectiveness (cost per unit of service), or liquidity (days cash on hand).
2. More than 80 percent of annual incentive plans include a clinical quality measure.
   - Quality measures vary significantly from one organization to another. The most common now is compliance with core measure standards established by the Centers for Medicare & Medicaid Services (CMS).
   - Many organizations have a quality improvement plan that focuses on high-priority quality-improvement initiatives each year; they tend to choose two or three of these initiatives for the incentive plan. Others develop a quality dashboard with a set of measures and incorporate all of them in a single composite measure representing the quality dashboard as a whole.
3. Approximately 70 percent of annual incentive plans use a patient satisfaction measure.
   - Most plans measure patient satisfaction as the percentage of positive responses (the top or top two responses) to a written questionnaire or phone survey.

- The new HCAHPS survey developed by CMS to introduce national reporting with a uniform set of survey questions is becoming the standard tool for measuring patient satisfaction, as it is one of the bases for Medicare reimbursement.

Number of Measures

Most annual incentive plans use far more than the three to five measures recommended by theorists. They often measure performance in three to five categories and use two or more measures in each category (e.g., patient satisfaction is often measured separately for inpatients, outpatients, and emergency department visits). Many annual plans include ten or more measures.

The number of performance measures has three important effects. First, the more measures used, the less award size will vary from year to year; the fewer measures used, the more they will vary. Second, the more measures used, the less time the compensation committee has to consider each of them, so the committee tends to cede more control of goal setting, performance measurement, and award calculation to management. Third, the more measures used, the more subjective the plan is likely to be, as relatively few measures are quantitative in nature.

Weighting Measures

Most organizations weight goals according to their overall importance, but some weight them more or less equally. In years past, hospitals and health systems typically emphasized financial performance, often by putting half or more of the total weight on it. Now organizations commonly weight patient satisfaction and clinical quality as much as or more than financial performance, so financial performance accounts for only a quarter or a third of award size.

Rewarding Executives for What They Can Control

In centralized multihospital systems, subsidiary hospital executives do not control or even exercise much influence over certain variables such as volume, market share, or even price of services because system executives control managed care contracts, pricing of services, billing and collections, and decisions about where the system places specialty programs. Entity executives should be evaluated primarily on variables they control or at least exercise significant influence over—given their mix of business, patients, and payers—and on doing what they can to ensure the success of the system as a whole. In most centralized systems, for example, entity executives do not control revenue, but they do control staffing and variable costs, so they should be rewarded for entity-level productivity and cost-effectiveness rather than revenue or operating profit.

Performance Measures in Long-Term Plans

Most organizations that use long-term incentive plans try to tie long-term awards to strategic success. Many intentionally avoid the types of measures typically found in annual incentive plans for being focused on incremental improvement of operations rather than the large-scale strategic changes required to strengthen the organization's competitive position or transform the way it delivers healthcare services.

The choice of performance measures for long-term incentive plans depends as much on the views of trustees and the CEO as on any other factor. Some boards insist that long-term awards be based largely on financial performance. Others insist that they be based largely on strategic achievements, expansion of market share, or permanent reduction in operating costs.

Most long-term plans employ just two or three performance measures. One is virtually always a measure of financial success. The others are often measures of competitive strength or corporate competencies (e.g., improvements in market share or in service quality, meaningful use of electronic medical records). Some organizations set goals related to timely and cost-effective completion of multiyear strategic initiatives, such as the development and introduction of a new electronic health record, completion of a new building, or development of a new service line.

Measures frequently used in long-term incentive plans include the following:

- Financial performance: return on equity or return on assets, cumulative earnings or growth in surplus, improving or maintaining credit rating
- Growth/market share: overall market share or share in specific niches or service lines, overall growth or growth in specific niches or service lines
- Cost-effectiveness: cost per case relative to peers, elimination of costs through reengineering, reduction in unnecessary admissions or length of stay
- Service quality: improvements in patient satisfaction, improvements in process and cycle time
- Clinical quality: improvements in clinical outcomes, ranking on CMS core measures relative to peers
- Community health status: demonstrable improvements in community health status (e.g., reduced frequency of hospitalization for chronic diseases)
- Strategic initiatives: completion or implementation of common, seamless information system for all entities or common electronic medical record for all entities; new services developed or acquired

SETTING GOALS

Goals for incentive plans are typically set as general business goals while budgets and the operating plan for the coming year are developed. Goals are vetted by the board and various committees as the budget and operating plan are refined and approved. Once the operating plan for the year is approved, management and the compensation committee should only need to select the goals that are most appropriate for the incentive plan, rather than set them, and decide how to position each goal on the scale used to link performance to award size.

Over time, organizations develop a fairly standard approach to positioning goals. Some routinely set all goals representing on-plan performance equal to target-level awards; others, using another scale, routinely set them all equal to maximum opportunity. And some set the budget for operating margin equal to threshold performance, on the principle that no awards should be paid for financial performance if operating margin is below budget. Some set threshold performance equal to the prior year's performance, on the principle that no award should be paid unless performance improves each year.

When organizations use a two- or three-point scale in their incentive plan, they need to decide where to set the bottom and top of the scale—not just a single point to represent the goal set in the budget or operating plan—and goal setting becomes more complicated. With a two-point scale, the budget for the year and any other goals borrowed from the operating plan are generally set at the top of the scale, where they will be worth a maximum award. With a three-point scale, they are generally set at the middle of the scale, where they will be worth a target-level award. Then management and the committee need to decide how far below the goal they should set the threshold level below which no award will be paid and, with a three-point scale, how far above the goal they should set the level representing outstanding performance, which will be worth a maximum award.

Deciding where to set performance standards for satisfactory and outstanding performance on a three-point scale is often more difficult and time consuming than deciding where to position the goal for on-plan performance. The goal for on-plan performance, as often as not, is determined by increasing the numbers on current performance by a modest amount. For example, assuming that costs will rise by, say, 6 percent, productivity (measured as full-time equivalent employee per admission) will need to be improved by reducing staffing by 1 percent.

The question of how much lower the threshold for an award should be set is challenging, as results even 1 percent below the threshold will eliminate an award on that measure. Trustees are often tempted to set threshold at current performance levels, in the belief that no award should be paid unless performance improves—even though management knows how difficult it was to reach current performance levels and how some unexpected event could make it impossible to maintain them. Likewise, trustees wonder why the standard representing outstanding performance should be set below a score representing ideal performance—why the standard for a maximum award for compliance with CMS core measure standards for pneumonia should be set at 99 percent rather than 100 percent, or why the standard for a maximum award for patient satisfaction should be set at the 86th percentile instead of the 90th percentile.

To make it easier for management to reach agreement with trustees on standards for threshold and outstanding performance (or minimum and maximum awards), many organizations develop standard patterns that position threshold and maximum exactly 1 percent or 1 percentile (or 2 percent or some other distance) above and below the goal for on-plan performance. For operating profit measured in dollars, a more volatile measure, threshold would be positioned exactly 20 percent above and below the budgeted figure (or some other ratio, such as 10 percent below budget for a threshold-level award for satisfactory performance but 30 percent above budget for a maximum award for outstanding performance). Determining where they should be set on a totally discretionary basis requires sensitivity analysis, intuitive estimations, or arbitrary decisions following an algorithm whereby the standard for a threshold-level award should be set at a point where the odds of success are about 80 to 90 percent and the standard for a maximum award, where the odds of success are 10 to 20 percent. Needless to say, management is likely to estimate the odds of achieving any particular result lower than trustees would. Data-based sensitivity analysis of past performance can be useful in refining these standards.

When setting goals, organizations consider past performance, anticipated changes in circumstances, and assumptions about what factors are unlikely to change. They are increasingly turning to external benchmark data, too, when it is available, for help in setting goals (e.g., "The goal is to achieve the 90th percentile"). External benchmark data are also used as a point of reference when setting goals based on internal improvement (e.g., "Our goal is a 1 percentage point improvement in raw scores above our current performance, which lies at the 88th percentile").

Data Needed for Goal Setting

Compensation committees rely on management for the information they need to decide whether to approve or modify the goals proposed by management and to determine whether the proposed relationship between performance and pay is appropriate. That information should include a record of past performance in the areas being measured, data showing trends that may affect performance in the coming year, a list of the challenges or opportunities expected during the coming year, external data showing performance elsewhere in the field, and benchmarks representing the best performance in the industry.

Most compensation committees do not receive this much information, however, when they are asked to approve goals for the incentive plan, making it difficult for the committee to judge how appropriate the goals are and leaving the committee to decide whether to rely on management's recollections or estimates or to delay approval of the goals until it gets the information it needs to be comfortable approving them.

Documenting Goals

Goals should be defined and documented clearly to provide a record of what was approved and how performance is to be measured or evaluated at the end of the year. Too often, goals are defined so loosely or documented so poorly that it is not clear a year later what was intended.

Without clear definition and good documentation of goals, the committee will need to ask management at the end of the year to explain what the goal means, what data are supposed to be used to evaluate performance, or what last year's performance was. Without contextual information about past performance and norms elsewhere in the industry, the committee may need to ask what the trend has been over the past three or four years, and at what percentile this year's performance puts the hospital relative to a national or regional peer group. Management should carefully document the definition of each goal and contextual information about trends and industrywide norms when the goals are proposed and when they are approved, and the documentation should be resubmitted to the committee at the end of the year when it evaluates performance and determines awards.

Approaches to Goal Setting

Goal setting involves answering three sets of questions:

1. Should we set goals at one level only or at two or three? If we set them at more than one level, which level is the real goal representing on-plan performance?

2. How difficult should the goals be? Should they be set so that they are very difficult to meet, or so that they can probably be met unless something goes wrong?
3. What benchmark should we use in setting goals? Last year's performance? Our best recent performance? Average performance in the field, or in our peer group? Seventy-fifth percentile performance in the healthcare industry or our peer group? Best performance in our peer group?

The decisions depend in part on (1) the scale and approach embedded in the structure of the plan; (2) the approach management or the compensation committee expects to use in evaluating performance and determining award size; and (3) the nature of the performance measure or the goal itself, as some goals fit neatly onto a sliding scale, while others are not metrical and can only be evaluated on a pass/fail or a subjective basis.

Hospitals and health systems may use the following guidelines to address these issues:

- Many organizations use a highly quantitative and tightly calibrated approach and, as much as possible, set performance standards at three levels, representing on-plan performance, acceptable performance somewhat below plan, and outstanding performance—or at two levels representing on-plan performance and acceptable performance somewhat below plan. Performance on these two or three markers is measured at year end, typically using a sliding scale that accommodates interpolation.
- Some use a highly subjective approach whereby they set goals at one level only that represents on-plan performance, and determine awards through an evaluation process much like performance appraisal. Performance is evaluated at year end using scores (e.g., 0-1-2-3) for performance more or less on-plan (2), acceptable but somewhat below plan (1), too far below plan to count (0), or outstanding performance

far above plan (3)—taking into account all known circumstances.

- Some use a pass/fail approach in which they set goals at one level only that represents on-plan performance. Performance is evaluated by counting the number of goals achieved.

Many organizations use all three approaches, as some goals fit a metrical scale, others are suited to a pass/fail approach, and still others are best handled with subjective evaluation.

Most organizations also use three benchmarks in setting goals:

1. Past performance, whether last year's performance, best performance over the past few years, or average performance over the last few years. Goals are often set to beat past performance but may be set to just maintain past performance if it was high enough.
2. Performance relative to a peer group, whether average performance in the peer group, 75th percentile performance, or 90th percentile performance. Goals are set to meet or beat these benchmarks, which may mean improving past performance or maintaining past performance.
3. A standard or an ideal, whether 100 percent compliance with a best practice or eliminating never events, winning recognition or meeting the requirements for a recognition (e.g., Baldrige award, Magnet nursing status), or completing a project on time and within budget. Goals may be set to meet the standard or to make reasonable progress toward meeting the standard.

The benchmark chosen depends in part on the type of measure and in part on prior performance, or prior performance compared to best in the field. Financial and patient satisfaction goals are usually set in relation to past performance and performance in one's peer group. Clinical quality goals take both into account and may also take into account ideal performance, or best-in-class performance.

Goals set for incentive plans rarely call for breakthrough performance—overcoming huge obstacles, making huge leaps in improvement, or reaching perfection—because they are unlikely to be met. Such goals may make sense in a five-year business plan or a vision for the future but not in an annual incentive plan. Participants would dismiss such goals as fantasies rather than strive to achieve them.

Typical Guidelines for Goal Setting

While guidelines should vary with the type of scale used, they typically call for setting goals at ambitious but also realistic levels. Pass/fail goals, for example, should generally be more realistic than ambitious, as no award is paid unless the goal is reached. Goals set equal to target-award level on a three-point scale should be both ambitious and realistic because smaller awards can be paid for performance below the goal and bigger awards can be paid for performance above the goal. Goals set equal to maximum award size should be more ambitious than realistic if the intent is to pay less than maximum, but they should be equally realistic and ambitious if the intent is to pay at maximum.

The following guidelines may be used to calibrate goals when the organization has in place a three-point scale running from threshold to target to maximum:

- Target goals should be achievable about 50 percent of the time (i.e., target or better performance should be achieved five or six of every ten years).
- Threshold goals should be achievable about 80 to 90 percent of the time (i.e., threshold or better performance should be achieved eight or nine of every ten years).

- Maximum goals should be achievable about 10 to 20 percent of the time (i.e., maximum performance should be achieved one or two of every ten years).

Organizations that define goals only at a single level tied to maximum opportunity and that intend to pay awards near maximum most years should set goals to be achievable about 80 percent of the time.

Goals should also reflect an organization's compensation philosophy. A hospital or health system whose compensation philosophy calls for positioning total compensation at the 75th percentile should presumably set goals that are tougher to achieve than those set by organizations whose pay is positioned at median.

An approach that is more common as comparative data become increasingly available is to set goals by benchmarking against performance in other organizations. For an organization that wants to position total compensation, on average, at median but is willing to pay up to the 75th percentile for outstanding performance, the guidelines would call for positioning the goal for on-plan performance at the median performance level in the appropriate peer group and the standard for outstanding performance at the 75th percentile performance level. For an organization that wants to position total compensation, on average, at the 75th percentile but is willing to pay up to the 90th percentile for outstanding performance, the guidelines would call for positioning the goal for on-plan performance at the 75th percentile level in the appropriate peer group and the standard for outstanding performance at the 90th percentile in the peer group.

Exhibit 5.8 shows how one organization proposes goals to its compensation committee. This organization provides the committee with all of the information it needs to set goals at the appropriate level. Each goal is supported by historical performance data and, if available, external benchmark data. The proposed goals are also supported by a rationale as to why they are appropriate for the organization.

Exhibit 5.8: One Organization's Method of Proposing Goals to Its Compensation Committee

FY2009 Annual Incentive Plan Performance Goals	FY2008 Performance Information	Comments
3. Patient satisfaction survey aggregate results: *Threshold:* Overall level of patient satisfaction ≥ 88.6% *Target:* Overall level of patient satisfaction ≥ 90.1% *Maximum:* Increase overall level of patient satisfaction by 1.5 percentage points to 91.6%	*Historical Performance on Overall Satisfaction* FY08 89.7% FY07 90.4% FY06 90.1% FY05 90.1% FY04 88% FY03 90% FY02 89% FY01 89%	• Maintaining a high level of performance in the 90th percentile requires consistent focus and attention • FY2009 target is equal to the 3-year average for overall level of patient satisfaction (90.1%) • To be statistically significant, a difference should be 1.5% (based on sample size of 2,400 inpatients), so threshold and maximum are 1.5% from target • 75th percentile score in Ohio is 88.5%; nationally it is 89.1

EVALUATING PERFORMANCE AND DETERMINING AWARDS

In any executive incentive plan, determining appropriate awards depends on four interrelated decisions:

1. Evaluating data and reports on performance relative to goals set for the year
2. Determining where performance lies on the scales used for each performance measure (if there are no scales, use the appropriate algorithm)

3. Calculating awards earned given the weights assigned to each goal and the scales or algorithms defined at the beginning of the year
4. Exercising discretion given all information known at the end of the year, paying particular attention to unforeseen changes in circumstances; board-approved changes in priorities; and the impact on financial results of unusual and nonrecurring events, such as retrospective Medicare settlements or gain or loss on sale of assets

The process for determining awards should demonstrate the ideal relationship between governance and management. Management collects the data the compensation committee needs to make an informed decision. The committee probes and asks questions, and management answers them. Management calculates and recommends awards. The committee verifies the calculations and determines whether to modify awards on a discretionary basis. Committee members exercise diligence by reviewing data and reports on performance, asking questions about them, expressing skepticism of any information it does not understand or agree with, and deciding whether to accept management's recommendations or modify them. Management does its best to help trustees understand management's point of view.

Incentive plans may or may not explicitly assign boards responsibility for evaluating performance or latitude for exercising discretion in determining award size, but IRS guidance on incentive compensation plans makes it clear that boards or compensation committees should exercise administrative control of any incentive plan the CEO participates in, and intermediate sanctions regulations require that boards or compensation committees approve awards for any participants subject to these rules.

Evaluating performance involves more than calculating award size or accepting management's reports at face value. It entails determining whether awards are appropriate, taking all facts into consideration, so that awards do not amount to a windfall or to private benefit, private inurement, excess benefit, or misuse of charitable resources. It also entails determining whether the awards and the resulting total compensation are reasonable compared to what is paid by other similar organizations.

Evaluation is different from measurement in that it involves discretion. Committees should be willing to take into account factors not covered by performance measures, especially their effects on performance of extraordinary and nonrecurring events, and any midyear changes in strategies or priorities.

The compensation committee's responsibility for exercising administrative control of the plan includes determining an award for the CEO and approving awards for other participants in the plan—even if it approves only the size of awards or the aggregate amount of awards paid. Determining only the scope of the CEO's award does not meet that responsibility, unless the goals are entirely team oriented and the same for all participants, so the committee's decision on the CEO's award amounts to determining the awards for all other participants. For incentive plans in which part of each award is tied to individual goals or goals at the business-unit level, the committee typically respects the CEO's right to manage, evaluate, and determine pay for subordinates—unless awards for individual performance are disproportionate to awards for institutional performance. The committee should then ask why the two seem to be mismatched.

With the emergence of governance standards calling for boards to exercise more diligence in governing executive compensation than in the past, and under the risk of intermediate sanctions for excessive pay, committees now tend to approve the total value of incentive awards for at least those senior executives who are "disqualified individuals," insiders subject to risk of intermediate sanctions.

RETENTION INCENTIVES

Retention incentives, or "stay bonuses," are agreements to pay an employee a certain amount of money only if the employee stays until the end of a designated retention period. A retention incentive is virtually always extra pay in addition to a fully competitive pay package and is intended to motivate the employee to decline any offer to take another job until after the retention period.

Retention incentives are increasingly common in not-for-profit healthcare organizations. Surveys of executive compensation report that stay bonuses are used with some regularity by 15 to 20 percent of hospitals and health systems. But the statistics on stay bonuses dramatically understate their prevalence because some employers also use them irregularly, as the need arises, and others may structure retention incentives as supplemental retirement plans, long-term incentives, deferred compensation, housing loans, permanent life insurance, severance, hiring bonuses, and employment agreements. For example, an employment agreement that promises one year's total compensation as severance on voluntary termination, retirement, death, or disability is a retention incentive disguised as severance. A hiring bonus that needs to be repaid if the executive does not stay for two years is a retention incentive with another name. An agreement to provide a paid life insurance policy worth $500,000 if redeemed at retirement (age 65) and $2 million at death is a retention incentive disguised as life insurance. A supplemental retirement plan that is cliff vested at age 62 or 65 is a retention incentive disguised as a retirement plan. Several of these scenarios are described later in this section.

Uses for Retention Incentives

Retention incentives address five types of risks:

1. Loss of an employee (to another employer) whose role is critical to the success of the organization and who cannot be replaced easily and quickly
2. Loss of an exceptionally talented employee (to another employer) who has the potential to take on major leadership roles in the organization

3. Loss of a number of employees at the same time, especially when the organization is facing major challenges, such as a merger or major reorganization
4. Loss of exceptionally good succession candidates when the organization is planning a transition in leadership
5. Loss of an employee to premature retirement when it is easier or preferable to retain the employee for another few years than to find and train a replacement

The circumstances and the type of retention risk have a bearing on the way retention incentives are designed and used, as described in the following paragraphs.

Major organizational changes. Organizations facing major changes—mergers, reorganizations, or leadership transitions—sometimes use retention incentives to discourage people from considering other opportunities before the changes are completed. Recruiters see organizations facing change as fertile grounds for recruiting, and employees facing likely loss of job and income are usually willing to move on sooner rather than later.

Completion of a project. Organizations investing a large sum of money in a new building or computer system sometimes offer a retention incentive to the executive in charge of the project to ensure management continuity until the end of the project.

Retirement. One of the most straightforward uses of retention incentives involves persuading employees to stay beyond normal retirement age, their intended retirement date, or the point at which they are fully vested in retirement benefits. Because many executives plan to retire earlier than age 65, some organizations have designed supplemental retirement plans to vest at full value at age 60 or 62. Once employees reach the point at which their retirement benefit will not increase (or not increase much) with additional years of service, they have little economic reason to continue working, unless the retirement benefit is insufficient to live on. This use of a retention incentive is especially common with high-ranking executives when no internal candidate can fill the job and the organization needs time to conduct an external search or spend a few years developing internal candidates.

Final CEO contract. Some organizations have offered a retention incentive to their CEO to encourage the CEO to renew her employment agreement. CEOs, like other executives, recognize that their best opportunities to change jobs are likely to come when they are between 50 and 55 years of age. Once they reach age 55, they want to know that they will have a reasonable degree of job and income security to ensure an optimal retirement income. Employers that are pleased with the performance of their CEOs want to keep them off the job market and are sometimes willing to offer them long contract terms and retention incentives to stay in their jobs, sometimes for the duration of their careers.

Hiring a new employee. Newly recruited executives often demand certain payments in addition to ordinary compensation and benefits as a condition of accepting a new job and moving to a new location. These payments may be in the form of a hiring bonus, a housing allowance or subsidy, or a buyout of deferred compensation they are leaving behind. Sometimes these payments are made at the start of employment, but they are often contingent on staying for a period of time and require the executive to repay the incentive if he leaves before the retention period expires.

Types of Retention Incentives

Retention incentives come in different forms. Some are easily recognizable as retention incentives, while some are disguised as additional payments in the form of supplemental retirement benefits, a hiring bonus, or a bonus for renewing an employment agreement, or even as a long-term incentive plan by tying the retention award to performance requirements.

The most typical structures for retention incentives are described below.

Stay bonus. A stay bonus is a simple promise to pay a sum of money at the end of a specific period. The sum may be defined as a dollar amount, a percentage of salary at the end of the period, or a series of annual credits plus accrued interest over the retention period. While this structure is an agreement to pay only if the person is still employed at the end of the retention period, it usually includes a provision for payment in full or pro rata payment on death, disability, or involuntary termination without cause before the end of the retention period.

Rolling stay bonus. Some retention incentives are structured as a series of annual grants that vest after two to five years, so that a participant would forfeit a significant amount of money upon departing voluntarily. These plans typically have a provision for early vesting on death, disability, or involuntary termination without cause, and sometimes on retirement. The annual grant or credit is defined either as a flat dollar amount or as a percentage of pay.

Duration-of-career agreement. A retention incentive intended to convince an executive to stay for the duration of his career is a stay bonus tied to retirement at a specific age. The retention period tends to be longer than that defined for most other types of retention incentives, often five or more years, to set the end of the agreement at age 62, 65, or beyond. The value is generally defined as a lump sum payable at retirement.

Supplemental retirement agreement. A retention incentive can deliver its value in the form of a supplemental retirement benefit. The retention period is defined as ending on the normal retirement date at which the participant qualifies for a full (or a reduced) retirement benefit. This structure differs from a straightforward stay bonus or a duration-of-career agreement in that it typically involves interest or investment income and often allows the participant some role in deciding how funds should be invested.

A defined-benefit supplemental executive retirement plan (SERP) can be an unusually effective retention benefit because

(1) the value it promises is large and (2) the value of the SERP rises dramatically from year to year as the participant gets closer to retirement. Because it is defined as lifetime income proportional to pre-retirement income, its value is often far more substantial than the value of a retention incentive tied to a shorter period.

Enhanced severance. Organizations contemplating a merger may offer executives enhanced severance as a kind of retention incentive to persuade them to stay as long as they are needed and to encourage them to work on the merger, even though it may result in the elimination of their jobs. Structuring the retention incentive this way is efficient because it helps retain all executives as long as they are needed but pays only to those who lose their jobs.

Value of Retention Incentives

To be effective, the retention incentive needs to be sufficient to motivate the recipient to forgo other job opportunities and remain with the organization for the time being. It must match or exceed other potential employers' offers of a signing bonus or a permanent increase in compensation. If the retention incentive is an enticement to delay retirement, it needs to be more attractive than what the recipient would gain by retiring earlier.

The value of stay bonuses ranges from 10 percent to 100 percent of salary per year. In terms of these incentives, value is defined as value per year because the duration of stay bonuses ranges from a few months to five and even ten years. A stay bonus of 10 percent of salary to stay for three months, for example, is worth 40 percent of salary per year, whereas a retention incentive of 100 percent of salary at the end of five years amounts to only 20 percent of salary per year.

Typical stay bonuses offer 20 to 30 percent of salary per year if they are defined for a period of a year or more. They tend to be higher—up to 50 percent, and some even 100 percent—for shorter periods because the total dollar value for a few months at, say, 20 percent of salary, would be modest at only 5 percent of annual salary, too little to entice an employee to stay in the face of another opportunity.

The size of stay bonuses tends to be larger for higher-paid employees than for lower-paid employees, just as incentive opportunity does under ordinary annual incentive plans. They also tend to be bigger under difficult circumstances than under a comfortable status quo. A stay bonus of 30 percent of salary per year for five years may be enough for a CEO of a successful organization to agree to a new contract, especially if the rest of the compensation package is fully competitive. But a stay bonus of 30 percent of salary per year to stay through a chapter 11 bankruptcy filing with the prospect that the executive will lose his job in another year or two is unlikely to convince him to turn down a more promising opportunity—unless it is supplemented with two or three years' full pay as a severance benefit.

Because retention incentives are extra compensation on top of a fully competitive compensation package, they pose a risk of making total compensation unreasonable. Because retention incentives are not related to performance, they do not offer the usual rationale for exceptionally high pay, which is exceptionally good performance. Boards approving retention incentives should be careful to articulate and document a sound and persuasive rationale as part of establishing a presumption of reasonableness.

ALL-EMPLOYEE INCENTIVES

Roughly 10 to 20 percent of hospitals offer some kind of all-employee incentive plan. The generic name for the plans is a misnomer, as the plans are almost always limited to employees who do not participate in a separate incentive plan for executives or managers.

Executives and trustees of hospitals and systems that offer an all-employee incentive plan find it useful in justifying an incentive plan for executives, as it allows executives to tell employees, "We're all in it together."

But an all-employee incentive plan may introduce unwelcome complications for an executive plan. First, in years in which the all-employee plan does not pay awards, it is difficult to justify paying awards to executives, even on measures not included in the all-employee plan. Second, when awards are paid to employees, the cost of an all-employee plan can pull operating income down enough to leave little room for paying awards to executives. Third, in a multi-hospital system, all-employee awards are generally determined at the hospital level, while awards for executives are determined in part, at least, at the system level; the all-employee plan might pay no awards to employees at one hospital even though the executive plan calls for paying awards to executives of the same hospital on the basis of systemwide performance. Fourth, any linkage between the all-employee incentive plan and the executive incentive plan puts the compensation committee in charge of an all-employee plan, taking it into what would otherwise be management's turf.

EQUITY-BASED INCENTIVES

A few not-for-profit health systems have implemented equity-based incentives in their for-profit subsidiaries. As long as these plans are limited to employees of the for-profit subsidiary, they should not run afoul of the prohibition against private inurement, even though the for-profit subsidiary is owned entirely by the nonprofit.

However, equity plans used in this way may tempt the parent organization to allow system-level executives who oversee a not-for-profit subsidiary to participate in the for-profit subsidiary's equity-based incentive plan or to develop a parallel plan for the nonprofit that rewards system-level executives for system-level success in venture capital management. Doing so runs a risk that the plans could involve private inurement. Using an equity plan for subsidiary executives but not for system executives also introduces a disparity in the organization's executive compensation program that can be disruptive to morale on the executive team.

BEST PRACTICES IN INCENTIVE COMPENSATION DESIGN

Balance Between Annual and Long-Term Incentives

- Use long-term incentives only if a compelling reason exists for doing so, they include enough people to make the administrative burden worthwhile, and the compensation committee is willing to put in the effort needed to make two incentive plans effective.
- If using both annual and long-term incentives, set incentive opportunity high enough in both plans to make them meaningful to executives. Do not use both plans if your compensation policy is conservative, because there will not be room in the compensation program for enough incentive opportunity to make both plans meaningful.

Eligibility

- Include all executives in the annual incentive plan. Use a separate plan for directors and managers so that the compensation committee does not need to oversee incentive compensation for mid-level managers.
- Include only senior executives in a long-term incentive plan. Limit eligibility to executives responsible for developing and executing the organization's strategic plans and initiatives.

Incentive Opportunity

- Set incentive opportunity high enough to capture participants' attention, but remember that it is the process—the strength of the planning and goal setting and the effectiveness with which goals are communicated repeatedly—that makes incentive plans effective, not the amount of money in the plan.

Structure

- Keep the structure simple enough that the plan is easy to communicate, understand, and administer.
- Set one or more hurdles or circuit breakers that must be surpassed before any awards can be paid. These hurdles should be fail-safe measures that prevent payment of awards only if some element of performance is so disappointing that it would be embarrassing to pay awards.
- Avoid features that make the structure a profit-sharing plan.
- Use a three-point scale to define performance expectations and incentive opportunity. Define a scale for each measure that represents the range of likely performance outcomes, from acceptable performance a bit below plan to outstanding performance far above plan. Use three markers representing on-plan performance, the lowest level at which awards would be paid, and the best performance likely to be achieved if performance was better than expected.
- Use probabilities in setting performance expectations, with a probability of 0.5 or 0.6 for on-plan performance, a probability of 0.8 or 0.9 for threshold, and a probability of 0.1 or 0.2 for outstanding performance.

Performance Measures

Annual Incentive Plans

- Choose performance measures and set goals that reflect the organization's priorities and its approach to managing operations.
- Choose measures that best represent overall performance of the organization; incorporate projects as measures only if they are extremely important.
- Use a balanced scorecard as the basis for selecting measures for the incentive plan if the organization uses one in planning and monitoring operational performance.

- Weight measures in a way that balances mission-related measures, such as clinical quality, patient satisfaction, and community benefit, with business-related measures, such as operating margin, growth, and market share.

Long-Term Incentive Plans

- Choose performance measures that represent major strategic goals that do not fit neatly into the annual plan because they have a longer timeline.
- Limit the measures to four, and keep them entirely team oriented and the same for all participants, unless geographic dispersion of operations calls for measuring some factors at the local market or entity level.

Governance of Incentive Compensation Plans

- The committee should follow a process that demonstrates that the plan is controlled by the committee, that it is not an annuity executives have a right to participate in, and that the plan's purpose is to support the organization's tax-exempt mission.
- The board or its compensation committee should formally approve the plan, select participants, and set incentive opportunity every year.
- The board or its compensation committee should set or approve performance measures and goals for the CEO and for the executive team as a whole; at year end, it should evaluate performance on those goals and determine or approve awards for the CEO and for other senior executives before they are paid.
- The board or compensation committee should periodically review the plan to ensure that it continues to support the organization's tax-exempt mission and that awards under the plan and resulting levels of total compensation are reasonable compared with pay practices at similar organizations.

NOTE

1. Private benefit occurs when an institution operates in whole or in part for the private benefit of individuals or when it provides greater benefit to private individuals than to the community served. For not-for-profit organizations, any private benefit must be incidental to the public benefit the organization provides. Activities of a tax-exempt charity must be primarily those that represent a public benefit. Private inurement occurs when an institution gives an insider a greater benefit than he provides to the tax-exempt organization in exchange or when it allows an insider to enrich himself at the expense of the tax-exempt organization.

   Private benefit and private inurement differ in that private benefit could involve any beneficiary of the organization whereas private inurement generally involves an insider (someone with special influence over the organization). In addition, no amount of private inurement is allowable, whereas a small amount of private benefit is allowable as long as it is incidental to the public benefit provided (IRS 1990).

CHAPTER 6

Benefits

INTRODUCTION

Benefits have long been a standard feature of compensation in the United States. Nearly every full-time employee who works for a large US employer—public or private—receives benefits as part of his compensation package. Benefits are less common at small employers, for whom providing benefits has become too expensive.

Employer-paid benefits became common in employee compensation packages during the late 1940s and early 1950s, when federal wage controls limited increases in pay. In response, employers introduced or increased the value of benefits. Over time, large companies began to use benefits as a tool to recruit and retain talent.

Since the 1980s, the rising cost of medical benefits and the transformation of the American economy in response to global competition have led to a decline in the prevalence of benefits and an expectation that employees will pay part or all of their cost when they are offered. Much of the responsibility for saving for retirement was shifted to employees following the introduction and rapid adoption of defined-contribution plans, such as 401(k) and 403(b) plans, signaling a widespread retreat from defined-benefit pension plans. And a similar shift was seen in responsibility for healthcare coverage when employers introduced managed care plans and health plans with cost-sharing features, marking a retreat from indemnity health plans, which covered all costs of care and were fully paid for by employers.

Most hospitals and health systems continue to provide a broad set of benefits to their employees because they need to attract and retain large numbers of high-caliber, specialized employees. Some segments of the healthcare arena, however, reflect the changes occurring in the rest of the US economy. Outsourcing of functions such as housekeeping and food services, for example, has moved employees into firms that pay less and provide only minimal benefits.

Yet at the same time that corporations have been cutting back on benefits for the workforce as a whole, they have been increasing benefits for executives. Over the last 30 years, large corporations, including large hospitals and health systems, expanded and enriched supplemental benefits for executives. Supplemental executive retirement plans (SERPs) became more widespread and richer than they had been before, supplemental life insurance became a standard feature of executive compensation packages, and severance benefits were increased. Many large private employers now offer supplemental life and disability insurance and enhanced vacation allowances, sick-leave programs, and even supplemental healthcare benefits to their executives.

In the aftermath of public dismay about the types of benefits General Electric provided to former Chairman and CEO Jack Welch as part of his retirement package and public disclosure of the types of benefits commonly provided to other executives, however, corporate America has begun to retreat a bit from providing generous supplemental benefit packages to executives.

In 2009 The Conference Board issued a set of recommendations on executive compensation, including one that corporations avoid "controversial pay practices," such as providing supplemental benefits and perquisites not provided to other employees (Conference Board 2009, 9, 11, 20–22). Two benefits singled out for special attention were supplemental retirement and severance. Two perquisites targeted by The Conference Board were reimbursement of expenses that would normally be paid by employees and "gross-ups," or bonuses to cover taxes due on benefits and perquisites. This report seems to condone the use of supplemental benefits that restore the benefits promised to employees on income above the limits set by legislation or insurance carriers, but it clearly discourages the use of supplemental benefits that are richer for executives than for other employees. If this recommendation gains wide acceptance, it will dramatically change the shape of executive benefit packages.

The disparity in pay between executives and employees has attracted much attention, but the disparity in benefits generally has not, because it is far less visible. Criticism has focused more on automobiles and severance than on retirement benefits. As a result, boards have not had to address much criticism of executive benefits.

Cutting Retirement Benefits for Workforce More than for Executives

A large hospital in the Midwest region froze its defined-benefit pension plan and moved its non-executive employees into a new cash balance plan. The change resulted in a significant reduction in retirement benefits for these employees and saved the hospital a significant amount of money. Prior to the shift, executives had participated in a restoration plan based on the now-frozen defined-benefit plan. In deciding how to modify the executives' retirement benefits, trustees kept the executives in the restoration plan on the premise that executives needed the plan to keep their retirement benefits competitive. As a result, retirement benefits were reduced far less for executives than for other employees. The committee approved the change without recognizing that the change favored executives.

Decisions about executive benefits have been driven largely by the board's desire to be competitive—to match prevailing practices. Benefits are generally regarded as contractual obligations, so boards are reluctant to change them. Boards are usually far more willing to trim employee benefits than to trim executive benefits, because board members are more exposed to the resulting discontent if they cut executive benefits.

OVERVIEW OF BENEFITS

Benefits are often divided into two classes—health and welfare benefits and retirement benefits. Health and welfare benefits include medical, vision, dental, and Medicare contributions; disability benefits, such as sick-leave, short-term disability, and long-term disability benefits; and life insurance or survivor benefits. Retirement benefits include retirement plans, savings plans, and Social Security contributions. Paid time off (PTO), including vacation, holidays, and sick leave, may be considered a third class or included with health and welfare benefits.

The concept of health and welfare benefits is built on the principles of insurance—spreading the risk of disaster or expense across a large population—and of providing security as an adjunct to employment by protecting workers and their families from disruption of income. Retirement benefits are based on the principle of deferral or saving—deferring a portion of pay to allow retirement with dignity. All three classes of benefits are built on a presumption of paternalism—taking care of employees (and their families) to encourage them to be loyal and productive.

A standard employee benefits package includes healthcare benefits, sick leave or short-term disability, long-term disability, life insurance, vacation and holidays, and retirement benefits. Most hospitals and health systems provide all these benefits to employees in one combination or another and to varying degrees.

Benefits packages now generally offer employees a number of choices, especially in healthcare and retirement benefits. Most offer a choice among health plans; a choice between individual, couple, and family coverage; voluntary retirement savings plans, often with a matching contribution, which allows employees to decide how much to save and how big a matching contribution to get; and a choice between taking vacation and taking an equivalent value in cash (or as severance or retirement benefit).

Standard benefit packages are designed for salaried and hourly employees, not for executives. Benefits tied to salary (paid as a percentage of salary) typically have limits, so that the benefits stop accruing after a certain level of salary. For most employees the limits are irrelevant because their salaries do not reach the limit. For higher-paid executives, however, these limits mean that they receive less benefit, as a percentage of salary, than other employees do.

Because standard life and disability insurance and retirement benefits do not fully cover salaries for higher-paid executives, most not-for-profit hospitals and health systems provide executives some form of supplemental benefits to cover income above the limits set on standard plans. The most common of these types of benefits is a supplemental retirement benefit. The next most common is supplemental life insurance, followed by supplemental disability insurance.

A supplemental benefits package for executives may also include salary continuation in lieu of sick leave, an executive vacation allowance, and an executive severance benefit. Some organizations provide a supplemental healthcare benefit covering deductibles and copayments.

Some organizations use supplemental benefits selectively, offering them only to senior executives or, sometimes, only to the CEO. A few provide them to all employees paid more than the limits set on standard benefits.

PURPOSE OF BENEFITS

Benefits serve two main purposes—one for employers, one for employees. From the employers' perspective, benefits help maintain the stability of the workforce. A generous package of benefits provides security to employees and helps maintain employee morale, and maybe even loyalty, by demonstrating that the organization is willing to take care of employees' needs when a crisis arises, such as illness, disability, involuntary termination, or inability to work due to infirmity of old age.

Healthcare and disability benefits promote well-being in the workplace by encouraging employees to stay home when sick, get medical treatment as needed, and get back to work as quickly as possible. Long-term disability and retirement benefits facilitate the discharge of employees when they can no longer work effectively, without being unfair, without paying severance, and without being exposed to litigation for wrongful discharge. PTO supports the organization's smooth operation by allowing employees to get the rest they need to come back to work with greater enthusiasm and productivity.

From the employees' perspective, benefits provide security that allows them to pursue their careers, attend to their families, and enjoy life without worrying unnecessarily about the risks associated with illness, disability, loss of income, and aging. Benefits help them take on responsibility for a family. Vacation, holidays, and sick leave allow time for rest, relaxation, and renewal without having to sacrifice income.

Benefits help employees' families, too. Healthcare benefits are designed to cover the healthcare costs incurred by employees' families as well as the employees. Life insurance provides a benefit to employees' families, and disability, retirement, and severance benefits provide income continuity to the family. Some employers offer child-care benefits, and many offer paid or unpaid leave to care for newborns or sick family members or for bereavement.

Why Offer Benefits?

While most employers believe they need to offer a competitive benefits package to recruit and retain the high-caliber employees they need, the question is worth asking why employers should provide benefits to employees. Benefits typically cost about 25 percent of payroll, which could otherwise be spent on higher salaries and wages. Why wouldn't employees want higher pay instead of benefits—some of which most employees never use (e.g., life insurance, disability insurance, severance)? Why wouldn't employers want to minimize the administrative costs associated with benefits and just pay employees higher salaries and wages?

The reason employers provide benefits rather than higher pay is twofold: competitive necessity and employee preference. Higher-wage employees, especially, want, expect, and can command competitive benefit packages. Employers that continue to provide generous, competitive packages tend to be large corporations that need large numbers of highly qualified employees—whether professional employees or skilled and semi-skilled workers—with a high commitment to quality. Employers that do not offer competitive benefits tend to be those that can easily replace workers.

Healthcare organizations tend to maintain fairly generous benefit packages. Because their labor costs are so high, however, they have had to find ways of trimming costs and must cut back on what were once even more generous benefits. Most hospitals and health systems have scaled back retirement benefits by replacing defined-benefit pension plans with defined-contribution matched-savings plans. As with employers in other industries, most healthcare organizations have shifted a significant portion of the cost of healthcare benefits to their employees. Many have introduced flexible benefit plans that give employees an allowance to pay for some, but not all, of the benefits that were previously provided free of charge. Many have also introduced PTO programs that allow employees to convert what were once sick days to vacation or personal days by reducing the total number of days off provided under separate vacation, holiday, and sick-leave policies.

There are two underlying economic reasons for providing benefits rather than additional cash compensation. First, the risks associated with illness, disability, and death are more easily managed on a group insurance basis than on an individual basis, and retirees are more likely to have adequate income with an employer-provided retirement plan than with the equivalent amount of additional compensation. Second, employers have an interest in stemming the impact of one employee's calamity on the morale of the workforce as a whole, on its productivity, or on its commitment to quality.

The principal reasons employers offer supplemental benefits to executives are the same. Supplemental benefits are so prevalent that hospitals and health systems find it difficult to recruit and retain executives if they do not offer them; executives, knowing how widespread supplemental benefits are, ask for them until they get them.

Benefits are a paternalistic solution to ordinary economic risks and seem incongruous with the preference many Americans show for self-reliance. Benefits are a holdover from the employment model of the last century in which most employees stayed with

---

Forgotten Benefit Incorporated into CEO's Salary

A hospital on the West Coast discovered that, unbeknownst to the compensation committee, it had been paying its CEO a benefit for 15 years. When the CEO had been hired many years before, the hospital had agreed to give her an annual cash payment in lieu of a contribution to a tax-sheltered annuity. The executive benefit program had been redesigned in the meantime, and the consultant retained to develop the new program had recommended eliminating this benefit. Not only was it not eliminated, but everyone except staff in the payroll department had forgotten about it. When the compensation committee learned about this situation, the committee decided to incorporate the stipend into the CEO's salary, without considering its effect on the competitiveness of retirement benefits or the reasonableness of total compensation.

the same employer for their entire careers and employers intended to retain most of their employees as long as they could. Employers could eliminate a lot of the expense and administrative burden associated with benefits if they got rid of them altogether, paid employees more, and told employees to manage their own risks.

Major parts of the US economy have shifted from the model of stable employment and no longer view benefits as a competitive necessity in attracting and retaining employees, especially employers who are content with unskilled, inexperienced, or part-time workers and willing to tolerate high turnover. Many employers offer few or no benefits to part-time workers and try to keep most of their workforce at part-time status to avoid paying for benefits. Some offer no benefits even to full-time hourly workers. And most have shifted to their employees some responsibility for paying for healthcare benefits and saving for retirement.

BENEFITS VERSUS PERQUISITES

Some surveys of executive compensation treat any supplemental benefit as a perquisite, but it is more common to distinguish between them based on whether the benefit is similar to one provided to other employees. In other words, supplemental life and disability insurance and supplemental retirement plans are usually considered benefits, whereas extra compensation, goods, services, or privileges offered only to executives as an acknowledgment of their rank or stature in the organization are considered perquisites.

Perquisites include noncompensatory items such as titles, offices (e.g., a corner office, a bigger office, a better-decorated office), and reserved parking spaces; the use of company-owned equipment not provided to all other employees, such as laptop computers, cell phones, smart phones, automobiles, and home office equipment; and the privilege of charging certain expenses to the employer—magazine subscriptions, membership dues for clubs and civic associations, business entertainment, and travel expenses and fees for out-of-town conferences—more often and more easily than other employees are permitted to do. Examples of compensatory perquisites are car allowances, financial planning allowances, and tax gross-ups on taxable benefits or other perquisites.

Because we view perquisites as something different from supplemental benefits, we discuss them in detail in Chapter 7.

QUALIFIED VERSUS NONQUALIFIED BENEFITS

Qualified benefits receive special tax treatment under Internal Revenue Service (IRS) regulations because they are generally provided to all employees in a nondiscriminatory manner. Nonqualified benefits are not eligible for special tax treatment under the rules for qualified benefits, usually because they are not provided to all employees in a nondiscriminatory fashion. Many supplemental executive benefits fall into this second category.

Qualified benefits generally allow a taxable employer to deduct the cost of the benefit in determining its income tax liability and allow employees to receive the benefit on a tax-deferred basis. Some qualified benefits are taxable when a benefit is paid but not while it is being earned (e.g., qualified retirement plans). Some defer taxation by allowing employees to reduce their taxable income through voluntary contributions to a tax-deferred savings plan [e.g., 403(b) plan, 401(k) plan]. Qualified retirement plans allow their underlying investments to accumulate earnings without being subject to corporate or individual tax until they are paid out. Over a 30- or 40-year career, this delay in taxation creates much of the value of the eventual retirement income stream.

Nonqualified benefits are not treated favorably under IRS rules. In both taxable and tax-exempt organizations, nonqualified deferred compensation and retirement benefits are generally sheltered from individual taxation as they are being earned and accrued, in part because they may never be paid. (They might be forfeited if a participant leaves before meeting vesting requirements or if the employer enters bankruptcy, and they could even be lost due to a change of control.) Some plans are structured under Internal Revenue Code (IRC) § 457(b), which defers taxation until the deferred compensation is distributed to the participant. Many plans are structured under IRC § 457(f), with no limits on the amount that may be deferred, but the plans are sheltered from taxation only if they are subject to a substantial risk of forfeiture, such as cliff vesting, and the deferred compensation in a 457(f) plan is taxed when it vests or when it is no longer subject to the risk of forfeiture, even if it is not yet paid.

ISSUES IN SUPPLEMENTAL BENEFIT DESIGN

The following questions reflect some of the issues that arise when deciding which supplemental benefits to provide and how to structure them.

- Why provide supplemental benefits to executives when the organization is trimming benefit costs for other employees?
- Why provide better benefits to executives than the organization provides to other employees?
- Why not limit supplemental benefits to a supplemental retirement plan and inform executives that they must purchase any additional life or disability insurance they wish to carry?
- Why provide supplemental retirement benefits to executives who leave voluntarily to pursue a career elsewhere?
- Why not use group policies instead of individual policies to provide supplemental life and disability insurance if it costs the organization less to do so?
- Why provide any post-retirement benefit other than the retirement benefit itself (e.g., post-retirement medical benefit, paid-up permanent life insurance, paid-up long-term care insurance)?
- Why provide any tax gross-up bonus for executives when the organization does not cover tax liabilities for other employees?

Each issue is discussed in the following paragraphs.

Health and Welfare Benefits

Health, Dental, and Vision

Health benefits usually cover most services provided by physicians and hospitals and by clinical practitioners employed by hospitals or physicians (e.g., physical therapists). Dental and vision benefits are sometimes included as part of the basic healthcare plan but more often are structured as separate benefit plans.

Originally, healthcare benefits were typically paid entirely by the employer. Now the cost of healthcare benefits is almost always shared, with employees paying part of the premium and part of the cost for each service provided, such as a physician visit, a lab test, an X-ray, a drug prescription, surgery, or hospitalization. Dental and vision plans usually pay for most or all of the costs of basic services, such as examinations, but only a portion of the cost of more expensive services, such as orthodontia, dental fillings and caps, and prescription glasses or contact lenses.

Most large employers offer several different health plans or several different levels of benefits. Some healthcare organizations provide post-retirement medical benefits to their employees, but many of those that do are gradually freezing or eliminating them because they are very expensive. Post-retirement medical benefits are provided less often in healthcare than in other industries.

Supplemental Healthcare Benefits

Supplemental healthcare benefits for executives are not common because organizations have no compelling rationale for providing them. Healthcare benefits treat executives the same as other employees because these benefits are not tied to income or capped in a way that limits their value to higher-paid employees. Supplemental plans for executives that reimburse the employee's share of premiums or out-of-pocket expenses are less common than they once were. Providing free physicals to executives is still common, however, because they are viewed as a program to keep executives healthy and productive and therefore represent as much benefit to employers as to the executive employees. Post-retirement medical benefits have become more prevalent for CEOs and their spouses over the past decade—even as they are being eliminated for the workforce as a whole.

Supplemental executive healthcare benefits are not so common that anyone could legitimately claim they are a competitive necessity. As employers shift more of the cost of medical benefits to employees and freeze or eliminate post-retirement medical benefits for the workforce, they recognize that they cannot insulate their highest-paid employees from the rising cost of medical benefits by covering their share of premiums or out-of-pocket costs or providing them with post-retirement medical benefits.

Life Insurance

Most employers provide employer-paid life insurance through a group term life insurance policy. Such a policy pays a benefit to the employee's beneficiary only if and when the employee dies and only if death occurs while the employee is still employed by the organization sponsoring the plan. A typical group life insurance benefit formula is one to two times salary to a limit of, say, $100,000 or $300,000. Some plans provide a flat benefit, such as $10,000 or $50,000. Sometimes the employer-paid basic benefit is paired with voluntary, employee-paid supplemental coverage.

A life insurance benefit is often coupled with an accidental death and dismemberment policy. This type of policy pays an additional death benefit if the employee is killed in an accident or pays a lower amount if the employee loses a limb, another body part, or her sight or becomes otherwise disabled in an accident. It may also be supplemented with a business travel accident and life insurance policy, which pays an additional benefit on death or disability caused by an accident while traveling for business.

Supplemental Executive Life Insurance

Most large hospitals and health systems provide supplemental employer-paid life insurance to their executives. The supplemental benefit generally provides life insurance at a higher multiple of salary than offered under the basic plan and with a higher maximum benefit or no cap at all. Some plans sponsor a special group term policy for executives, others purchase individual term insurance, and still others provide permanent individual insurance.

The presence of this supplemental benefit is driven by competitive standards, which are higher for executives than for other employees. The competitive norm for executives is three to four times salary in employer-paid life insurance.

Supplemental executive life insurance serves three purposes in an executive compensation package. First, it provides income continuity to the executive's family if the executive dies while employed with the organization. Second, if it is permanent insurance, it enhances retirement income by allowing the executive to draw down retirement assets at a faster rate (as a single life annuity rather than as a joint annuity) than if there were no life insurance to provide income continuity to a surviving spouse. Third, it may be used to hold retirement assets themselves, or to build additional assets for retirement, by allowing for tax-deferred growth of cash value.

Over time, supplemental life insurance has become accepted as an almost essential element of a competitive executive compensation program to assure executives that an adequate or appropriate benefit will be provided for their family.

Until recently, one common way of providing supplemental life insurance to executives was through a permanent individual life insurance policy using a split-dollar arrangement, with some aspect of the policy shared between employer and employee. Regulatory changes have made the split-dollar arrangements significantly less attractive, so this approach has fallen out of favor and most of the policies remaining under split-dollar agreements are grandfathered.

Permanent individual life insurance was once the preferred way to provide supplemental life insurance to executives because it offers more value and flexibility to executives than term insurance does. Permanent insurance allows executives to continue the coverage on their own after retirement to enhance the value of retirement benefits or to protect their estates. It often provides some cash value in addition to the death benefit; it is sometimes structured to be fully paid up at retirement. It is portable, too, so executives can take it with them if they are terminated involuntarily or become disabled or decide to change jobs.

Organizations have three good reasons to provide permanent individual policies rather than group or individual term policies. First, group term insurance ends when employment ends and cannot be replaced easily or inexpensively; individual term insurance becomes too expensive to maintain after retirement. Second, permanent life insurance offers income continuity even during a period of unemployment, and few employers want to see the families of their most important leaders left with no protection if the executive dies shortly after being laid off or becoming disabled. Third, permanent life insurance enhances the value of retirement benefits by about 25 percent (the difference, roughly, between a single life annuity and a joint and survivor annuity), doing so at a much lower cost than increasing the retirement benefit by that amount.

Now term policies are becoming as common as permanent individual policies as the preferred approach to providing supplemental life insurance to executives, because term insurance, whether through individual or group policies, is generally less expensive than permanent individual policies. This shift coincides with a change in thinking about supplemental benefits. In the past, decisions about supplemental benefits for executives were shaped more by a concern that benefits were competitive than that they represented a wise use of the employer's resources. They were also shaped by consultants, who promoted permanent individual life insurance policies, partly because of the higher commissions on permanent individual policies.

Permanent individual insurance is still a better benefit than term insurance, and it may still be the most appropriate way to provide supplemental life insurance to executives, as long as the rationale for doing so is clear.

Disability Benefits

Most large employers provide two or three types of disability benefits, one to cover short-term periods of sickness or disability and one to cover long-term disability, and sometimes one to cover short-term disabilities longer than the typical illness. Sick leave is now often combined with vacation under a PTO policy.

A typical sick-leave benefit for hospital employees might give employees six or so days a year of sick leave, but because most employees do not use all the days allotted to them, unused sick days are usually allowed to accumulate until they reach a limit. When an employee becomes sick, he is paid the same as if he were working until he has exhausted his accumulated sick leave.

A long-term disability benefit is a group insurance policy that promises to pay a disabled employee a benefit—typically set at 50 percent to 66 $2/3$ percent of salary, up to a limit—for the duration of the disability or until normal retirement age, when the benefit usually ceases. Sometimes the employer pays for a basic level of coverage (e.g., 50 percent of salary up to a monthly benefit of $5,000 a month) and offers employees additional coverage at their own expense. Some employers offer only a voluntary employee-paid benefit. Long-term disability policies do not begin to provide a benefit until the employee has been disabled for 90 or 180 days.

A short-term disability benefit is intended to cover the period between a few days of sick leave and the point at which a long-term disability policy begins to pay a benefit. A short-term disability policy typically requires employees to use accumulated sick leave first then pays salary at a reduced level for a period proportional to the employee's years of service.

Some states mandate providing a short-term disability benefit under a plan designed and administered by the state. These plans generally provide a very modest benefit, perhaps $100 a week for 26 weeks.

Supplemental Executive Disability Benefits

Many hospitals and health systems provide supplemental disability benefits in one of two forms. The first is a supplemental short-term or midterm disability benefit—an extended sick-leave plan that keeps income whole while the executive is out sick or disabled, without limiting it to the number of sick days she has accumulated over time.

This first form, often called "disability salary continuation," promises continuation of salary for 90 or 180 days (sometimes as long as 360 days) in conjunction with or in place of sick leave and short-term disability benefits. Some employers provide this benefit informally by not keeping track of executives' sick days. Others provide it under a formal policy. The rationale for a policy that keeps their salary whole is twofold—the organization does not need to replace the executives when they are out sick or disabled for a short period of time, and the executives often do some work while they are sick. This rationale could be applied equally well to many salaried employees and mid-level managers, of course.

The second form is a supplemental long-term disability benefit intended to cover income above the limit set on the basic group long-term disability plan. It often follows the same formula used by the basic group plan, but the amount of coverage available is still capped by carriers, frequently at a level too low to cover the entire income of high-paid executives.

Sometimes this supplemental long-term disability benefit is more generous than the basic benefit. If the basic plan promises disability income of 50 percent of salary, for example, a supplemental benefit for executives may promise disability income of 60 or 65 percent of salary (up to the carrier's maximum) to bring it up to a fully competitive level.

Supplemental long-term disability benefits are provided either through individual policies or through a special group policy for executives. Individual policies have been preferred, as an executive can take over the policy on termination to provide protection during a period of unemployment.

Long-Term Care
Some hospitals and health systems offer employees the opportunity to buy a long-term care benefit at their own expense through

a group or individual policy. Long-term care policies provide a benefit if the policyholder becomes disabled enough to need to be cared for by someone else. Few employers provide an employer-paid long-term care benefit for all employees. Those that do provide a modest benefit on an employer-paid basis and offer employees the opportunity to buy additional coverage at their own expense.

Even though some employees need long-term care while they are still of normal working age, long-term care policies are typically exercised at an advanced age, often long after retirement. For this reason, they need to be structured as individual policies, not as group benefits for employees. The advantage of buying a permanent individual policy at a young age is that the policy should still be affordable after retirement, while a policy purchased at retirement might not be.

Executive Long-Term Care Benefits
Some hospitals and health systems provide employer-paid long-term care benefits to executives only. They are sometimes offered as part of a flexible benefit program whereby participants can select it as a benefit. Long-term care policies were not widely available at the time when boards were willing to add new benefits and perquisites to executive compensation programs, so this type of benefit did not become a competitive standard.

Vacation, PTO, Personal Days, Holidays
Vacations, holidays, personal days, and sick-leave days are forms of PTO—days on which employees get paid for not working. While they were traditionally separate benefits, organizations now commonly combine vacation, sick leave, and personal days into a single PTO benefit in recognition that employees sometimes called in sick when they wanted or needed a day off. The combined structure allows people to take the day without fibbing about being sick.

Hospitals and health systems generally recognize fewer holidays per year—six or seven—than employers in other industries do (perhaps up to 11 paid holidays per year) because paid holidays are expensive to cover for organizations that operate every day of the week. To provide the necessary seven-day-a-week coverage, they allow employees who work on holidays to take another day off instead.

Healthcare organizations typically grant new employees two weeks' vacation time, which increases to three and four weeks with 10, 15, or 20 years of service. When vacation, holidays, and sick leave are combined in a single PTO allowance, the total number of days off is often lower than if they were provided separately. A beginning employee's PTO allowance, for example, might be 19 or 20 days off a year, instead of ten days' vacation, six holidays, and six to eight days of sick leave.

For hourly employees, the vacation or PTO allowance is often defined as a certain number of earned-hours-off per pay period. Some employers impose a use-it-or-lose-it policy for vacation and PTO (the employee forfeits any time off accrued that was not taken during the year), to avoid incurring liabilities for unused PTO. Most, however, allow employees to hold unused vacation or PTO days over into the following year in a vacation bank, often up to a designated limit. Because employees' vacation time off is costly to the organization, hospitals and health systems tend to grant additional vacation or PTO at a slower pace than do industries that are less labor intensive.

Supplemental Executive PTO Policies

Most hospitals and health systems offer a special vacation or PTO allowance for executives. A typical executive vacation allowance starts at four weeks and may increase over time to five or six weeks. Executives also often receive PTO in forms other than those already mentioned. For example, a disability salary continuation program provided in lieu of sick days gives executives an unlimited number of sick days. When disability salary continuation is offered in addition to a PTO benefit that includes sick days, sick days are converted to additional vacation days. Another example is accommodation for travel. When executives attend out-of-town conferences, they can arrange travel schedules to give them extra time away from work.

On the other hand, many executives do not use their full vacation or PTO allowances. The PTO days they accumulate can generally be converted to additional compensation at termination. Some organizations even allow employees to convert unused PTO to additional compensation each year. The problem with converting unused PTO days to compensation at retirement is that days accrued when a young executive earned a modest salary are converted to compensation at the rate of the executive's salary at the end of his career—at a rate perhaps five or ten times higher than the salary in force when the days were earned.

The principal rationale for providing executives additional time off is competitiveness. Candidates for executive-level positions have already worked elsewhere for 10 to 20 years and are likely unwilling to accept a new position that offers just two weeks' vacation, as it would be akin to starting their career all over again.

Two additional rationales support the practice:

- Because executives are not replaced while they are off, allowing them to take additional time off does not incur an additional cost (unless, of course, the executives convert unused time off to additional compensation).
- Executives often make up for some part of their time off by putting in extra hours before and after vacations.

But many executives do not use all their PTO, so some of it is eventually converted to additional compensation in the form of cash, additional severance, or additional retirement income, which was never intended when the executive PTO policy was approved. Little analysis is conducted to determine how much unused PTO executives accrue, and boards tend not to pay much attention to PTO when reviewing benefits. As a result, little thought goes into designing or critiquing executive PTO policies.

Trustees should consider the following questions when reviewing the executive PTO benefit:

- If the extra time off is eventually converted to compensation, does the executive really need that much time off?
- If she really does need the additional time away, should the policy eliminate the possibility of converting it to compensation?
- If executives are eligible for unlimited sick leave under a disability salary continuation policy, why should the first few days of leave not be deducted from their PTO allowance?
- Is there a good rationale for increasing executives' vacation to five or six weeks after long-term service, or does that extra vacation time just end up getting converted to extra compensation, severance, or retirement benefits?

One trade-off for granting executives more PTO than is given to other employees is to limit or eliminate executives' option to convert unused PTO to additional compensation.

Retirement Benefits

Most employers provide three types of retirement benefits. The first is a qualified retirement plan that serves as the foundation of the retirement benefit for all employees. The second is Social Security, half of which is paid by the employer and half by the employee through payroll tax. The third is a voluntary savings plan, which allows employees to place some of their income in a tax-deferred savings account. Some savings plans offer a matching contribution from the employer.

All qualified retirement plans are subject to limits, such as on the amount of income that can be counted in determining retirement benefits and the amount that can be contributed annually. They are also subject to regulations covering their administration, the fiduciary responsibility of the plan sponsor, contingencies related to withdrawal of funds before retirement and rollover of funds to other retirement plans, assurances of nondiscrimination between highly paid and lower-paid employees, integration with Social Security, and so on. The rules and regulations vary from one type of plan to another in ways that are not altogether consistent and that change over time. They are too numerous for anyone but a retirement plan specialist to master, and discussing them in detail is beyond the scope of this text.

Albeit with many variations, qualified retirement plans come in two basic forms: defined-benefit plans and defined-contribution plans. Defined-benefit plans promise employees a specific benefit at retirement. Defined-contribution plans promise employees a specific contribution each year to an account maintained for each employee. (Cash-balance plans are a form of defined-benefit plan that looks like a defined-contribution plan; these are also briefly discussed later in this section.) Defined-benefit plans are usually funded entirely by the employer and rarely allow additional contributions by the employee. Defined-contribution plans frequently allow, and may require, employee contributions (sometimes in a separate, parallel plan).

Under the social contract in place in the 1950s and 1960s, employers were largely responsible for providing employees' retirement benefits, and defined-benefit pension plans were the standard approach for doing so. During the inflationary 1970s, however, American social policy began to shift some of that responsibility to employees through tax-sheltered savings plans, such as 401(k) and 403(b) plans, and now defined-contribution plans have become the norm.

Defined-Benefit Plans
Defined-benefit plans still survive in hospitals and health systems, although they have in many cases been closed to new participants and replaced by defined-contribution plans. Defined-benefit plans are more common in public hospitals than in private ones, more common in unionized environments than nonunionized, and more common in healthcare than in many other industries.

Even most organizations that maintain defined-benefit plans, however, have introduced tax-sheltered savings plans to encourage employees to save for retirement. These plans may be funded entirely by voluntary employee contributions or may include employer-matched savings.

In defined-benefit plans, the employer is responsible for contributing enough money to the plan each year that it has adequate funds to pay the promised benefits to employees when they retire. The federal government, through the Pension Benefit Guarantee Corporation (PBGC), guarantees some portion of that benefit. Employers are also responsible for managing the investments made through the plan and any investment-related risks.

The traditional defined-benefit pension plan promised employees a retirement benefit defined as a percentage of final-average pay (or occasionally career-average pay) proportional to years of service and to pay, and subject to caps on years of service and pay. Final-average pay is often defined as the average of the last five years' pay, the average of the five highest of the last ten years' pay, or the average of the last three years' pay. Pay is typically defined as salary or wages before voluntary salary reductions or as taxable income before voluntary salary reductions, including overtime pay and annual incentive awards but excluding long-term incentives, distributions of previously deferred compensation, and other extraneous payments, such as hiring bonuses, car allowances, and imputed income on fringe benefits.

Typical formulas for calculating the amount of retirement benefit are 1 percent of final-average salary times years of service capped at 35 years, with a maximum benefit of 35 percent of final-average pay, or 1.5 percent of final-average pay times years of service capped at 30 years, with a maximum benefit of 45 percent of final-average pay. In these scenarios, adding the employer-paid portion of Social Security, total employer-paid retirement benefits would be 50 to 60 percent of final-average pay for typical hourly employees.

The formula for some plans explicitly integrates the retirement benefit with Social Security. One such formula is 1 percent of final-average pay up to the Social Security wage base ($110,100 in 2012) and 1.5 percent of final-average pay times years of service above that integration point.

Cash-balance plans are defined-benefit plans that look like defined-contribution plans because they promise a specific contribution each year and track account balances for each employee. What makes them a defined-benefit plan is that the employer promises a fixed investment return, has responsibility for investing the funds, and manages the funds as an aggregate. The defined benefit is the account balance, which is more or less guaranteed by the employer. As a defined-benefit plan, a portion of the account value is also guaranteed by the PBGC.

Defined-Contribution Plans

Defined-contribution plans are retirement savings plans in which each participant has an individual account that holds employer and employee contributions plus investment returns, minus fees charged for administering the account or for managing the investments. Investment of the funds in the account is usually directed by the employee from a selection of investment choices offered to participants by the employer. The investment options are usually a set of mutual funds, but the choices can include other investment vehicles, such as specific stocks or bonds. For-profit firms often offer their own stock as an investment choice.

The two most common types of defined-contribution plans are 401(k) plans and 403(b) plans. The latter were authorized for public school systems and 501(c)(3) organizations long before 401(k) plans were enacted into law. There is now little difference between 403(b) and 401(k) plans, except for technical regulations.

Both 401(k) and 403(b) plans can be established as voluntary savings plans, allowing employees to reduce their taxable income in exchange for pretax contributions to a tax-deferred savings account. When these plans are offered in combination with a defined-benefit plan, they are often funded entirely by employee salary reductions.

When these plans are used as the principal employer-sponsored retirement plan, the employer usually offers to match employee contributions, in whole or in part, to a certain limit. They also may offer a contribution in addition to the match. Some plans establish that contribution or the match or both as discretionary, which makes the plan a "profit sharing" plan. Others define the exact contribution each year.

The level of employer contributions varies enormously. An average employer contribution to a defined-contribution plan is about 5 or 6 percent of pay per year; some plans contribute as little as 1 percent of pay per year, and others contribute as much as 10 percent per year.

Employees can defer up to $17,000 (in 2012) of their own pay into a 401(k) or 403(b) plan, even if the employer matches only a portion of that amount. A participant over 50 years of age can make an additional, catch-up contribution of $5,500 (in 2012).

Employees can also defer compensation on an after-tax basis in a Roth 401(k) or Roth 403(b). The principal advantage of Roth 401(k) and 403(b) plans is that withdrawals or distributions, including investment returns, are tax free as long as the withdrawals begin after the participant reaches 59½ years of age and at least five years after the first after-tax deferral. These plans have not yet become popular, though, perhaps because people can save or invest after-tax dollars more easily on their own, without the restrictions imposed on a qualified retirement savings plan.

Nonqualified Retirement Plans

Most large hospitals and health systems provide some kind of supplemental retirement benefit to their executives. Qualified retirement plans are subject to caps that do not allow organizations to cover the entire income of highly paid employees, so they provide nonqualified plans (e.g., SERPs) to overcome this limitation. (Some employers also use nonqualified plans to provide executives with richer benefits than are offered to other employees.)

In tax-exempt institutions, nonqualified deferred compensation is generally structured under IRC § 457 as a 457(f) plan, a 457(b) plan, or a combination of the two.

To keep nonqualified deferred compensation in a 457(f) plan sheltered from current taxation, it must be subject to a substantial risk of forfeiture (SRF). While for years the IRS tacitly accepted noncompete and post-retirement consulting agreements as SRFs, it has announced that it will issue new rules indicating that the only risk of forfeiture substantial enough to shelter deferred income in a 457(f) plan from current taxation is cliff vesting.

The most logical SRF for a nonqualified retirement plan is cliff vesting at retirement age, say age 65. One might expect employers to choose this SRF, as it would help them retain executives. Few employers use a cliff vest at age 65, however, for three reasons. First, any executives who retire before age 65 or who leave their job before age 65 to work for another employer would forfeit their deferred compensation. Second, the plan would not do much to retain or satisfy younger executives, as they would question whether they would ever receive it. Third, the age-65 vesting date would discourage early retirement, retain executives who are no longer the best people for their positions, make it difficult to encourage them to move on or retire early, and delay an employer's revitalization by keeping it from bringing in new leadership when appropriate to do so. Accordingly, some organizations set vesting at an earlier age, such as 62, 60, or even 58.

But executives and employers have wanted to discover and use other approaches that make it less likely that executives would forfeit their retirement benefits, and this led to experimentation with other risks of forfeiture. With the IRS insisting on cliff vesting, however, employers are now taking one of two principal approaches to structuring their deferred-compensation plans: providing supplemental retirement benefits on an after-tax basis, with no risk of forfeiture, or using a series of cliff vesting dates with vesting periods of four or five years' duration.

The after-tax approach generally amounts to paying whatever the employer would have contributed to a nonqualified plan as an extra allowance—paid in cash but intended for retirement savings. It is by far the simplest approach because no rules constrain this plan's design. It has two weaknesses, however:

1. It is difficult to distinguish a supplemental retirement benefit paid in cash from a salary or a special stipend intended for any other purpose, and participants are likely to forget that this allowance is intended for retirement savings unless the employer frequently reminds them.

2. Paying a supplemental retirement benefit in cash has no retention value for the employer, and retirement benefits are essentially the only effective retention device used in executive compensation programs. Boards have wanted executive compensation programs to include retention-oriented features and have been reluctant to give up vesting requirements. Why should they provide supplemental retirement benefits to an employee who leaves for another job, they wonder, rather than staying until retirement?

Paying SERP as Cash Compensation Hampers Retention

A multihospital system in the Northeast restructured its supplemental retirement plan by paying annual contributions in cash, rather than deferring them, on the premise that the board should not care how the benefit is structured as long as total compensation remained the same. A month later, when the chief financial officer left for another opportunity, the compensation committee wanted to implement "golden handcuffs" that would make executives think twice before leaving, having realized it had just eliminated the only element in the compensation program that helped retain executives.

Paying supplemental retirement benefits as current cash compensation may turn out to be just an interim approach as the industry decides on the best way to provide supplemental retirement benefits.

The approach that sets a four- or five-year vesting period for each year's credit to the plan means that participants would generally forfeit four or five years' credit if they left voluntarily. (Except on a day that a credit vests, or during the days before a new credit is granted, four credits would always be unvested in a plan with four-year cliff vesting, and five credits would be unvested in a plan with five-year cliff vesting. See the exhibit in the sidebar titled "Vesting.") A variation on this approach uses a series of cycles, for example, four-year cycles, with four years' credits vesting all at the same time every four years. To give participants some flexibility in retirement planning and to make sure they do not forfeit contributions when they retire, the plan typically designates a vesting age at which all remaining account balances vest and beyond which all annual credits are fully vested and payable in cash.

Some employers continue to use end-of-career vesting, however, on the premise that supplemental retirement benefits should not be paid to anyone who leaves to work elsewhere. Some of these end-of-career cliff-vested plans vest at age 65, but organizations tend to move the vesting age up to 62 to allow people to retire at least a few years early without forfeiting supplemental retirement benefits. Another approach uses partial vesting at, say, ages 60, 62, and 65, to provide even more flexibility.

A 457(b) plan (described below) is the one kind of nonqualified deferred compensation plan that does not require SRF. For this reason, some employers use it to hold supplemental deferred compensation, at least up to the limits set on the plan, and put any remaining benefits in a 457(f) plan. The 457(b) provision allows highly compensated individuals to defer more compensation voluntarily than is allowed in a 403(b) or 401(k) plan.

Congress and the IRS have intentionally made it difficult for tax-exempt organizations to offer their executives deferred

Vesting

Under IRC § 457(f), compensation deferred in nonqualified savings or retirement plans offered by tax-exempt organizations is taxable as soon as benefits are no longer subject to SRF. A vesting requirement is well accepted as an SRF.

Vesting can be defined in many ways. However it is defined, any compensation subject to a vesting requirement is contingent on fulfilling that requirement. A typical vesting requirement entails continued employment for a period of time. One example for a series of annual contributions to a deferred compensation plan is to set a five-year vesting period for every year's contribution. Under this approach, the first contribution would vest at the end of the fifth year, and thereafter another contribution would vest each year. So that participants would not forfeit otherwise unvested contributions at retirement, the plan could also specify a date (e.g., age 62) when any remaining unvested contributions would vest and after which future contributions would be paid annually in cash. The graphic that follows shows five-year vesting on each year's contribution.

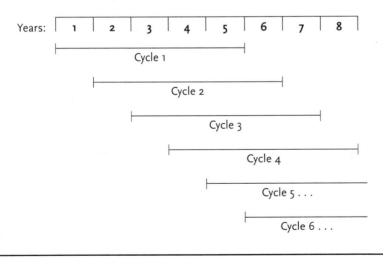

compensation above the limits set on qualified plans. Why, then, do hospitals and health systems put so much effort into designing nonqualified SERPs and deferred compensation plans? And why do executives want nonqualified deferred compensation as part of the executive compensation package? Employers could, after all, provide the same amount of compensation as additional taxable cash compensation.

Employers offer SERPs and other forms of nonqualified deferred compensation on the following premises.

- Supplemental retirement benefits are so widespread that they have become an ordinary part of the executive compensation package, and executive compensation is not considered competitive if it does not include some kind of nonqualified retirement benefit.
- Over a 30- or 40-year career, interest and investment returns are more substantial if they compound on a tax-deferred basis, so many people believe that deferring income and paying taxes later is better than paying taxes now and saving or investing on an after-tax basis. This effect is diminished or disappears entirely for shorter deferral periods.
- Many executives often do not spend all their income, they want to save some of it, and they prefer to receive at least some of it in plans that are sheltered from current taxation.
- Some executives believe that their income in retirement will be low enough to put them in a lower tax bracket, so they will be able to keep more of their retirement benefit if they defer it until retirement.

Six types of plans are commonly provided, albeit with many variations: pension restoration plans, defined-benefit SERPs, defined-contribution SERPs, target-benefit SERPs, capital accumulation accounts in flexible executive benefit plans, 457(b) plans, and life insurance policies.

Pension Restoration Plans

A restoration plan is a nonqualified retirement plan that provides the same retirement benefit on income above the legislative limit that the qualified plan provides on income below that level. In other words, it restores the benefit promised by the qualified plan on income above the legislative limit ($250,000 in 2012).

A restoration plan follows the same formula as the qualified plan. If the qualified plan is a defined-benefit plan, so is the restoration plan; if it is a defined-contribution plan, so is the restoration plan. If the qualified plan provides a reasonably competitive retirement benefit, so does the restoration plan, especially if the plan uses total cash compensation (including incentive awards) as the basis for determining retirement benefits. On the other hand, if the qualified plan provides only a modest retirement benefit, a restoration plan will not bring executives' retirement benefits up to a competitive level.

A restoration benefit is the easiest kind of supplemental retirement plan to provide, as boards readily understand why they should adopt it, participants quickly learn how it fits with the qualified plan, and employers find it easy to explain. It is also the easiest kind of supplemental executive benefit to justify to third parties, as its intent is explicitly to overcome the mandated limits on qualified plans.

Why, then, do so many hospitals and systems not have restoration plans? One reason is that a restoration plan will not deliver a fully competitive retirement benefit to executives unless the qualified plan is generous. Another is that a restoration plan on a defined-benefit pension can be expensive, especially if the plan is open to all employees paid over the limits on qualified plans.

Defined-Benefit SERPs

A defined-benefit SERP promises a retirement benefit proportional to final-average pay and years of service, as does a defined-benefit pension plan. The difference is that the value of this SERP is based on executives' entire salary or total cash compensation, not just the portion below the legislative limit. A SERP is usually defined as the total retirement benefit paid by the employer, counting all other employer-paid retirement benefits, such as the qualified plan and the employer-paid portion of Social Security.

Even though employers are moving away from defined-benefit retirement plans for the workforce as a whole, they continue to offer them to senior executives, especially CEOs. For example, they may be provided to newly recruited CEOs to make up for retirement benefits forfeited when they left the previous employer, to provide a richer retirement benefit than the qualified plan delivers, or to bring the retirement benefit up to a competitive level for a long-service CEO toward the end of her career.

The great advantage of a defined-benefit SERP is that it defines fairly precisely what the retirement benefit will be at a particular age, or at a particular combination of age and years of service, in proportion to pre-retirement pay at the end of an executive's career. It also allows the organization to base retirement benefits on all years of service at retirement, even those before introduction of the plan, thereby enabling the organization to promise a better benefit to an executive promoted toward the end of her career than it could provide using any approach not based on final or final-average pay.

Some defined-benefit SERPs do not count every employer-paid retirement benefit as an offset to the SERP, sometimes intentionally, and other times through an oversight. Either way, the result is a richer retirement benefit to the executive than the board had intended to provide. Because the only compelling rationale for offering employer-funded deferred compensation is to provide a supplemental retirement benefit, failing to count all employer-funded deferred compensation as an offset to a defined-benefit SERP is difficult to justify.

Sometimes the defined-benefit SERPs apply retirement benefits from previous employers as offsets. Most employers, however, calibrate the retirement benefit in terms of the years of service to the current employer only. This approach is practical, considering retirement benefits earned early in a career at a different employer are based on much lower income than an executive has at retirement, and often on relatively few years of service.

The principal problem with defined-benefit SERPs is that they commit the employer to an uncapped liability. They promise a benefit based on final-average pay, and no one can anticipate what final-average pay will be. The following examples are scenarios that may result in extraordinary expense to the employer using a defined-benefit SERP:

- A promotion from chief operating officer to CEO at age 60
- A change in compensation philosophy from setting salaries at median to setting salaries at the 65th percentile, if the SERP is based on salary

- An increase in incentive opportunity, if the SERP is based on total cash compensation
- Exceptional performance in the last few years of an executive's career, if the SERP is based on total cash compensation

Because the lump-sum value of a retirement benefit is roughly 10 or 11 times the annual retirement benefit, salary increases during the last few years before retirement cost 6 or 7 times as much as the salary increase itself, if the SERP replaces 60 percent of final-average pay.

The employer needs to assume the entire risk of the plan, which includes interest-rate risk, investment risk, risk related to the total amount of salary increases over time, and risk related to promotions toward the end of an executive's career. Any estimate of the cost of the plan is based on current facts and assumptions, one of which is that nothing will change much over time. All too often, this is a faulty assumption.

SERP as a Retention Incentive

The board of a healthcare organization hired a new CEO who had accrued, but was not vested in, supplemental retirement benefits at his previous employer. To make up for what the CEO had to give up to accept the new job, the board gave the CEO a fully competitive retirement benefit under the condition that she stay for the duration of her career. In essence, the board agreed to pay in just 10 years the amount of benefit that would normally be accrued over 20 or 25 years. While this arrangement was extraordinarily expensive it was structured as a retention incentive, so the new CEO would receive no retirement benefit unless she stayed for ten years.

This disadvantage is the primary reason defined-benefit SERPs are used mostly for CEOs, not for broad groups of executives. Any broad-based plans that are still in place are generally old plans that are likely frozen and closed to new participants.

Defined-Contribution SERPs

A defined-contribution SERP is an account-balance plan to which the organization makes contributions in the form of credits (essentially accounting entries) on a fixed schedule. The account balance, and thus the value of the retirement benefit, reflects the accumulated contributions plus or minus the results of investment performance over time.

To keep these plans from being subject to all the rules set by the Employee Retirement Income Security Act of 1974 (ERISA), defined contribution SERPs and deferred compensation plans are intentionally left unfunded. They are structured as a set of phantom individual accounts owned by the employer, not the participant, and subject to creditors' claims in event of bankruptcy. As such, the accounts are liabilities, which most employers hedge by investing funds representing each account in the investments chosen by participants.

Like a cash balance or 401(k) or 403(b) plan, a defined-contribution plan maintains a set of individual accounts, credits interest or investment returns to the account periodically, and may offer participants the right to "direct investments" by deciding what mutual funds will be used to determine investment return on the account. To keep them sheltered from current taxation, the account balances are subject to SRF.

These plans often use the same contribution formula, defined as a percentage of salary, for all participants. Some plans use a two- or three-step scale, with larger contributions made for higher-paid executives and smaller ones for lower-paid executives, to provide roughly comparable retirement benefits as a percentage of final-average salary, taking into account the limits on qualified retirement plans and Social Security benefits. A few plans have a service-based scale with credits that increase with service.

The contribution rate, or schedule, is usually set by determining the amount of money a typical executive retiring at age 65 with 20, 25, or 30 years of service would need, in addition to qualified retirement plans and Social Security, to obtain a certain level of retirement benefit.

The contribution required to bring total retirement benefits to a reasonably competitive level varies with the value of qualified retirement benefits and the amount of salary or total cash compensation paid above the legislative limit for qualified plans. If qualified retirement benefits are reasonably competitive, contributions to the nonqualified retirement plan do not need to be as high as if the qualified benefits are modest. The higher-paid the executive, the larger is the contribution needed, as Social Security covers only about the first $100,000 in income ($110,100 in 2012) and qualified plans cover only about the first $250,000 in income ($250,000 in 2012).

Over the past decade many tax-exempt hospitals and health systems have introduced 457(b) plans, or "top hat" plans, to give highly compensated employees an opportunity to defer more income than they can in a 401(k) or 403(b) plan. A 457(b) plan is a tax-deferred savings plan like a 401(k) or 403(b) plan except that it is nonqualified. To be eligible for tax advantages, plans offered by tax-exempt organizations (as opposed to government entities) may not be funded. They are called "top hat" plans because eligibility for these plans must be limited in the tax-exempt sector to a few higher-paid employees.

Through these eligible top-hat plans, employees can save another $17,000 (in 2012) and, if they are within three years of normal retirement age, they can make an additional catch-up contribution equal to the standard limit, but only to the extent that they did not take full advantage of 457(b) deferrals in previous years. It is rarely the first choice for deferrals, as any deferrals are subject to creditors' claims in event of bankruptcy. In many organizations, few employees other than the CEO use the top-hat 457(b) plan, as few reach the limit on deferrals in the qualified 401(k) or 403(b) plan.

Employers may contribute to 457(b) plans. Some hospitals and health systems use them as a vehicle for holding supplemental retirement benefits to avoid the risks of forfeiture required in 457(f) plans. More are likely to do so in the future, as the IRS makes it more difficult to defer income in 457(f) plans.

Nonqualified defined-contribution plans are simpler than defined-benefit SERPs in that they are easy to understand, explain, and administer. They are similar enough to 401(k) and 403(b) plans that executives can easily grasp how they fit together. They can be designed to provide a fully competitive total retirement to career-service executives, in combination with whatever qualified plans the employer offers, and the retirement benefit adjusts automatically to reflect years of service, years of plan participation, and pre-retirement earnings. Employers like them because their obligation is limited to making annual credits to the plan. Participants like them because they have the opportunity to direct the investment of funds in the account and the ability to monitor account balances at any time.

Target-Benefit SERPs

A target-benefit SERP is a defined-contribution SERP with annual credits calibrated to deliver a specific, clearly defined retirement benefit. These plans have become more common than defined-benefit SERPs over the past few decades with the growing popularity of defined-contribution retirement plans. The idea is to provide a retirement benefit comparable to that provided under a defined-benefit SERP but to shift most of the investment risks to the employee and limit the employer's obligation to making a fixed annual credit to the plan. The target-benefit SERP tracks account balances like a 401(k) or 403(b) plan, and the value of the account at retirement is based on cumulative credits and investment results.

The ability to shift most of the risks associated with a defined-benefit SERP to participants is this plan's principal advantage. The advantage to participants is the opportunity to direct investment of the funds in the account and the ability to monitor account balances at any time. The disadvantage to employees, of course, is the exposure to investment risk and timing risk—the risk that market values will decline just before retirement.

Like defined-benefit SERPs, target-benefit SERPs typically aim to provide a retirement benefit based on final-average pay proportional to years of service. For that reason, target-benefit SERPs can be as expensive as defined-benefit SERPs. When a new plan covers executives who have substantial prior service, providing a benefit proportional to years of service means providing credit for all years of service, including those before introduction of the plan. If that cost is prohibitive, the board may decide not to cover past service. Like defined-benefit SERPs, target-benefit SERPs are used more often for CEOs than for other executives; unlike defined-benefit SERPs, however, target-benefit SERPs may also be provided to broad groups of executives.

Credits are determined independently for each participant based on age and years of service and using assumptions about future salary growth and investment return. Annual credits differ so much from one participant to another that it is difficult to explain to participants why they vary so much. Contributions are generally defined as a percentage of salary, so that actual contributions rise over time as a participant's salary increases.

Some target-benefit plans call for periodic recalculation of the annual contribution to account for salary increases that may be different from the assumptions used in designing the plan and determining the initial contribution level. Other plans allow for recalculation but do not require it; some are silent on the issue, suggesting that the plan was approved on the assumption that the initial target contribution would be sufficient and would not be recalculated as circumstances changed.

Target-benefit SERPs are attractive to participants when stock values are rising because they achieve better-than-expected investment returns and therefore a higher retirement benefit than the employer would have promised if it had used a defined-benefit approach. These SERPs are not as attractive to participants when stock values fall or are stagnant because lower-than-expected investment returns generate a smaller retirement benefit than the employer would have promised under a defined-benefit approach.

Employers find target-benefit SERPs more attractive than defined-benefit SERPs because the liability involved is clearly defined as a set annual cost, instead of the uncapped, unpredictable liability of a defined-benefit SERP. Boards sometimes make decisions that undermine the advantages of target-benefit SERPs, however. Some boards, for example, recalibrate the SERP shortly before an executive's retirement to make sure the retirement benefit is adequate, while others require regular recalibrations to account for larger-than-expected salary increases or unanticipated changes in qualified plans or Social Security—which, while seemingly appropriate, moves the target-benefit SERP one step closer to being a defined-benefit SERP by basing the intended retirement benefit on final-average salary, instead of an initial estimate of final-average salary when an executive first becomes eligible for the plan. Some boards actually make up for investment results, or adjust the assumption for future investment return when the market is flat; these decisions, in effect, make the employer responsible for investment return.

The principal advantage of target-benefit SERPs is that they can be calibrated to deliver essentially the same retirement benefit as a defined-benefit SERP and treat people with the same tenure fairly, without taking on the uncapped, unpredictable liability of a defined-benefit SERP. The principal disadvantage of target-benefit SERPs is that it is hard to explain and justify the different contributions for each participant, as they do not seem fair.

Capital Accumulation Accounts in Flexible Executive Benefit Plans
A capital accumulation account in a flexible benefit plan is similar to a defined-contribution retirement plan except that the contribution is defined as the amount left of the plan allowance after

deducting the cost of any other benefits, rather than a specific contribution dedicated to retirement.

Although the board may structure this type of plan to allow longer deferrals, capital accumulation accounts typically require only short-term deferral (e.g., for two years), to give optimal flexibility to participants. Requiring only short-term deferral implies that the plan is not intended to function as a retirement plan and often leads to participants' withdrawing the funds as soon as they can.

Nonetheless, a steady stream of credits to a capital accumulation account can provide a fully competitive supplemental retirement benefit over 20 or 25 years, assuming that the allowance is generous enough to allow for credits of 8 or 10 percent of salary and that participants save most of their allowance for retirement.

Life Insurance as Vehicle for Funding Deferred Compensation

Some supplemental retirement benefits and deferred-compensation plans are funded in life insurance, and some life insurance policies build up cash value over time to allow executives to accumulate funds that can be converted to additional retirement income. Changes in tax regulations have made it less attractive to use life insurance in this way.

In years past, life insurance was commonly used as a vehicle for sheltering deferred compensation from current taxation, as life insurance did not need to be subject to SRF. Split-dollar arrangements were often used, so that employers advanced funds to the policies' premiums that were large enough to generate investment returns to produce the intended retirement benefit and leave enough cash value to return the premiums to the employer when the executive retired or died. When the market declined unexpectedly, many employers and participants were disappointed that the policies did not perform as expected, and split-dollar insurance acquired a bad reputation. Now it is being reintroduced with investment returns determined by investment indices with minimal returns guaranteed.

The principal advantage of using life insurance as a funding vehicle for supplemental retirement benefits or deferred compensation is that it can shelter from taxation the contributions and even withdrawals taken in the form of loans from the policy. The amounts reportable as deferred compensation are lower than if they were credited to a 457(b) or 457(f) plan. The principal disadvantage of using life insurance as a retirement vehicle is that it is not intended primarily for retirement, so unusual and complicated modifications need to be made to convert a policy to a retirement vehicle. Providing a retirement benefit through a split-dollar insurance plan, for example, requires unusually high premiums and unusually high death benefits, often with such high leverage that the risk of the program not performing as expected is high.

Funding and Trusts

To keep them from being subject to all ERISA rules, supplemental retirement benefits provided by tax-exempt organizations must be *unfunded,* meaning that the benefits appear as a general liability on the employer's books. Any funds reserved to pay the benefits belong to the employer and are subject to creditors' claims in the event of bankruptcy. Nonetheless, many of these plans are informally funded—that is, funds are set aside to make sure they are available to pay the liabilities when they come due.

Nonqualified account-balance plans allowing participants to choose how investment returns will be determined are generally hedged, with the employer buying mutual funds chosen by the participant. This approach helps organizations determine the account balance and the amount of the liability at any time because it matches the value of the mutual funds in the participant's account. The plan is still technically unfunded, however, because the mutual funds belong to the employer and are subject to creditors' claims in event of bankruptcy.

Considering the participant's right to the benefit is secured only by the employer's promise to pay, even if memorialized in a plan document that amounts to a contractual obligation to pay, participants typically want additional assurance that the benefit will be paid when it is supposed to be paid. It has become standard practice to set funds aside in a rabbi trust,[1] which prohibits the employer from using the funds for any purpose other than paying the deferred compensation. The rabbi trust still leaves the funds subject to creditors' claims in event of bankruptcy, but it protects the accounts from "change of heart" and "change of mind," which could be especially important after a change of control.

Target-benefit SERPs, defined-contribution SERPs, capital accumulation accounts, and other types of nonqualified deferred compensation accounts are typically protected by rabbi trusts. Less common is to establish rabbi trusts for defined-benefit SERPs, as these plans do not typically involve individual accounts or give participants a choice of investment vehicles to use in determining investment return.

FLEXIBLE BENEFIT PLANS

About 20 percent of large and midsize hospitals and health systems in the United States use a flexible approach to providing executive benefits. Like flexible benefits plans provided to the workforce as a whole, flexible executive benefit plans start with an allowance and a menu of benefits from which to choose. Flexible benefit plans allow participants to allocate the allowance to the benefits they value most.

Flexible benefit allowances may be taxable or tax sheltered. A recent regulatory change has narrowed the choices available under a tax-sheltered plan, making these plans less attractive than they once were. As a result, some organizations now offer flexible benefit plans in a taxable format, which expands the number of choices available. Others are abandoning the flexible benefit plans altogether.

Flexible executive benefit plans come in two types. One is an allowance dedicated only to supplemental benefits, and it is provided in addition to the basic benefits provided to all other employees. The other is a larger allowance intended to cover all benefits, including Social Security and the basic benefits provided to all employees.

When the allowance covers all benefits, the cost of basic benefits is subtracted from the allowance, the cost of any supplemental benefit given to all executives (e.g., a pension restoration plan) is subtracted from the allowance, and the remainder is the flexible portion of the benefit allowance. The allowance for this type of flexible benefit plan (often called a "full-flex plan") is set at about 40 percent of salary when it includes all PTO, or at about 30 percent of salary when PTO is not included.

When the allowance covers only the set of supplemental benefit choices (often called a "flat-flex plan"), it is typically set at about 8 to 12 percent of salary.

Flexible executive benefit plans are provided for the same reasons flexible benefit plans are provided for the workforce as a whole:

- They are economically efficient, as they require participants to use the funds for benefits they value most.
- They control costs at a fixed percentage of salary, which does not increase as healthcare premiums rise.
- They correct for the limits on Social Security and qualified retirement benefits by allowing higher-paid executives to defer more income than lower-paid executives can.
- They allow participants to modify their benefits as they age and their family circumstances change.
- They focus attention on all the caps and limits that keep the basic group benefits from covering the full compensation of the organization's leaders and provide an easy way to see that the benefits promised to all other employees are extended to cover executives' income.

Tax-sheltered flexible executive benefit plans are significantly more difficult to administer than plans with the same benefits for all executives, and they require more effort to communicate to participants. Most organizations with such plans use a third-party administrator to help with communication and administration of benefits. Communication of benefits is discussed in greater detail later in the chapter.

PREVALENCE OF SUPPLEMENTAL EXECUTIVE BENEFITS

Statistics on prevalence of supplemental benefits for executives vary from one peer group to another and change from year to year, as regulations change and new trends develop. The information presented here is based on multiple sources[2] and is intended to give only a general idea of the prevalence of various types of supplemental benefits for executives. It represents a restricted universe of large, private, tax-exempt hospitals and health systems that use consultants regularly and participate in national surveys. Prevalence for most supplemental benefits is much lower in small, independent hospitals, especially rural ones, and in public hospitals.

Medical

Supplemental medical benefits that reimburse executives for medical expenses not otherwise covered by basic medical plans (the employee portion of healthcare premiums, copays, deductibles) are becoming rare, except for executive physicals, which are still fairly common. At one point as many as 10 percent of large hospitals and health systems had plans that reimbursed executives for all out-of-pocket medical expenses, sometimes even employees' usual share of premiums. Few organizations now cover the executive's share of premiums, but the practice survives for some CEOs under their employment agreements.

Post-retirement Medical

Post-retirement medical plans for CEOs (and often their spouses) have become more common over the past decade, even as post-retirement medical plans for the workforce as a whole have been disappearing. About 15 or 20 percent of large hospitals and health systems now provide lifetime post-retirement medical benefits to their CEOs; only about 5 percent of healthcare organizations provide this benefit to executives other than the CEO. Prevalence is higher for pre-Medicare coverage for early retirees, but these plans cover only the period between early retirement and eligibility for Medicare.

Disability Salary Continuation

Formal disability salary continuation plans that substitute for sick leave and short-term disability plans are found in about 30 percent of large hospitals and health systems. Informal practices at another 10 percent of the industry provide the same benefit to executives by not formally tracking sick days.

Long-Term Disability

About 60 percent of large hospitals and health systems provide supplemental long-term disability benefits. About half of these use a special group policy for executives; the other half use individual policies.

Long-Term Care

Approximately one-third of all large hospitals and health systems offer long-term care benefits to executives. More often than not, they are offered as a choice within a flexible benefit plan or as a voluntary employee-paid benefit. While less than 10 percent of the industry offers employer-paid long-term care benefits to all executives, the prevalence of this benefit has risen dramatically over the past decade.

Life Insurance

About two-thirds of all large hospitals and health systems provide supplemental life insurance to executives. In the past, most of this benefit was provided in permanent, individual policies, often under split-dollar agreements. Split-dollar arrangements have fallen out of favor, however, and term policies are increasingly seen as the preferred vehicle for supplemental life insurance for executives. Excluding grandfathered plans under split-dollar arrangements, supplemental life insurance benefits for executives are split evenly between permanent individual life insurance and term insurance using individual term policies or special group term policies for executives.

Retirement

Most large hospitals and health systems provide some kind of supplemental retirement benefit. About 30 percent of the industry uses a restoration plan to restore the benefit promised under the qualified plan on income above the legislative limit. More than half of the industry provides an employer-paid defined-contribution supplemental retirement plan. Defined-benefit and target-benefit SERPs are provided by nearly half of all large hospitals and health systems, counting SERPs intended for CEOs only; the prevalence drops to about a fourth of the industry, counting only plans for a broader group of executives.

Vacation

At least half of the industry uses a special vacation or PTO schedule for executives, which gives them an extra week or so of PTO above the schedule for other employees. In practice, the prevalence is much higher, as many organizations do not carefully track days off for executives.

Flexible Executive Benefit Plans

About 20 percent of large hospitals and health systems use a flexible benefit plan that allows executives to choose the supplemental benefits they want or need most. Prevalence is declining, however, as the plans are no longer as attractive as they once were.

COMMUNICATING BENEFITS TO EXECUTIVES

Given their importance and expense, benefits are too little understood and too little appreciated by participants. Although most employers recognize the need to communicate benefits carefully and well, communicating benefits remains an ongoing challenge because employees do not really need to understand them in any detail until they must use them.

Supplemental benefits for executives are often more complicated, and therefore more difficult to explain, than benefits for the workforce as a whole. It takes a special effort to communicate benefits well to executives (or to employed physicians), but it is generally worth that effort to increase executives' satisfaction with the benefits they receive. Why spend a lot of money on supplemental benefits only to have them be underappreciated because they are not well understood?

One common complaint executives express about supplemental benefits is that these benefits are too complicated and difficult to understand. In part the confusion is due to the rules and constraints that tax law imposes on benefits, but it is due equally to the good intentions of benefits designers who aim to provide elegant solutions to the issues raised by the rules and constraints. If supplemental benefit plans were simpler, they might be appreciated more, but they are complicated, so it is important to remind participants at least once a year how they work, why they are provided, and how valuable they are.

Toward this end, three messages are important to deliver: the value of the supplemental benefits; the terms and provisions of the benefits and the relationship between basic and supplemental benefits; and executives' responsibility in determining and understanding the risks that benefits address and deciding how best to protect themselves, their families, and their incomes from those risks. These issues are addressed in the following paragraphs.

Value of Benefits and of the Total Compensation Package

Most employees, and even most executives, have no idea what benefits cost or the value they add to the total compensation package. To communicate their worth, the board should prepare total compensation exhibits for executives (or for all employees) to help them appreciate the benefits' value. Furthermore, the value message should go beyond the employer's cost, because that perspective lowers the perceived value of the benefits. It should stress that many benefits would cost more for executives if they had to purchase them on the open market and that the true value of such benefits as long-term disability, long-term care, life insurance, and severance is realized only when they are needed. The message should also focus on the risks and consequences of disability, death, and involuntary termination—the reasons the benefits are offered in the first place—and the value of the benefits if and when they are used.

Terms and Complexities of Supplemental Benefits

Nonqualified benefits, with the exception of deferred-compensation and retirement plans, do not need to be formally documented. Some employers document all supplemental executive benefits thoroughly to protect the interests of participants and the employer, to memorialize the terms of the benefits, to explain how disputes and claims will be resolved, and to clearly communicate the terms of the benefits to participants. Others document supplemental benefits only informally, in meeting minutes, employment agreements, offer letters, or straightforward descriptions of the executive compensation program. Regardless of whether or how the plan is documented, the employer still has some responsibility for communicating and explaining the benefits to participants. Because supplemental benefits typically complement or surpass basic benefits, the relationship between the two is often as important as the terms of the supplemental benefits. Some supplemental benefits are subject to complex rules, and no one wants to memorize them all. With that limitation in mind, the employer may communicate just a few important concepts:

1. Under what circumstances do participants qualify to receive the benefits?
2. What are the limits on the basic benefit, and how does the supplemental benefit override those limits?
3. What is the value of the benefit, when is it paid, and how long does it continue to be paid?
4. What decisions does the participant need to make now? And when and how can initial decisions be changed?
5. Does any decision the employee makes now change the value of the benefit?

Employee Responsibility

Employer-paid benefits are paternalistic. The employer presumes to know what benefits should be provided to employees, which ones it should pay for, how much of the cost it should share with employees, and which benefits should be offered on a voluntary basis at employee cost. But ultimately, the employee is responsible for understanding the benefits provided by the employer. Considering these factors, and because benefits rarely cover every contingency, communication of benefits should emphasize employees' personal responsibility for deciding what risks are worth managing through insurance or personal savings; what additional insurance or savings employees may need to accumulate beyond the value of the benefits provided by the employer; and how employees' personal or family circumstances should affect their decisions about benefits, retirement savings, and insurance. The personal responsibility message should not focus exclusively on which benefits are provided by the employer but also on the issue that any employer-provided benefits may not meet the employee's needs. The executive is responsible for saving enough money for retirement and obtaining whatever insurance he needs to cover any risks he may face, beyond whatever benefits the employer provides. He should know not to expect the employer to take care of every contingency or to provide any more benefit than what its plan documents say it will provide.

ADMINISTERING SUPPLEMENTAL BENEFITS

Any employer that provides supplemental benefits should see that they are administered properly. The regulations pertaining to supplemental benefits are different from those pertaining to basic benefits, and they change frequently. To expect the staff member charged with administering employee benefits to administer supplemental benefits as well may be unrealistic. If the organization chooses to shift supplemental benefits administration to a separate individual, it may be wise to give that responsibility to the chief human resources officer because of their often confidential nature.

The administrator of the supplemental benefits needs to have ready access to legal counsel, tax advice, accounting help, and benefits consultants to make sure that benefits are appropriately documented to reflect the latest regulatory changes, responsibly administered to stay in compliance with regulation, accurately recorded and communicated to participants to avoid legal liability, and handled responsively to avoid frustrating the organization's leaders. Having one party responsible for administering the executive benefit program as a whole is best, rather than leave each benefit in the hands of a separate party—the insurance carrier, the trust administrator, the broker, the record-keeper, or the participants. Many organizations use a third-party administrator to manage the program as a whole. Others use an insurance broker for insured benefits and another vendor for retirement benefits.

A few hospitals and health systems give their executives a taxable benefit allowance and let them deal with supplemental benefits on their own. This approach relieves the organization of the need to administer the program; all it needs to do is distribute the allowance, pay the withholding taxes, and report the benefit accurately. Other healthcare employers have agreed to pay for insurance policies an executive owned at the time she was hired. The advantage of providing an allowance or reimbursing premiums for personally owned policies is that it avoids the need for the organization to establish, administer, and communicate supplemental benefits. It may become more common in the future, considering that the IRS is making it more difficult for employees to defer income on a tax-sheltered basis, certain supplemental benefits now must be disclosed in more detail than before on IRS Form 990, and some employers have already begun to provide some or all supplemental benefits on an after-tax basis.

The principal weakness of providing an allowance or reimbursing the costs of premiums for an executive's existing policy is that the employer is providing an allowance with which executives can do what they want. They do not have the opportunity to take advantage of the employer's purchasing power to obtain a benefit they may not be able to get on their own or on cost-effective terms. The allowance is nothing more than additional salary, unless its use is restricted to reimbursement of premiums for supplemental insurance. The employer may as well pay higher salaries and stop providing supplemental benefits.

Some challenges of administering supplemental benefits are discussed below.

Compliance with regulation. Supplemental benefits are subject to many types of regulations—insurance, securities, tax, employee benefit, accounting, privacy, and other regulations. Although some rules remain constant for years, others change frequently.

Customized individual service. Executives often expect special treatment when they encounter the kind of circumstances that require administrative action related to supplemental benefits. They are more likely than other employees to grouse when matters are not handled well. It may be easier for a firm that specializes in providing customized customer service to do this well.

Recordkeeping. Some supplemental benefits, especially retirement benefits and split-dollar life insurance policies, require special record-keeping systems, as systems designed for qualified retirement benefits generally cannot handle supplemental benefits well. Recordkeeping for supplemental deferred compensation is unusually difficult, especially when it involves keeping track of individual accounts invested in mutual funds and multiple vesting dates.

Accruing liabilities. Organizations generally obtain regular annual actuarial evaluations of defined-benefit SERPs to determine accruals and liabilities. Any retirement or deferred compensation plan with individual accounts needs careful calibration of annual accruals, investment returns, and account balances or liabilities.

Reporting. Now that supplemental benefit costs must be disclosed in detail on IRS Form 990, it is more important than ever to maintain accurate records of benefit costs and their impact on taxable income. The IRS requires organizations to restate inaccurate reports, so to avoid this inconvenience, hospitals and health systems should ensure they are reporting supplemental benefits accurately the first time.

Timeliness. Securities regulations require timely implementation of investment decisions. A delay in processing an insurance application can lead to litigation if the applicant dies or becomes disabled. A delay in distributing deferred compensation after it has vested can lead to claims or litigation if the value of assets declines in the meantime.

Communication. Participants need to be told when regulations change; reminded of deadlines for making decisions about deferrals; informed of their choices when deferred compensation vests; alerted when supplemental insurance policies are transferred to employees; and taught how to handle benefits when employment is terminated. They need to be reminded repeatedly of the tax consequences of benefits—in writing and in plain English—or they may claim they were told the benefit was tax free and press the employer to cover their taxes.

Taxation. Employers need to make sure that taxes are withheld, paid on time, paid in the right amount, and reported accurately for almost every kind of supplemental benefit.

BEST PRACTICES IN EXECUTIVE BENEFITS

The following is a list of best practices in supplemental executive benefits:

- Establish the principles that guide decisions on supplemental benefits for executives. These may include (1) providing the same benefits to all executives, (2) using a flexible benefit plan that allows executives to allocate an allowance to the benefits they value most, (3) providing all benefits at a fully competitive level to all executives, (4) using supplemental benefits only to restore executives' benefits on income above the limits set on the basic benefit for the workforce as a whole, (5) providing supplemental benefits only to the CEO, or (6) providing supplemental benefits only as needed to recruit new executives.
- Keep supplemental benefits for executives reasonably consistent with basic benefits for other employees to simplify communication and to minimize risk of criticism.
- Avoid giving executives benefits that are notably better than those for other employees, unless the enhanced benefits are

needed to recruit or retain executives or the logic underlying the design of basic benefits does not apply to executive positions (e.g., executives do not need to be replaced when they are out sick).

- Design supplemental benefits in a way that is best for the organization, rather than base decisions principally on what is best for participants.
- Avoid assuming responsibility for executives' tax obligations on benefits by letting preferential tax treatment determine benefit design or by paying bonuses to cover any part of taxes due on benefits.
- Avoid assuming responsibility for post-retirement health or life insurance or long-term care benefits for executives, unless these benefits are consistent with those for other employees.

NOTES

1. The first rabbi trust was established by a rabbi, hence the name. Rabbi trusts are used to protect a participant's right to the assets in the trust, which are subject to SRF and creditors' claims.

2. Based on standard surveys of executive compensation in the healthcare industry, published by the Hay Group, Integrated Healthcare Strategies, and Sullivan Cotter, and on surveys of executive benefits and perquisites published by the Hay Group, Integrated Healthcare Strategies, Mercer, and Towers Watson.

CHAPTER 7

Perquisites

INTRODUCTION

A perquisite is a special privilege or benefit given to an executive in recognition of the executive's status in the organization. Perquisites are relics of an era during which privilege was as important as profitability and executives viewed themselves as proprietors of the businesses they managed. Before global competition emerged, American businesses were less concerned with maximizing profits for their shareholders than they are now. Country club memberships, luncheon club memberships, martini lunches, and first-class travel—all perquisites—were standard privileges for executives and, as such, easily explained as a cost of doing business.

Prior to managed care and diagnosis-related groups, when reimbursement was more generous so hospitals did not need to focus relentlessly on cost control, perquisites were provided to hospital executives because their peers in private industry had perquisites, they did not cost much, and they were not yet regarded as visible representations of excess. They afforded status to executives who were not at that time paid nearly as well as their counterparts in the for-profit sector.

At one time, executive compensation was a well-guarded secret, and few people were aware of which perquisites were provided to executives, other than the obvious—titles, large offices with impressive furnishings, executive dining rooms, and reserved parking spaces, among others. Boards thought that perquisites were appropriate favors accorded to executives because that was the way business was conducted. Stakeholders and other observers had little basis on which to criticize executive perquisites.

Now much of this information is public. Schedule J to IRS Form 990 asks tax-exempt organizations to indicate whether they provide loans to executives or trustees, pay for first-class travel or spouse travel, provide a housing allowance or reimbursement for business use of an executive's residence, reimburse an executive for personal services (e.g., chef, housekeeper), or pay dues for membership in a health club or social club (e.g., luncheon club, country club).

Recognizing the incongruity between asking the public to increase reimbursement for Medicare and Medicaid, for example, and paying for automobile or club memberships for its highest-paid employees, trustees have begun to eliminate perquisites.

OVERVIEW OF PERQUISITES

Perquisites are generally restricted to a privileged few—the CEO and perhaps a few executives. Those that are offered to all employees, such as continuing education, health club memberships, or subsidized cafeterias, are better regarded as benefits than as perquisites because they are not limited to executives.

Some perquisites have no economic value, such as a title, yet their perceived value is high because of the prestige they convey. Others, such as large offices with good furniture and art, entail significant cost but provide only modest economic value to executives and do not result in taxable income to the employee because they can be treated as ordinary business expenses.

Employer-provided cell phones and smart phones have a clear economic value but do not result in taxable income as long as they are reserved for business use. While these items are ordinary business expenses, they are also considered perquisites because the employer does not provide cell phones and smart phones to all employees.

Perquisites such as memberships in luncheon and country clubs have a clear economic value and do result in taxable income to the extent that they are used for personal enjoyment or convenience. They are also considered a legitimate business expense when they are provided and used to support business development, business meetings, or other business entertainment.

Employers provide cars and car allowances to executives strictly as a privilege of rank. Employers typically expect employees, even those who travel for work, to buy their own cars, and they reimburse those employees for business mileage. Hospitals that expect home health nurses who travel all day to buy their own cars have little business justification for providing a car or car allowance to an executive, other than to make the executive feel privileged.

Some perquisites are provided to help executives learn and become more effective in their jobs. Most hospitals and health systems encourage executives to join professional societies and pay for those memberships. They encourage executives to attend professional and industry conferences and pay their expenses even for national conventions, while they typically cover the expenses of other employees only if those staff members attend local or in-state conferences.

Perquisites Versus Supplemental Executive Benefits

Perquisites can be distinguished from supplemental benefits in the following ways:

- A supplemental benefit enhances a benefit provided to the workforce as a whole, whereas a perquisite is given only to executives by virtue of their rank.
- A supplemental benefit typically has relatively high economic value, whereas a perquisite typically has little

economic value (but significant perceived value, as only executives qualify for it).

- Supplemental benefits may be relatively easy to defend as similar to benefits provided to all other employees; perquisites are difficult to defend because they are special deals for executives who could afford to pay for the perquisites themselves.

Some authorities and surveys overlook the difference between supplemental benefits and perquisites, lump them together, and label them all perquisites in their analyses. This practice obscures an important distinction between items that affect the organization and the executive in economic terms (benefits) and privileges that rarely carry much economic value (perquisites).

Finally, supplemental benefits serve an important role in attracting and retaining leadership talent. Perquisites generally do not.

Perquisites Versus Business Expenses

The distinction between perquisites and business expenses is harder to draw than that between perquisites and supplemental executive benefits. The principal difference is that ordinary business expenses do not result in taxable income for the executive, whereas many perquisites do. Any expense that an employer would reimburse to any employee who incurred the expense is clearly an ordinary business expense. One that would be reimbursed only to an executive is clearly a perquisite. A business expense that can be incurred only by an executive with authority to incur the expense may be a perquisite (e.g., subscription to a professional journal, membership in a professional society). When perquisites are reported as taxable income, the employee generally may not deduct the cost as a legitimate job-related expense.

Many perquisites are both ordinary business expenses and perquisites; some are part business expense, part taxable personal income. For example, an employer-provided cell phone is an ordinary business expense as long as its use is restricted to business purposes; when it is used at all for personal calls, it is a perquisite. Similarly, allowing an employee to use a fleet car for business travel is an ordinary business expense, but allowing the employee to use an employer-owned car for commuting or personal travel is a perquisite.

PURPOSE OF PERQUISITES

The usual rationale for providing perquisites to executives is to facilitate the organization's work: helping executives be productive, giving them tools to use their time well, or assisting them in promoting business development. This rationale holds for cell phones, smart phones, memberships in professional societies, attendance at industry meetings, laptop computers, home office equipment, offices big enough to accommodate a conference table, luncheon and country club memberships, airline club memberships and first-class travel, even use of private planes for transportation to meetings in far-flung locations. It does not apply for cars or car allowances, financial planning allowances, custom office furnishings, titles, or tax gross-ups on supplemental benefits and perquisites.

The rationale works best when the organization provides the same perquisite to many people, because many people in any organization could be more productive with several of these perquisites.

Perquisites convey a privilege to one or a small number of executives to spend money that other employees are not allowed to spend. They are an exception to any organization's focus on cost control for the following reasons:

1. Boards' decisions to provide perquisites are primarily driven by their need to satisfy executives and secondarily by their desire to be competitive with other potential employers. Those concerns evidently outweigh their concern for cost-effectiveness.

2. Executives generally like their perquisites. They rarely volunteer to give them up, even in the midst of major cost-cutting initiatives.
3. Boards often get some satisfaction from giving perquisites to executives. They like having the CEO be a member of the same clubs they belong to, as it develops a social bond with the CEO. They want the CEO's office to be at least as impressive as the boardroom, as it enhances their impression of the organization they govern.

Perquisites generally can and do enhance executives' productivity. The gradual disappearance of the most controversial perquisites—cars and country club memberships—indicates that the business rationale is not strong enough to overcome the criticism these perquisites attract.

Exhibit 7.1 demonstrates the prevalence of executive perquisites in hospitals and health systems during 2006–2007. The following sections discuss each major perquisite found in tax-exempt organizations and the degree to which they are generally used.

AUTOS AND AUTO ALLOWANCES

Employer-provided automobiles and automobile allowances are among the most common and most economically valuable perquisites. They typify the public's and the press's conception of perquisites.

In general, an organization does not have a compelling business rationale for providing a car or a car allowance to an executive unless the executive is a member of a religious order, with no personal income, whose job entails meeting with executives and board members of geographically dispersed hospitals. Because executives can presumably afford to buy their own cars, autos and auto allowances are good examples of perquisites that are difficult to defend from criticism.

Form of the Perquisite

Employer-provided cars and car allowances come in two forms. The most common form is a straightforward allowance. The allowance is presumably dedicated to purchasing and maintaining an automobile, but it is fungible, so it could be used to purchase any other item. The allowance is fully taxable, except to the extent that the executive claims a deduction for business mileage on his personal income tax return.

The next most common form is the use of an automobile leased or owned by the employer. Often the executive is allowed to choose the car; sometimes the employer leases a fleet of cars and allows executives to use one of them for personal as well as business use.

Some large healthcare systems lease a fleet of cars and allow executives and other employees to use a fleet car when needed for business travel. This form does not qualify as a perquisite because use of a fleet car is not limited to executives and the car cannot be used for commuting or for personal travel.

Value of the Perquisite

The size of car allowances and the value of employer-provided cars varies enormously. Some car allowances are sufficient to cover the full cost of a leased automobile, plus insurance, gas, and maintenance. Others merely cover the cost of an inexpensive lease. Employer-leased cars for CEOs tend to be moderately expensive sedans, while cars purchased or leased for fleets tend to be more modest.

A typical car allowance for a CEO is about $800 to $1,000 a month. A typical car allowance for other senior executives is $500 to $700 a month. A modest allowance may be $200 to $400 a month.

When employers provide automobiles for executives, they generally cover the cost of the lease and of operating, maintaining, licensing, and insuring the car.

Exhibit 7.1: Prevalence of Executive Perquisites

	CEO		COO	
Perquisite	*n*	*%*	*n*	*%*
Perquisite Allowance	***	***	***	***
Loans	507	3.7%	377	2.1%
Housing Allowance	508	2.4%	377	1.1%
Executive Vacation Policy	534	54.5%	387	43.9%
Professional Subscriptions	527	61.1%	382	55.2%
Car Purchased	534	21.3%	386	6.5%
Car Allowance	535	52.5%	386	40.9%
Luncheon Club	509	19.1%	377	9.8%
Health Club	509	15.9%	374	10.7%
Country Club	526	43.0%	382	14.7%
Financial Plannning Allowance	517	28.2%	380	19.7%
Legal Services Allowance	508	7.5%	376	4.8%
Home Computer	513	34.9%	379	29.3%
Cell Phone	509	58.0%	373	50.4%
Blackberry	277	41.5%	197	38.1%
Transportation Allowance	229	3.5%	167	1.8%
Parking Allowance	498	25.1%	372	20.4%
First Class Travel	507	7.5%	377	2.9%
Spouse Trips	516	17.6%	379	5.8%
VIP Lounge	506	4.5%	376	2.1%
Dependent Tuition	511	8.4%	379	6.9%
Sabbatical—Full Pay	506	4.5%	376	4.3%
Sabbatical—Partial Pay	505	1.2%	375	0.5%

Note: n = number of organizations responding; % = percentage of respondents reporting the perquisite.

Source: Reprinted with permission from Integrated Healthcare Strategies, Survey of Perquisites in Hospitals and Health Systems, 2006–2007.

CFO		Other Direct Reports		Other Executives	
n	%	*n*	%	*n*	%
***	***	***	***	***	***
470	2.8%	447	2.7%	420	2.9%
470	1.5%	447	1.8%	420	1.2%
486	51.9%	467	50.1%	433	48.3%
475	58.1%	456	57.7%	421	54.9%
484	7.2%	455	4.0%	419	2.6%
484	37.2%	458	34.3%	423	30.7%
471	5.7%	447	8.3%	418	5.3%
469	11.3%	444	11.0%	418	10.3%
471	13.0%	451	11.1%	420	5.7%
473	20.3%	450	20.4%	420	18.1%
469	4.5%	446	4.9%	419	3.8%
471	31.2%	447	28.9%	419	27.7%
466	50.9%	446	48.7%	413	47.7%
258	39.9%	249	38.2%	229	35.4%
215	2.3%	209	1.0%	195	0.5%
461	21.0%	441	18.6%	409	15.4%
470	3.2%	447	2.0%	419	2.6%
471	7.0%	451	6.9%	420	4.5%
469	3.0%	447	3.1%	419	2.1%
472	6.6%	451	6.7%	420	6.2%
469	3.8%	446	3.6%	419	3.8%
469	0.9%	446	0.9%	418	1.0%

CLUB MEMBERSHIPS

Employer-paid memberships in country clubs and luncheon or business clubs are fairly common perquisites for healthcare executives because they provide good venues for off-site business meetings. The business rationale for providing country club memberships is more compelling in a small community than in a big city with multiple venues for business entertaining. Conversely, the rationale for giving executives luncheon club memberships is more compelling in a large city than a small town, and luncheon clubs are generally less expensive than country clubs.

Organizations can offer two good reasons for paying for executives' club memberships. First, membership in a country club or luncheon club supports the local business community. Second, the clubs are among the best places in any community for hospital executives to build relationships with other community leaders. Providing club memberships to executives also gives the trustees ready access to hospital executives and affords them the opportunity to help newly hired executives establish relationships with community leaders and thereby represent the hospital more effectively.

Form and Value of the Perquisite

Employer-paid club memberships entail three types of expenses: initiation fees, membership dues, and business entertainment costs. The most expensive payment is often the initiation fee, which can range from a few thousand dollars to $100,000 and more for exclusive country clubs in major metropolitan areas. Membership dues generally range from $1,000 to $5,000 a year for a luncheon club and from $5,000 to $10,000 a year or more for a country club.

Country Clubs

Country clubs are golf clubs, and their principal utility as a business perquisite is for entertaining business associates—physicians, board members, local business and community leaders, and other healthcare executives. While golf may be the principal activity, members may also conduct business meetings over lunch or dinner at the club.

The value of country clubs as a perquisite is in their exclusivity. Through this perquisite, executives and their families gain ready access to a prestigious private club for golf, swimming, social events, and other entertainment.

Like cars and car allowances, employer-paid country club memberships attract criticism because hospitals pay for memberships only for the employees who could most easily afford to buy their own memberships.

Business or Luncheon Clubs

Business clubs are eating clubs and athletic clubs, and their principal utility as a perquisite is giving executives easy access to local business and community leaders. Some hospitals and health systems use these venues for meetings—especially board committee meetings—over breakfast or lunch. Executives' membership can signal that the hospital or health system is an important participant in the local business community. Luncheon clubs often allow easier access to business and community leaders than country clubs do.

Airline Clubs

Airline clubs are used for working while traveling. They provide access to work stations and wireless capability. At a few hundred dollars per year, they are relatively inexpensive.

Membership in an airline club conveys no particular prestige, but these clubs are similar to first-class travel in that they provide members with comfortable waiting rooms. They are particularly useful for frequent air travelers, but beyond that utility, their value is marginal—primarily a matter of convenience.

Providing a convenient place for executives to work while waiting for a flight can enhance productivity. As memberships in airline clubs are relatively inexpensive, one might expect hospitals and health systems to pay the membership dues for any executive (or any manager or professional) who travels often enough by air to make good use of the club. Employer-paid memberships in airline clubs are not a common perquisite, however. The systems that do pay for airline club membership are those that are geographically dispersed enough to require executives to travel frequently for work.

PROFESSIONAL MEMBERSHIPS

Paying for executives' memberships in professional societies is an ordinary business expense. It is barely identifiable as a perquisite, and not at all identifiable as one if the employer pays dues for all professional employees and managers. Only a pattern of restricting the number of memberships paid makes professional memberships a perquisite.

The business rationale for paying membership dues for professional societies is to promote continuing education and professional development. Membership in professional societies is relatively inexpensive, and the dues should be regarded as an investment, not an expense, because the investment is expected to be repaid many times as employees apply what they learn to solving the hospital's problems and improving its performance.

Professional Societies

Professional societies exist to provide education to members and to advance knowledge in the field. They publish professional journals, organize educational conferences, and offer training programs to members. Memberships in professional societies are a form of continuing education.

Individual Membership Associations

Associations differ from professional societies in that their purpose is to promote the interests of their members. Memberships in individual membership associations have some value in offering continuing professional education and other services that can enhance professional effectiveness, but insofar as they are oriented to protecting and advancing the economic interests of a profession, the business rationale for subsidizing membership is less strong than for a professional society.

Individual Memberships in Trade Associations

Some trade associations have individual members as well as institutional members. Because hospitals and health systems join a number of industry associations, executives of those organizations do not generally join trade associations as individual members, unless they choose to join a trade association that their employer does not join.

CONTINUING EDUCATION

Continuing education for executives is largely about keeping up with the latest developments in the industry—learning how to deal with the latest regulatory changes, how to apply the latest technological developments, what innovations are improving performance elsewhere—and less about earning degrees or credentials or taking standard management courses.

Attendance at professional meetings and industry conferences can easily cost several thousand dollars for a few days, with the combination of registration fees and travel expenses.

All-Employee Benefit

Employers provide continuing education for employees in three ways: internal training programs generally provided on-site during work hours; tuition reimbursement programs that allow employees to attend courses at local trade schools and colleges, often as part of a program to obtain a degree or professional certificate; and reimbursement for expenses of attending educational programs offered by professional membership societies, state and local hospital associations, and commercial training and education programs. This benefit is intended to enhance job- or career-related knowledge and skills. Organizational policies typically specify the types of education that are covered. The all-employee continuing education benefit usually does not cover travel expenses, so employees are effectively restricted to local training programs.

Professional Conferences and Training Programs

Professional societies offer a wide variety of educational programs through national conferences, educational programs held around the country, local chapters, online training, and on-site training. Virtually every professional and administrative discipline in healthcare has its own professional society that offers such programs. Because conferences and programs are generally held in big cities, attendance usually requires travel expenses in addition to tuition reimbursement. Participation is expensive, and attendance is often limited to higher-level managers and professionals.

Industry Conferences

The healthcare industry sponsors numerous trade associations at the local or regional, state, and national levels. They represent hospitals, nursing homes, medical practices, home health agencies, and specialty healthcare organizations. All these associations hold conferences and offer other types of educational programs. Because most of the conferences entail travel, attendance is often limited to higher-level managers and professionals.

FINANCIAL PLANNING

Employers provide basic information about benefits to all employees as part of their benefit program. Thirty percent or more of large hospitals and health systems offer access to professional financial planners and attorneys as a perquisite for executives (Integrated Healthcare Strategies 2010). They do so for the following reasons:

- Recognizing that executives are often too busy dealing with business issues to attend to their own affairs, organizations encourage executives to take care of personal issues such as retirement planning, estate planning, and tax planning through this perquisite.
- Recognizing that basic benefits often do not meet the needs of higher-paid employees, employers use this perquisite to educate executives about the limits on basic benefits.

- Recognizing that supplemental benefits and the rules pertaining to them are complicated, organizations aim to keep executives well-informed through this perquisite.
- Recognizing that executives' higher incomes present special challenges, such as lump-sum taxation of nonqualified deferred compensation and opportunities to voluntarily defer significant portions of their income, employers know that they, too, can benefit from helping executives learn how to optimize the value of their compensation packages.

Form of the Perquisite

Some hospitals and healthcare organizations provide an allowance with which the executives may choose their own planners and decide how to use the allowance. Others hire a financial planner to provide planning services and advice to executives. Still others provide education related to financial planning as part of annual reenrollment in benefits to help executives make decisions about supplemental executive benefits.

Financial Planning

Financial planning in this context is essentially retirement planning—determining how to invest savings, how much one should save while working to increase one's retirement income, and how much income one will have in retirement. This decision-making process dovetails with making decisions about how much income to defer in tax-sheltered retirement savings accounts and how much more to save on an after-tax basis, considering the anticipated amounts of qualified and nonqualified employer-paid retirement benefits and how long one intends to work before retiring. It also entails deciding whether and how to protect family income against the risks of death and disability by buying life, disability, and long-term care insurance.

A financial planning allowance pays the cost of working with a professional to develop a customized financial plan, which can then be used to guide decision making about savings, investments, and insurance. It also pays for periodic reviews of the plan, progress in implementing it, and any alterations needed due to changed circumstances.

Estate Planning

Estate planning aims to protect one's estate from unnecessary taxation and deliver as much of it as possible to the designated beneficiaries in the preferred form (e.g., nontaxable death benefits from life insurance, joint and survivor annuities, income from a trust). Through such planning, executives decide how to package assets to maintain flexibility in their use during their lifetime while preserving the value of those assets for beneficiaries, largely through the use of trusts and insurance.

A financial planning or legal services allowance pays for the cost of developing an estate plan, a will, and a trust, which can then be used as a guide for deciding when and how to shelter assets or protect them with insurance. As with financial planning, it also pays for periodic reviews of the plan, progress in implementing it, and any alterations needed due to changed circumstances or change of mind.

Tax Planning and Tax Return Preparation

Tax planning helps executives decide when to recognize investment gains and losses and whether to defer income voluntarily to avoid current taxation. Tax return preparation allows executives to identify all deductible expenses and tax liability on each type of income to protect current income from unnecessary taxation.

A financial planning allowance pays for the cost of having a tax professional help determine when and how to recognize income and expenses to minimize tax liabilities. It can also be used to pay a tax adviser to prepare and file a tax return for the executive.

Value of the Perquisite

A financial planning allowance typically runs from $1,000 to $5,000 a year. The initial allowance for a financial plan is often higher than the allowance in subsequent years because the bulk of the work in financial and estate planning takes place early on as the planner and the executive determine the goals and structure of a financial plan. A separate legal services allowance, if offered, typically falls within the same value range.

TRAVEL PERQUISITES

Employers recognize that business travel is inconvenient and burdensome, so they often allow certain executives the privilege of flying first class, staying in a first-class hotel, bringing a spouse along on one or more business trips each year, and using an airline club at employer expense. Other employees who travel on business are generally expected to take advantage of the lowest available airfare and patronize modest hotels and restaurants, often subject to limits on hotel and meal expenses. Allowing executives to travel in comfort is a real privilege and a highly valued perquisite.

Because healthcare executives generally do not travel a lot, travel perquisites are not common in tax-exempt healthcare organizations and are often limited to the CEO. Geographically dispersed multihospital systems, however, often require a lot of travel for a few executives, and they may be exempt from the usual rules on travel.

The business rationale for travel perquisites is that they help executives be more productive when traveling on business. Flying first class and having access to an airline club provide more time to get work done.

The rationale for spouse travel perquisites is that they bolster support for family, making business travel less of an emotional burden than it would be otherwise. Some systems, notably those sponsored by Catholic religious orders, allow all executives to bring their spouse along on at least one business trip each year.

RELOCATION EXPENSES

Employers pay moving expenses for executives under two circumstances: when they recruit new executives from a distant location and when geographically dispersed systems ask executives to move to another location. In either case, moving expenses that cover the cost of transporting household goods and other personal possessions are considered a necessary business expense rather than a perquisite.

However, relocation expenses often cover more than the cost of moving household possessions and as such may have value as a perquisite. Employers often pay for several house-hunting trips and temporary housing. Sometimes they cover transactional costs for sale of a house (e.g., Realtor's commission, closing costs). Occasionally they cover losses on the sale of a house or, in locations where housing is unusually expensive, provide a housing allowance to subsidize the incremental cost. Some employers even give newly recruited executives a relocation allowance above the transactional costs it reimburses to pay miscellaneous expenses related to resettling a family in the new location.

While all of these expenses can be thought of as part of the cost of recruiting a new executive or persuading an executive to accept a transfer, they are treated under tax law as additional taxable income for the executive. What makes reimbursement

> **Covering a Loss on Housing**
>
> A large system with a hospital in a resort area provided a housing subsidy to allow the new CEO to buy a house in the community. The system structured the arrangement as a joint investment with the CEO. By the time the CEO moved on to another of the system's hospitals, the market value of the house had fallen. The system bought out the CEO at the original value because it had asked him to move both times. Even though the CEO would have seen the value of his home decline if he had never moved in the first place, the system covered the executive's loss because it had asked him to move both times. Then, because the system had to report the loss it covered as imputed income for the CEO, it decided to pay him a bonus to cover the taxes due, too.

for relocation expenses a perquisite as well as a business expense is that it represents special treatment of executives. Employers sometimes cover moving expenses for other employees, but they generally do not cover all the other costs of relocation.

COMMUTING EXPENSES

A number of large, geographically dispersed health systems have begun to reimburse executives for commuting expenses if they do not live near their workplace. A few single-market health systems and hospitals have also done so.

Most employers have historically required executives to live in the community, as they are expected to participate in community events that may occur outside normal work hours. This requirement makes less sense for a geographically dispersed system than for one whose operations are primarily in one urban area, especially if the system-level executives are not actively involved in managing a local operation close to system headquarters.

To recruit first-choice candidates for leadership positions, systems have found that they may need to allow executives to commute long distances. Some organizations limit this allowance to an initial employment period or cap the number of trips they will cover; others make it a permanent arrangement, as when a candidate cannot or prefers not to move her family to the new location. In these cases, employers sometimes agree to cover the cost of commuting every week to allow the executive to return home every weekend.

TAX GROSS-UPS ON SUPPLEMENTAL BENEFITS AND PERQUISITES

Tax gross-ups, described in Chapter 6, are rarely provided as a matter of policy, but they are sometimes promised in employment agreements or as part of a hiring package. While not common, some hospitals and health systems agree to pay cash bonuses to cover the taxes due on employer-provided cars and car allowances, club memberships, housing allowances, and supplemental benefits for one or a few senior executives.

No good business rationale can be offered for providing tax gross-ups on supplemental benefits or perquisites; they are used only to satisfy executives' expectations. Employers do not cover tax obligations for other employees. Any supplemental benefit or perquisite that incurs taxation is like salary, and executives do not expect employers to cover tax liability on cash compensation. Among the reasons employers cover taxes on supplemental benefits and perquisites are that executives do not always have the choice to decline taxable benefits or perquisites and that a change in plan design or in tax regulations can make a previously tax-sheltered benefit or perquisite taxable.

> ### Moving Perquisites into a Taxable Benefit Allowance
>
> A large medical center in the Midwest folded all perquisites into a taxable benefit allowance. Executives pointed out that this move represented a reduction in value because certain perquisites now covered by the allowance had not been taxable before. Despite the fact that the most valuable perquisites had always been taxable, the medical center agreed to increase the allowance by 40 percent to cover taxes due on the allowance. This increase almost doubled the amount of executives' taxable income attributable to perquisites and positioned the allowance above the 90th percentile for perquisite values in its peer group.

OFFICE SPACE AND FURNISHINGS

Offices and office furnishings are among the most visible and most valued perquisites given to executives. The business rationale for providing executives with a larger-than-average office and comfortable furnishings is that they accommodate meetings and signal status to emphasize the importance of those meetings. The CEO's office, for example, should be large enough to host meetings with groups of people—an entire committee of the board, a group of executives, and so forth. It should also be impressive enough to signal status on a par with board members and major donors.

In reality, as long as the hospital has adequate meeting room space near the administrative office suite, the extra money spent on executive offices is almost pure privilege, with relatively little business rationale.

Size, Location

Offices of the highest-ranking executives are typically isolated in an executive suite. Sometimes the suite is big enough to accommodate all or most executives, but it may be reserved for just the CEO and one or two other executives. Corner offices are often designated for the highest-ranking executives.

Accoutrements

Office furnishing for mid-level managers are generally of standard industrial quality—sturdy, plain, modest, and relatively inexpensive. Office furnishings for executives are often distinctly better and notably more expensive—a high-quality wood desk and bookcase, an extra table, comfortable and stylish wooden chairs with custom upholstery, and attractive lamps. The CEO's office may also feature a high-quality carpet and original artwork, such as paintings or sculpture.

TITLES

The assignment of a title, too, is one of the perquisites most highly valued by executives. Titles carry no economic value, unless they are used as criteria for defining eligibility for incentive compensation, supplemental benefits, and perquisites. They carry a lot of psychic value, however. Directors want to be named vice presidents; vice presidents want to be named senior vice presidents; and senior vice presidents want to be named executive vice presidents.

Because titles cost nothing, some organizations use them liberally. Others use them sparingly, which may irritate executives who have lesser titles than their peers in other organizations.

PUBLIC RELATIONS RISKS

Perquisites attract criticism—especially visible perquisites with significant monetary value, such as cars and car allowances and country club memberships, but also visible ones with only symbolic value, such as reserved parking places and fancy offices. They are difficult to justify to physicians and employees when staff are facing cuts to basic benefits and adjusting to reduced staffing and expenses in their own departments.

Boards and CEOs need to decide if their desire to satisfy executives' expectations of perquisites outweighs the criticism the perquisites inevitably attract.

TAXATION OF PERQUISITES

Perquisites are taxable personal income to the extent that they represent additional, quantifiable compensation. They are not taxable to the extent that they represent ordinary business expenses.

Allowances for any purpose are taxable personal income except to the extent that they are deductible as a business expense on an individual tax return. The employee is responsible for keeping track of business use and deducting the expense from personal income.

Business use of an employer-provided car, a cell phone, a smart phone, or other equipment is not taxable and therefore not reportable as income for the executive, but personal use of these items is taxable and reportable, and the employee and employer both are responsible for estimating and reporting the value of personal use as taxable income for the executive. The same is true for business and personal use of employer-paid memberships in country clubs and luncheon clubs.

Perquisites that are most closely related to job requirements are not reportable as taxable income to executives. Employer-paid professional memberships and subscriptions, continuing education, and attendance at professional and industry meetings are not taxable or reportable. Paying for first-class airfares for executives does not need to be reported as taxable income, but paying for spouse travel does.

CHANGING PATTERNS IN USE OF PERQUISITES

Employers are slowly moving away from perquisites, especially those that have a significant economic value for the executive. This trend began in general industry, as boards reacted to criticism of excessive perquisites at publicly traded companies. Trustees brought this trend to hospitals and health systems and began encouraging them to eliminate employer-paid cars, car allowances, and country club memberships.

When boards have eliminated these perquisites, they have generally increased salaries by the same amount as the perquisites' value—which actually provides incremental income to executives, as the additional salary counts as part of the base for incentive compensation and benefits. Some boards have instead converted perquisites to a perquisite allowance or a taxable benefit allowance to avoid building the value into salary.

The IRS Form 990 requires tax-exempt hospitals and health systems to disclose whether they pay for first-class travel, spouse travel, tax gross-ups, club memberships, or housing allowances. It does not require disclosure of employer-provided cars and car allowances, but it does require their value to be reported. The need to disclose perquisites has reinforced the trend to abandon them.

A similar trend to reduce the value of supplemental benefits has emerged, although it has not yet had much impact on their overall prevalence or value.

Boards are not retreating from paying executives well. Their movement away from visible perquisites reflects their sensitivity to community and stakeholder concerns about the appropriate use of corporate resources. As public criticism of executive compensation continues to press boards to justify the way they pay executives, we should expect to see a decline in the prevalence of perquisites that result in taxable income—cars, car allowances, and club memberships. The trend will not likely affect the employer-paid use of cell phones, smart phones, professional memberships and subscriptions, continuing education, or attendance at professional and industry meetings.

BEST PRACTICES IN USING PERQUISITES

The following is a list of best practices in using executive perquisites:

- Limit perquisites as much as possible to those that have a strong business rationale.
- Avoid perquisites that are especially difficult to justify and those that need to be disclosed on Form 990.
- Replace perquisites that are not clearly justifiable as reimbursable business expenses with a taxable benefit allowance or a salary increase.
- Avoid taking responsibility for the tax consequences of executive perquisites by paying a bonus to cover taxes due on them.

CHAPTER 8

Employment Contracts
and Severance

INTRODUCTION

Employment agreements are nominally used to memorialize the terms of employment agreed to by employer and employee in negotiation over a new job or extension of employment. Most employers try to limit employment agreements to just one or a few executives, and many try to avoid using them altogether. Most employees, of course, do not have employment agreements and seem to have no difficulty getting along without them.

Why do most hospitals and health systems enter into employment agreements with CEOs but not with other executives? Why do some hospitals and health systems enter into employment agreements with all their executives? If these agreements are needed to document terms of employment for the CEO at most hospitals and health systems, how do the other organizations get by without using them?

The answer is surprisingly straightforward—but it entails two answers. First, employment agreements are used when they promise something outside the usual bounds of the executive compensation program. CEOs often negotiate special deals outside the general structure of the executive compensation program, and the terms of those deals need to be documented. Organizations that negotiate special deals with other executives often use employment agreements to document their terms, too. Organizations that do not offer special deals to their executives find that they have less need for employment agreements because compensation, benefits, and other terms of employment are documented in other ways.

Second, CEOs encounter more risks to their employment security than other employees do for the following reasons:

- Every year, some trustees and board leaders turn over; the trustees who hired the CEO could all have left the board five years later. Board turnover leaves the CEO vulnerable to changing expectations.
- The CEO's role is to lead change. She must be willing to challenge the board and medical staff to overcome their reluctance to change processes that have worked well in the past. When the medical staff gets upset, the CEO is usually the first to be blamed and the first to be asked to leave the organization.
- When a hospital loses money several years in a row, the CEO is held accountable and eventually fired.

The presence of these risks helps explain why CEOs of independent hospitals and systems are more likely to have employment agreements than CEOs of subsidiary hospitals and systems. A multihospital system is unlikely to provide special deals to the CEO of one hospital but not to others. The CEO of a subsidiary hospital is less exposed to risk of termination, as accountability for performance is more dispersed among a number of executives and as authority to terminate a subsidiary CEO generally rests with the system CEO or COO, not with a subsidiary board.

It is worth noting that an employment agreement has more value for an executive than for an employer. It guarantees the severance payable on involuntary termination without cause. It not only documents all the special deals a CEO manages to negotiate but also makes any reduction in compensation or benefits (or any reduction proportionately greater than for other executives at the institution) a contractual violation.

An employer gains relatively little value from an employment agreement. Provisions that are meant to benefit the employer include the executive's agreement not to compete against the employer for a period of time, not to disclose confidential information, and not to solicit its employees for employment elsewhere. However, none of these prohibitions is readily enforceable. The employment agreement also documents the executive's commitment to stay on the job for the duration of the term of the agreement, but neither employer nor employee has any obligation to keep that commitment, as employment agreements almost invariably include provisions for termination with appropriate notice. The employer essentially gets a promise from the executive to provide 60, 90, or 180 days' notice before resigning.

Furthermore, an employment agreement limits the organization's ability to change compensation and benefit programs or redefine an executive's job in the aftermath of a merger or reorganization. This limitation is particularly disadvantageous to employers

---

Severance on Voluntary Termination

The board of a new system formed through the merger of a public and a private hospital expressed concern that the political environment might be hostile and its executives would not be able to handle the pressure. It approved a severance policy that would allow executives to collect severance even on voluntary termination within 12 months of the merger. When a newly recruited chief operating officer quit after two weeks on the job and collected a year's severance, the committee changed its policy to allow payment of severance only on involuntary termination.

because most employment agreements now renew automatically unless notice is given.

PURPOSE

Employment agreements have two principal purposes: to define a period for which both parties can agree to work together and to define the terms by which employment can be terminated by either party. Because both parties to an employment agreement have the right to terminate the agreement at any time, the more significant purpose is the agreement on what happens when employment is terminated. Any other employment-related issue can be handled without an employment agreement and is sometimes better handled without one.

An employment agreement nominally offers an executive employment security for a period of time. What it really offers, though, is a guarantee of income security in the form of severance payments if the employer does not keep its promise to employ the executive for the specified period of time.

Some employers use employment agreements for other purposes that may or may not be valid in practice:

- To clarify job responsibilities and performance expectations (but these should be documented instead in a job description, so that minor changes in responsibilities or performance expectations do not amount to contract violations)
- To liberate executives to pursue risky endeavors that could result in the loss of their job (but this can be accomplished with a severance policy or a severance agreement and does not require an employment agreement)
- To document agreements on compensation and benefits to clarify exactly what the employer is willing to pay and the employee is willing to accept

- To offer a foundation for making decisions on how to deal with unanticipated changes due to merger, reorganization, and change of control

Employment agreements are often used to recruit an executive (or a physician), especially to persuade the candidate to give up a secure position elsewhere to accept the new position, which may not be secure and may not be a good fit for either the person or the organization. A severance policy or severance agreement—addressing what the employer will pay if it terminates the executive—provides the same income security an employment agreement does. An offer letter that specifies the severance benefit for the position also achieves this purpose.

Employment agreements are often used to persuade a mature CEO to spend the duration of his career with the current employer. At age 50 or 55, executives recognize that they have plenty of opportunities they will not have five or ten years later, so they are in an ideal position to ask for and get employment agreements that will persuade them to ignore other opportunities and stay with the employer until they retire. The same effect could be achieved with a retention agreement, a new supplemental executive retirement plan (SERP) agreement, or an amendment of an existing SERP agreement.

Another good use of an employment agreement is to document special benefits or perquisites the employer has agreed to provide to the executive, those that lie outside the existing executive compensation program and will not be provided to other executives. CEOs, for example, are often given supplemental benefits and perquisites not provided to other executives and, for that reason, not otherwise documented. This might seem to be the best reason for using an employment agreement, especially considering that the IRS encourages tax-exempt charities to document every benefit and perquisite they provide executives in an employment agreement.

Clarity of Terms

Given that employment agreements are contracts and that contract violation exposes the parties to liability for damages, all the crucial terms in an employment agreement should be expressed clearly. Many agreements, however, include vague terms, and some are so complicated that it is difficult to figure out what they mean. The longer and more detailed the contract, the more likely it is that some terms will be unclear, opening the door to misunderstandings and disagreements, which in turn lead to claims and litigation.

It is incumbent on all parties responsible for the agreement to test it for consequences under various scenarios. What does it say or imply the consequences will be if this happens, or if that happens? Too often, the terms need to be renegotiated at the time a situation arises because the employer and the executive cannot agree on what the terms mean.

By far the most important terms in an employment agreement are those that define different types of termination and their requirements and consequences. Most differences in interpretation of other terms can be worked out as long as these terms are clear—if only because they provide for a cure of what may seem to one party or the other to be a violation of contract terms and because they provide for liquidated damages in the form of severance.

The terms that especially need clarity are those pertaining to involuntary termination for cause, constructive termination, termination subsequent to change of control, and termination on disability; the requirements for giving notice of voluntary or involuntary termination; and rules for curing any apparent violation of contract terms, severance payable on the different types of termination, and other types of payments due on termination (e.g., pro rata payment of incentive awards or deferred compensation, early vesting of deferred compensation). One provision that requires special attention is the consequence of not renewing an employment agreement, as nonrenewal may or may not amount to termination without cause and may or may not require payment of severance.

Definitions of Cause

The reason to define *cause* carefully is to establish limits on the circumstances under which the employer can refuse to pay severance on involuntary termination. Executives, of course, want the term defined as narrowly as possible so that employers have virtually no basis on which to claim cause other than intentional misrepresentation, conviction on a felony charge, or causing irreparable harm to the employer's reputation. Provisions in the employment agreement that allow time for the executive to correct an action that appears to be cause for involuntary termination can make it even harder for an employer to terminate an executive for cause and avoid paying severance. For example, some agreements give an executive 30 days to retreat from a position appearing to be insubordination.

PRINCIPAL ELEMENTS OF EMPLOYMENT AGREEMENTS

The principal elements of employment agreements are listed below and discussed in the sections that follow.

Term (Duration)

Often the first section of an employment agreement, the section titled "Term" sets the start date and the end date for the agreement.

Position Responsibilities

The second section of the employment agreement describes the responsibilities of the position in general terms.

Compensation, Benefits, and Perquisites

The compensation and benefits section of the agreement defines the starting salary for the position and usually includes a provision for future salary increases. It typically says that the executive will participate in whatever incentive compensation plans the employer offers its executives. It also usually states that the executive will be eligible for whatever benefits and perquisites are provided to all other employees or to all other executives, or it lists any special benefits and perquisites provided and describes them in general terms.

Termination

The section discussing termination of employment defines different types of termination as well as *cause* for purposes of determining whether an involuntary termination has occurred for a reason that would relieve the employer from the obligation to pay severance (i.e., involuntary termination for cause). It specifies what notice is required for voluntary and involuntary termination.

Severance Benefits

This section defines the employer's liability for paying severance benefits on involuntary termination without cause.

Noncompetition, Nondisclosure, Nonsolicitation, and Nondisparagement

In this section or sections of the agreement, the executive promises not to compete against the employer for a specified period after termination, disclose proprietary information, solicit employees for employment elsewhere, or disparage the employer after termination.

Severability of Terms

This section states that the contract as a whole will remain valid even if any section of the agreement is declared invalid.

Legal Jurisdiction and Arbitration

This section of the employment agreement identifies the state in which disputes will be resolved and in accordance with whose laws the contract will be enforced. Some agreements have separate sections calling for resolving disputes through arbitration.

Amendments

The process for amending the employment agreement is specified in this section. It always calls for mutual agreement between the parties.

TERMS AND PROVISIONS FOR RENEWAL

Because employment agreements almost always are limited in duration, the provisions for renewal and nonrenewal must be specified. Employers and employees alike think of their jobs, with rare exceptions, as continuing on indefinitely until retirement. Nonetheless, to preserve flexibility and avoid long-term commitments, employers usually do not agree to contract duration longer than three years.

On the other hand, neither employers nor executives want to renegotiate contracts every few years. For this reason, some agreements leave the duration of the agreement indefinite, making the contract more or less perpetual until terminated by one party or the other. Other agreements are "evergreen," with the contract term automatically extended, often a year at a time, unless notice is given of either party's intent not to renew the agreement.

In practice, there is little difference between a perpetual agreement with no specified duration, an evergreen contract with automatic extensions, and an agreement with a fixed, finite term with provisions for renewal. An employment agreement can be terminated at any time by either party, with appropriate notice, so the duration of the agreement is largely irrelevant. And even a contract with a finite one-year term can be renewed indefinitely if both parties agree to that. However, it is important to be familiar with the language used in these types of provisions.

Finite Terms

Some employment agreements have finite terms, with or without provision for automatic renewal. The typical duration for an employment agreement is two or three years. Initial terms are sometimes longer, as are final terms.

Employment agreements with CEOs are often longer than those for other executives. The initial term for a CEO is often three years in duration while those for other executives are often only one year long. Employment agreements with physicians are often one year in duration.

The one advantage to a fixed-term contract with no automatic extensions is that it requires the two parties to talk about renewing the agreement and the terms of the contract. Employment agreements with automatic extensions or with no fixed duration can become obsolete as changes occur in the compensation program or in titles or names.

Automatically Renewable Terms

Some employment agreements provide for automatic extension of the agreement for one or more one- or two-year terms, unless one party decides not to renew. They may have sunset provisions or set limits on the number of automatic renewals so that the employer has no obligation to pay severance if it asks the executive to retire.

Evergreen contracts are an example of automatically renewing agreements. In effect, they are perpetual or career-long agreements, terminable at any time by either party but requiring severance payments on involuntary termination without cause.

Duration of Agreement Versus Duration of Severance Period

No necessary or logical relationship exists between the duration of an employment agreement and the duration of a severance benefit. Ideally, the severance benefit should be defined independent of the duration of the employment agreement so that the consequences are the same regardless of when the executive is terminated—at the beginning or the end of the agreement or sometime in between— and the same in the initial contract period or after the employment agreement has expired or been extended.

Sometimes the severance period is defined as the balance of the contract term. In this case the economic value of the contract must

---

Choose Severance Terms with Care

A new system formed through the merger of three local hospitals developed an employment agreement with its CEO that promised severance for the duration of his five-year employment agreement, with no offset for other employment. The CEO was 60 and recognized that he could collect almost as much in severance as he could by working for another five years. He deliberately took actions that caused the board to terminate him involuntarily, and he collected almost five years' severance after having been on the job for only three months.

---

be paid in full, regardless of how long the executive has worked. Tying severance to the contract term in this way is unusual for two reasons. The term is not long enough to result in a meaningful severance benefit if the executive is terminated in the last few months of an agreement, and it could be too long if the executive is terminated in the first few months of a three- or five-year contract.

Effect of Nonrenewal

Employment agreements generally treat an employer's decision not to renew the agreement as termination without cause. Unfortunately, some employment agreements are ambiguous, leaving the question of whether severance is payable open to different interpretations when the employer chooses not to renew a contract. Because termination without cause requires payment of severance benefits, and because every employment agreement will eventually not be renewed, it is important to explicitly state whether severance is payable when the contract is not renewed so that both parties know what to expect.

JOB RESPONSIBILITIES

The description of the position's responsibilities in an employment agreement is usually general, even vague (e.g., "will perform all the duties required of the chief executive officer," "will perform the duties of the chief executive officer as specified in the corporation's bylaws," "will perform the duties assigned to the position from time to time"). The agreement rarely provides a comprehensive description of the job or a list of accountabilities, and it rarely fulfills the claim that the purpose of the employment agreement is to define or clarify the responsibilities of the position and the performance expectations set for it.

The parties have good reasons for not specifying responsibilities in an employment agreement. Developing a comprehensive list of the responsibilities for a position is nearly impossible, and responsibilities change as the organization changes. Listing specific responsibilities in an employment agreement gives the incumbent the right to think that any responsibilities not mentioned in the contract are not responsibilities of the position.

The proper place to clarify job responsibilities is in the job description, and the proper places to clarify performance expectations are in the job description, the goals and performance expectations set in the performance management and appraisal process, and the goals and performance expectations set in the incentive plan.

COMPENSATION, BENEFITS, AND PERQUISITES

The employment agreement typically documents the starting salary for the position and indicates that both parties expect the salary to increase over time. It documents the executive's right to participate in whatever incentive compensation plans the employer offers its executives and sometimes defines the incentive opportunity for the position. When no incentive plan is currently in place, it may promise to provide an incentive plan, even if only for this executive.

The employment agreement usually states that the executive will be eligible for whatever benefits and perquisites are provided to all other employees or to all other executives. If the executive is promised benefits or perquisites not given to other executives, the employment agreement usually lists them and describes them in general terms (e.g., life insurance covering three times salary) without specifying the structure of the benefit.

Employment agreements are not the best place to document compensation and benefits and perquisites, however, as they change over time. The proper places to document them are in incentive and benefit plan documents and in the payroll system or a memorandum from the chair of the compensation committee to the executive who oversees the executive payroll.

Certainly, exceptions to compensation and benefit programs need to be documented in a manner that clearly overrides other documentation of the standard executive compensation and benefit program, and the employment agreement can be an effective place to do this. Most, but not all, of the customization of compensation packages pertain to CEOs, and most CEOs do receive certain benefits or perquisites that fall outside the parameters of standard executive compensation programs.

The problem with using an employment agreement to document every benefit and perquisite promised to the executive is that each term then becomes a provision that is difficult to change. The executive may argue that any such change amounts to a contract violation warranting payment of severance. It also opens the entire contract to renegotiation every time the employer wants or needs to change the structure of benefits promised in the employment agreement.

TERMINATION AND SEVERANCE BENEFITS

The section on severance benefits is the principal reason for having a formal employment agreement in place. It establishes, before termination occurs, the circumstances under which damages are payable if the agreement is broken.

Severance benefits are intended to provide a financial bridge to carry the employee from one job to the next. They presume that the affected employees have been terminated through no fault of their own but also that they might sue the employer for wrongful termination or discrimination. On the basis of the latter presumption, employment agreements and severance policies typically require the terminated employee to sign a release from claims in exchange for severance payments.

Why do people find severance benefits distasteful? The answer is that severance benefits are payments for not working, generally after having failed in some fashion.

Executives face a higher risk than other employees of being terminated for failures beyond their control, such as the following:

- Failing to impress or please certain key members of the board
- Failing to placate the medical staff
- Failure to impress or please a new boss, especially one who wants to bring prior associates into the organization
- Failure of a merger or a new clinical program to meet the expectations established at the time the merger or new program was approved by the board
- Failing to resolve an intractable problem caused by regulators or third-party payers

They can also be terminated for pursuing policies and strategies supported by the board but rejected by the medical staff, or for pursuing expansions that lead to excessive leverage or other risks that result in poor financial performance when external circumstances change unexpectedly.

Failures by executives are rarely due to lack of effort or good intentions. They often occur after the executive is well established in a successful career and may be the result of nothing more than slowness to adapt to changing circumstances. Therefore, severance benefits have long been a standard and essential part of executive compensation programs in every industry, including the public sector.

Purpose of Severance Benefits

Although terminated employees are generally eligible for unemployment benefits, major employers pay severance benefits for a number of reasons:

- The employer can obtain a release from all other claims (such as age discrimination) in exchange for payment of severance benefits.
- The employer can maintain morale among continuing employees by signaling that it treats terminated employees fairly or even generously.
- The employer can overcome any reluctance to terminate an employee if it feels it is treating the employee fairly or generously.

One more reason for paying severance to terminated executives is that unemployment benefits are capped at such a low level that they do not begin to provide income continuity for high-paid executives.

Severance benefits serve the same function as sick leave, disability benefits, life insurance, and retirement benefits in that they provide a certain level of income security to employees and their families in the event employment is disrupted. Their principal purpose is to provide income continuity for a period while the employee is looking for other work.

For this reason, the duration of severance benefits is typically tied in some way to the length of time required to find another position. It typically covers several weeks for hourly and salaried workers, several months for middle managers, and up to a year or more for executives.

Form of Severance Benefits

The severance benefit is often nothing more than continued payment of salary for a number of months. It sometimes includes a cash payment in lieu of incentive compensation. If the section on severance calls for continuation of certain benefits as well, the agreement will typically list them. It may state that the severance benefit includes continuation of all benefits that can legally be continued; sometimes it calls for payment of cash in lieu of benefits that cannot be legally continued. In the rare instances in which perquisites are included in the severance benefit, they are mentioned specifically. When the severance benefit includes out-placement services, these services are described in general terms, often with a specific limit on their duration or cost.

Severance payments may be guaranteed in full, but they are often suspended or reduced if the executive obtains other employment.

Severance is typically payable over time. Sometimes, however, severance is payable in a lump sum, often in conjunction with termination following a change of control. Now that tax regulations treat severance over a set limit (two times $250,000 in 2012) as deferred compensation, which becomes taxable immediately on termination, employment agreements may begin specifying whether a portion of severance will be payable as a lump sum.

Relationship to Years of Service

Severance benefits are sometimes related to length of service on the premise that an employer owes more security to a long-term employee than to a new one. Severance schedules for nonmanagerial employees, for example, often increase by a week or two for every year of service from a base of two weeks. Those for executives may increase by a month for every year or two of service from a base of 6, 9, or 12 months, to a maximum of 18 months.

For executives, involuntary terminations are more common in the first year or two than after 5, 10, or 20 years and more common for new employees than for those promoted internally. These terminations may be the result of a flawed selection and screening process in which both the employer and the employee make a decision that does not turn out well. When, for example, an employer has recruited an executive from another reasonably secure position and moved him across country only to find that hiring him was a mistake, the employer has as much obligation to treat that executive fairly as another who has put in five or ten years of service. Severance, after all, is not a form of deferred compensation that grows over time but a form of insurance intended to provide income security while the executive finds another position.

Organizations have no reason to assume that long-service executives will take longer than recent hires to find the next job. On the other hand, if we look at severance as a form of liquidated damages or as payment for release from claims of wrongful termination, providing more severance to a long-service employee than to a recent hire may be wise, especially if the long-service executive has performed well over that time and the termination may not have been entirely justifiable—or may not appear to be if a claim were tested in court. Looking at the severance benefit as a release from claims of wrongful termination, however, we would expect to see more severance given to people in protected classes, especially older workers (involuntary termination may amount to forced retirement for an older executive). We do not see this, though. Severance rarely varies with the potential economic damage of termination. Severance is, for example, no higher, on average, for a 62-year-old employee than for a 32-year-old with the same years of service and with the same rank.

Tenure-related severance schedules for executives typically start with a low base, often just six months, which is generally not an adequate period for a high-paid executive to find another comparable position. The justification for providing additional severance to a long-service executive, then, is that the base level is not adequate to ensure income continuity. Providing additional severance to longer-service executives when the base level is already adequate, as with 12 months' severance, makes less sense.

Release from Claims

Employment agreements usually require a release from all claims as a condition of receiving severance benefits. This requirement shifts severance from an insurance-like benefit to a settlement for damages or a payment for release from claims, or at least buys the employer something of value in exchange for payment of severance.

The release is primarily from claims of unlawful discrimination under state and federal civil rights laws. For these releases to be enforceable, they must meet a number of specific requirements set forth by the Age Discrimination in Employment Act (ADEA) of 1967 that demonstrate the releases are "knowing and voluntary" (knowingly and voluntarily entered into by the employee). The release must be clearly written so it can be easily understood by the terminated employee, explicitly refer to claims under the ADEA, advise the employee to consult an attorney before signing the waiver, give the terminated employee 21 days to consider the offer, give the employee 7 days to revoke the waiver, and exclude any rights or claims that may arise after the waiver is signed. These requirements serve as a template for release agreements signed as a condition of receiving severance.

Termination Without Severance

Not every type of termination warrants payment of severance. Severance is generally payable only on involuntary termination without cause, or some variation of that, such as constructive termination or termination due to change of control. It is not normally payable on voluntary termination or termination for cause. However, given the utility of severance in obtaining a release from all claims, many employers prefer to pay severance rather than terminate someone for cause, and they are often willing to label involuntary termination as voluntary, even though that may mean paying severance on voluntary termination.

Likewise, severance is generally not payable on termination due to death, disability, or retirement. Income security for these terminations is normally provided through life insurance, disability insurance, and retirement benefits, so there is usually no need or justification for paying severance in these cases.

TYPES OF TERMINATION

Because the amount and duration of severance benefits vary by type of termination, it is important to define types of termination clearly in the agreement.

Voluntary

Voluntary termination is voluntary for the employee. Because it is the employee who is breaking the employment contract or deciding not to renew it, the employer owes the terminating executive no severance benefits. The employee is only entitled to compensation for work completed as of the date of separation, payment of any benefits payable on termination, and payment for any accrued but unused paid time off.

Involuntary Without Cause

Cause is often defined as willful misconduct or gross negligence that causes or is likely to cause significant harm to the organization, refusal to follow orders or written directives, intentional breach of company policy, or commission of a felony or conviction of a crime involving moral turpitude. The definition sometimes includes willful and continued failure to perform the responsibilities of the position, but this interpretation is usually accompanied by an opportunity to cure the situation. It may also include behavior that causes or is likely to cause harm to the employer's reputation or it may refer to fraud, embezzlement, or theft of company assets.

Poor performance is either explicitly or implicitly excluded from the definition of *cause* because performance is subjective, can be constrained by circumstances, and can be difficult to prove in court.

Involuntary termination without cause is termination by the employer and hence involuntary for the employee. The majority of terminations are for performance below expectations, in recognition of a mismatch between the demands of the job and the talents of the incumbent, or in acknowledgment that the job has changed and requires a different type of leadership. *Without cause* does not mean without good reason; it only means that the reason for termination does not meet the narrow definition of *cause*.

Many employers choose to label involuntary termination as voluntary, to protect the reputation of the terminated executive, but still pay severance to obtain a release from other claims or an agreement not to disparage the employer or solicit other employees to work elsewhere. If the employer wants to label a termination voluntary and still pay severance, it should develop and document a good rationale for it, as it amounts to giving charitable assets to the executive as a parting gift on voluntary resignation. This kind of parting gift exposes the terminated executive to intermediate sanctions.

Involuntary with Cause

Involuntary termination with cause is also termination by the employer, but for a reason that meets the definition of *cause*. Termination for cause generally does not call for paying severance to the terminated executive, presumably because the threat of disclosure of the reason for the termination is sufficient to convince the terminated employee to sign a release from claims of unjustifiable termination. On the other hand, the employer, too, often wants to avoid adverse publicity about the cause for termination and sometimes agrees to pay severance to keep the reason secret—which transforms the termination into one without cause.

Constructive Termination

Constructive termination is voluntary termination "for good reason." The employee has good reason for resigning because the employer has in some important way broken the employment agreement. Constructive termination is usually defined in terms of reduction of responsibility or in pay or benefits (sometimes expressed as disproportionately greater reduction in pay or benefits than any reduction for other executives). Constructive termination clauses are not often used with executives other than the CEO. Constructive termination for a CEO would include any reorganization that gives the CEO any role other than that of the chief.

Constructive termination allows the executive to claim severance for involuntary termination without cause because the employer has in effect terminated him involuntarily by taking away his job or by reducing his pay to the point that he is likely to quit. Employment agreements almost always include a provision for curing the issue by requiring the executive to submit a written complaint and giving the employer an opportunity to fix the situation.

Elimination of an executive benefit or some part of the executive compensation program does not amount to constructive termination if it is even-handed and affects all executives to the same degree. It can be difficult to eliminate a benefit that is provided only to the CEO, however, without it being considered constructive termination, unless the employer substitutes another benefit of equal value.

Change of Control

Termination pursuant to a change of control is also voluntary termination for good reason—the good reason being that the position has been significantly altered by a change in reporting relationship, in the nature of the organization, or in the nature of job responsibilities. Change of control usually arises from a merger, an acquisition, or a joint venture agreement in which the executives of one of the organizations involved are no longer the executives of the new organization. It can also arise from a turnover in board membership, as when half or more of the elected or appointed board members are replaced, or when one faction of a board forces another faction to resign and replaces it with trustees who agree with the controlling faction.

Provisions for termination on change of control fall into three types: single trigger (voluntary), double trigger (constructive), and double trigger (involuntary).

- Single trigger (voluntary) termination provisions allow an executive to resign, claim constructive termination, and collect severance solely on the basis of a change of control. This type of termination provision is generally limited to CEOs, as theirs is the job most affected by a change of control.
- Double trigger (constructive) termination provisions allow an executive to resign, claim constructive termination, and collect severance only if job responsibilities are diminished or compensation is reduced following a change of control. This type of termination provision is sometimes extended to a few executives in their employment agreements, but it is more often added to employment or severance agreements or a severance policy as a special provision at the time an organization is contemplating a merger or sale, and it is often limited to the circumstances contemplated at that time.
- Double trigger (involuntary) termination entitles an executive to severance if she is terminated or her job is eliminated after a merger or sale (or other change of control)—even if she is offered another job in the new organization. Sometimes the distinction between termination without cause and termination for cause is eliminated for a year or so following a change of control to enhance the security of executives who are likely to be displaced. The change-of-control provision may be limited to a specified period following the change of control.

CEO contracts often have single-trigger change-of-control provisions. If the CEO survives the change of control to serve as the CEO of the parent organization or if he is content with the position he is offered after the change of control, even if it is diminished in some way, he will presumably keep the job and not exercise the right. But if the change of control leaves the CEO in a position he finds untenable, the provision allows him to claim constructive termination and collect severance. Employment agreements usually limit the time during which the CEO can claim constructive termination to 6 to 12 months following the change of control.

When change-of-control provisions are used with executives other than the CEO, they are often confined to mergers, sales, or joint ventures (as opposed to change in composition of the board), and they generally do not allow executives to claim severance unless the executives are involuntarily or constructively terminated within a set period following the change of control.

Severance following a change of control is often enhanced in one way or another to encourage executives to support changes that may be in the best interests of the organization, even if not in the best interests of the executives themselves. It is not uncommon to see the duration of severance benefits increase, for example, by half or to see the basis for severance payments enhanced by the addition of a benefit or incentive not otherwise counted.

Nonrenewal

Termination for nonrenewal may be either voluntary or involuntary termination, depending on who decides not to renew the agreement. If the executive decides not to renew, her action is considered the same as any other voluntary resignation. If the employer decides not to renew the agreement, that action is essentially the same as any other involuntary termination without cause.

Most employment agreements require advance notice of a decision not to renew. If the contract provides for automatic extensions, the notice period is sometimes as short as 90 or 120 days, but more often it is 180 days or one year. If the contract does not provide for automatic extensions, the notice period is generally 180 or 360 days. The notice period is typically longer for CEOs than for other executives, and it is typically longer for multiyear contracts than for single-year contracts.

Retirement

Termination due to retirement could be either voluntary or involuntary, but it is usually assumed to be a voluntary, intentional withdrawal from career-oriented employment at typical retirement age that allows an executive to begin drawing retirement benefits from a qualified or nonqualified retirement plan.

More and more executives seek flexibility in determining when they retire and in defining what retirement entails. As a result, the notion of retirement has become ambiguous. Executives who retire early often go on to other careers or even accept executive positions at other hospitals or systems. Executives who continue working, or need to do so to amass additional retirement benefits, sometimes work to age 68 or even 70.

If the employer decides when the executive is to retire, the employer is in effect terminating the executive involuntarily without cause, unless the employment agreement clearly requires retirement at a certain age or date or allows the employer not to renew the agreement without paying severance after a certain age or date. Forced retirement at age 63 with little or no advance warning, for example, is clearly involuntary termination without cause, whereas nonrenewal of an employment agreement after age 65 or 68 may not be.

Some institutions find it necessary to ask an executive to retire early because they want new leadership. They may offer the executive an enhanced retirement package, a transitional employment opportunity, or a consulting arrangement. More often, they pay severance, even enhanced severance, in recognition that retirement assets grow significantly in the last few years before retirement and that it can be difficult for an executive to obtain a comparable position after age 60.

Death or Disability

Employment agreements typically mention termination due to death or disability to make it clear that no severance is payable on death or disability. They sometimes state that the benefit payable at death is life insurance and on disability, long-term disability insurance.

PAYING SEVERANCE AT RETIREMENT

Any employment agreement, severance agreement, or severance policy that is open-ended promises severance on any involuntary termination without cause. Unless the organization has a mandatory retirement age for executives or a sunset clause on the promise of severance, an executive who is willing to work can continue to do so until being asked to retire, which amounts to involuntary termination without cause and entitles the executive to severance. Because many executives are now choosing to work beyond normal retirement age, it is becoming more common for executives to be paid severance when they retire.

Boards' emphasis on succession planning is driving some portion of this trend. Once boards begin planning for CEO succession, they sometimes decide to install the successor on a timeline that differs from the CEO's intended retirement date or from the term of the CEO's contract. That action often leads to asking the CEO to retire earlier than planned and results in paying severance at retirement. If severance is one year's salary, it may not be a significant issue for the organization, but in cases where severance is three years' salary or total compensation, it can be expensive.

When boards sign employment agreements with CEOs or approve severance policies, they do not expect to pay severance at retirement—especially if they sponsor a supplemental retirement plan designed to provide a fully competitive retirement benefit at age 62 or 65 proportional to years of service. Once a retirement benefit has matured to a fully competitive level, the hospital or health system has no good reason to pay more than a minimal amount of severance, even if a board asks the CEO to retire a bit earlier than he had wanted to retire. The best rationale for paying a modest amount of severance is to obtain a release from claims.

Few employment agreements should explicitly address the question of whether severance benefits are payable to executives of retirement age. Some attorneys believe that making any distinction in severance benefits related to age is essentially age discrimination. Others believe that making such a distinction for executives is permissible. One approach to avoiding unexpected claims for severance at retirement is to have a sunset clause in an evergreen contract that ends automatic renewal past a certain date or age or after a certain number of automatic extensions, then negotiate a final term of employment with an explicit retirement date, after which no severance is payable. Another approach is to reduce the amount of severance payable on involuntary termination without cause to zero or to a modest amount after a certain date or age coinciding with normal or expected retirement age.

AMENDMENTS

Employment agreements virtually always make some provision for amendments so that the agreements do not need to be replaced in their entirety when modifying one term or another. Amendments require documentation of any change in writing and signatures indicating the approval of both parties to the agreement.

The more specific the terms of an employment agreement, the more likely it will need to be amended. CEO agreements are amended more often than agreements with other executives because the former tend to be more specific and to have terms that do not apply to the executive group as a whole.

The terms that most often call for modification are those relating to severance and retirement benefits. Supplemental retirement benefits are frequently described in their own agreements, and those benefits can be changed by amending the plan document without amending the employment agreement. Any change in severance benefits typically calls for an amendment to the employment agreement.

Employment agreements become obsolete over time as circumstances change. Automatically renewable evergreen agreements are more likely to become obsolete than agreements with a fixed term, as their fixed term is likely to expire before they become obsolete. However, any multiyear agreements should be reviewed periodically to identify amendments that should be made to keep them from becoming obsolete.

DOCUMENTING SERPS AND RETENTION AGREEMENTS

Supplemental retirement plans and retention agreements must be documented as well, and even though they pertain only to payment of a benefit, they resemble employment agreements in certain ways. They deal with length of service rather than term of employment, termination and pro rata payment of the benefit rather than severance, and sometimes agreements not to compete after retirement.

Retention and SERP agreements can easily be documented in the employment agreement if their structure is straightforward and uncomplicated. More often than not, however, they are just complicated enough to warrant separate documentation. In these cases, the provisions in the employment agreement mention the benefit as part of the promised compensation package, describe it briefly, and refer to the formal document governing the plan.

SEPARATION AGREEMENTS

Separation agreements typically document the date of termination, all types of compensation and benefits payable, and severance benefits. They document any provisions for outplacement assistance and call for return of all employer-provided equipment. These agreements also require a release from all claims; offer the terminated employee time to consider the offer and time to rescind acceptance of the offer; suggest—albeit subtly—that the employee consider having an attorney review the agreement; include non-compete, nonsolicitation, nondisparagement, and nondisclosure agreements; and often require that the terms of the separation agreement be kept confidential.

Most of these terms can usually be found in an employment agreement, but obtaining a separate release in exchange for severance payments helps reinforce the other agreements at the time of termination. Institutions often develop separation agreements to obtain a release from claims regardless of whether or not severance is payable. If severance is payable, the separation agreement typically includes an agreement not to compete while severance is being paid as a condition for obtaining the benefits.

If an executive does not have an employment agreement and is not covered by a written severance agreement, a separation agreement represents a final opportunity to obtain signed noncompete, nonsolicitation, and nondisclosure agreements, as well as a release from claims.

Separation agreements can be useful even when no severance is payable, as, for example, when an executive is terminated for cause and both the executive and the employer prefer not to disclose the reason for termination or the terms of any settlement. Even when no severance is payable, a separation agreement can be used to obtain a release from claims and an agreement not to disparage the other party. It can even be useful on voluntary termination to remind executives of prior agreements not to compete and not to disclose confidential information. (Some kind of payment will likely be required, however, to persuade an executive to voluntarily sign an agreement with new constraints, like a new noncompete agreement.)

SEVERANCE POLICIES, AGREEMENTS, AND PRACTICES

Many employers have general severance policies covering the workforce as a whole. Some do not, however. Their lack of a policy does not mean that they never pay severance, only that they decide on a case-by-case basis whether to pay severance and how much to pay. Some hospitals and health systems have severance policies covering executives only and avoid a broad policy covering the workforce as a whole.

Some employers use severance agreements as a substitute for employment agreements. Like an employment agreement, a severance agreement represents a contract with an individual, but one focused only on termination and severance. It offers executives just as much protection as an employment agreement.

Severance practices do not, however, as they leave unanswered the question of how much, if any, severance will be paid until it is negotiated at the time of termination.

The differences among severance policies, severance agreements, and severance practices are discussed in detail in the following paragraphs.

Policies

Severance policies prescribe when severance will be paid and how much will be paid to which employees. These policies sometimes distinguish between general layoffs and other types of termination but rarely go into the types of distinctions found in employment contracts.

When these policies apply to the workforce as a whole, they often use a sliding scale related to tenure—a base level of severance and an incremental level for each year of service up to a maximum (e.g., two weeks plus a week per year of service to a maximum of eight weeks). The policies sometimes use different scales for hourly and salaried employees, managers, and executives.

Many hospitals and health systems have a severance policy that covers executives specifically. The policy clearly defines which positions are eligible, under what conditions severance is payable, how much severance will be paid (defined as a number of months of salary continuation and whether benefits will also be continued), and whether severance will cease on reemployment or be offset by other earned income.

Severance policies for executives typically require that the executive sign a release from all other claims and an agreement not to compete for the duration of the severance period as conditions of receiving severance. Severance policies often prescribe the same severance benefits for all executives, although the scale sometimes varies with rank or years of service (e.g., a longer severance period for senior vice presidents than for vice presidents, or an extra month for every year of service over 10 years up to a maximum of, say, 18 months).

Agreements

Severance agreements are special agreements dealing only with severance. They are not unlike employment agreements, except that they are usually not customized for position or incumbent. They are, in effect, short versions of employment agreements that are focused only on the consequences of terminating employment. These agreements typically have no set term, as they do not entail an agreement to employ the executive for a period of time.

The agreements clearly distinguish involuntary termination without cause from other types of termination—voluntary termination,

termination for cause, termination due to death or disability—because it is the only circumstance under which severance becomes payable. The agreements sometimes require notice for voluntary termination, involuntary termination, or both. They may address constructive termination and allow payment of severance benefits if the complaint of constructive termination is not resolved. They sometimes also address what severance is payable on termination following a change of control.

More often than not, severance agreements require executives not to compete with the employer during the severance period as a condition of receiving severance benefits. They may include nondisclosure, nonsolicitation, and nondisparagement requirements as well.

Executives are generally more comfortable with severance agreements than with severance policies because signed agreements are contracts and seem to provide additional security, but they ultimately serve no purpose that cannot be handled by a severance policy.

Practices

Severance practices are those patterns and precedents that emerge as a result of decisions the organization makes about severance in the absence of a policy. If the pattern is reasonably consistent, it becomes a precedent and takes on one characteristic of a severance policy—providing prima facie evidence of discrimination if the severance paid to a member of a protected class is less than that typically provided to other employees. If an organization avoids setting severance policy to maintain flexibility, it should also avoid establishing a standard practice, or it risks losing that flexibility as the standard becomes a clear precedent.

Discretionary Negotiation

Discretionary negotiations for severance are individual discussions to establish agreement on the amount of severance to be paid, either in the absence of or in addition to that which is called for by the policy or agreement.

Some boards object to severance policies because they view them as the starting point for executives to negotiate more than what is promised by policy. Boards that prefer to determine severance on a case-by-case basis, however, open the door to negotiation. If they gain flexibility by not having a policy, so do executives. Executives often know how much severance other executives received upon termination, and they can cite the most generous settlement among those provided to their former colleagues as a starting point in their own negotiations.

Of course, boards that establish a pattern of negotiating additional severance instead of adhering to their severance policy essentially encourage executives to negotiate for more than the policy promises. Employers that establish a policy and stick with it typically do not have difficulty enforcing the policy.

Circumstances do arise in which severance needs to be negotiated. These situations are generally related to handling benefits that fall outside of the standard severance package, rather than about the duration of salary continuation. The following are examples of such circumstances:

- An executive terminated shortly before a SERP vests is likely to negotiate payment in lieu of the SERP benefit she would have received if the termination had occurred after the SERP vested.
- An executive terminated in the last year or two before normal retirement age may negotiate additional severance to maintain income prior to drawing down retirement benefits.
- A new executive terminated soon after moving and buying a house is likely to negotiate some additional severance pay to cover moving expenses or transactional costs related to selling the house.

None of these negotiations are meant to enrich the basic severance benefit. Instead, they are special arrangements for dealing with a situation in which additional damages help offset the economic harm caused by the termination.

Discrimination Risks

Most executives fall into one or more protected classes. Almost all are over 40 years of age and therefore protected against age discrimination; a significant portion are female and thus protected against sex discrimination; more than a few have disabilities; and some are members of racial or religious minorities.

Sooner or later, in the course of basing severance on negotiation or subjective judgment, an employer will make the mistake of offering less severance to a member of a protected class who will be able to substantiate a claim of employment discrimination. A policy followed consistently is an effective bar to that type of claim.

BEST PRACTICES IN EMPLOYMENT AGREEMENTS AND SEVERANCE POLICIES

Following is a list of best practices in employment agreements and severance policies:

- Avoid using employment agreements except when essential for recruiting a new high-level executive. Use a severance policy instead, or use offer letters for new recruits and a retention agreement when needed to retain a senior executive.
- Identify elements of the compensation and benefit program, including perquisites, in an appendix to employment agreements, rather than in the body of the agreement, and make it clear that the board may change incentive opportunity and benefits from time to time, so that changes in the program do not break the agreement.

- Avoid binding the organization to any obligation future trustees would not be willing to meet or would not want to defend to the public.
- Avoid binding the organization to any liability that is indeterminate because of the duration of the commitment (e.g., a defined-benefit SERP for an executive with more than 15 years to normal retirement age).
- Use a sunset clause on any evergreen or open-ended employment agreement to give both parties the opportunity to renegotiate terms as the executive approaches retirement age (e.g., at age 60).
- Define severance as a specific benefit rather than as continuation of compensation and benefits for the duration of the agreement.
- Keep commitments to severance modest; limit severance to 24 months for the CEO and to 12 months for other executives.
- Keep the base for severance limited to salary and medical benefits and life and disability insurance.
- Define severance so that it declines to a modest level at retirement age.
- Make severance payments contingent on not having found other comparable employment, and offset severance by other earned income, at least in the second half of the severance period.
- Set the duration of post-termination noncompetition and nonsolicitation agreements the same as the duration of the severance benefit.

CHAPTER 9

Governance of Executive Compensation

It's not clear whether charitable board members are doing their due diligence and independently scrutinizing the justification for these compensation packages, or whether they are blindly accepting the recommendations of outside consultants. I've seen many boards rubber-stamp compensation recommendations from these consultants that might be considered excessive by the general public.

—Senator Charles E. "Chuck" Grassley

INTRODUCTION

Boards tend to view their CEO as a colleague and as the undisputed expert on all things related to healthcare. They tend to follow the CEO's lead in most areas, which essentially amounts to approving the CEO's recommendations. Even when members of the board disagree with the CEO on an issue, they generally accede to the CEO's wishes in the end. But governing executive pay is about saying no as much as it is about saying yes.

To achieve the right balance between agreeing to and rejecting executive compensation requests, between paying enough and paying too much, and between the board's responsibility to govern executive compensation and the CEO's need to pay enough to recruit and retain talented executives, the board must exercise a measure of control by establishing a policy and process for the compensation committee to follow. In approving the compensation philosophy and the charter for the compensation committee, the board defines the committee's responsibilities, the process the committee is expected to follow, and its obligation to report specific information related to executive compensation to the board.

Regardless of how much direction the board gives the committee when it delegates this responsibility, the board as a whole is accountable for seeing that executive compensation is governed well. The Internal Revenue Service (IRS) has ruled that boards of tax-exempt organizations cannot completely delegate the governance of executive compensation to a committee. Therefore, the board should make sure it

- is comfortable with the process the compensation committee follows,
- requires periodic reports on the process and results,
- requires assurance that the committee is following best practices to ensure that the institution complies with laws and regulations, and
- obtains assurances from the committee that the organization will not be publicly embarrassed by any decision the committee is making.

A Cautionary Tale in Lack of Governance

The CEO of a small system received $9 million from a supplemental executive retirement plan (SERP) when he retired. How had he come to be awarded such an extraordinary retirement benefit? Here's how it happened.

The SERP had been approved by the system's board 25 years earlier, and right from the start the board had promised a generous retirement benefit of 80 percent of salary, well above average for the mid-1980s. Over the years, the

→

---

board's compensation committee made several adjustments to the SERP at the CEO's request but did not apprise the entire board of the details. Fifteen years after the SERP was first approved, the CEO persuaded the compensation committee to change the basis on which the SERP was calculated from salary to total cash compensation (salary plus incentive award). This adjustment made sense to the committee because the CEO's compensation was highly leveraged with above-average incentive opportunity. What neither the committee nor the CEO acknowledged at the time was that the change put the retirement benefit even further above average. Several years later, the CEO convinced the committee to base the retirement benefit on a higher level of total cash compensation than he was being paid by redefining salary as 15 percent above a 75th percentile salary. His argument was based on two factors: that the compensation policy called for paying him at the 75th percentile and that a long-service CEO should be paid in the upper part of the salary range. Although the CEO's proposal had some basis in logic, the committee likely did not understand how much this salary redefinition distorted the relationship between the CEO's retirement benefit and his pay while working. Finally, shortly before retirement, the CEO persuaded the compensation committee to increase incentive opportunity in exchange for making the incentive plan riskier by tying awards more closely to the organization's financial performance. The board gladly agreed because it had wanted to encourage executives to increase operating profits. The committee got exactly what it wanted—a much better operating margin—but at the cost of substantially increasing the CEO's generous SERP. This time, too, the committee did not understand how much this change in incentive opportunity would affect the CEO's SERP.

$\longrightarrow$

As the CEO's retirement date approached, the compensation committee began reviewing its liability for the SERP and was surprised to find that the CEO's retirement benefit amounted to $9 million. The committee had no recollection and no understanding of how the SERP had grown to be so rich.

Because the compensation committee had shared only general information about executive compensation with the entire board, the changes in the formula for calculating the SERP benefit had never been approved by the board. Furthermore, the CEO had been accustomed to leading the committee's deliberations, and the committee had not hired a consultant to help it analyze and understand the CEO's proposals. Because the organization's performance was good and the CEO was recognized as a successful leader, the committee had found it difficult to deny any of the CEO's requests.

The size of the liability for the SERP was the result of a failure of governance. The compensation committee had not insisted on using an objective third party to help it understand the CEO's proposals; had not understood the ramifications of the changes it approved; had not sought the board's approval for these changes; had not asked for regular annual evaluations of the liability for the SERP; had not made any effort to establish a presumption of reasonableness by evaluating the CEO's total compensation; and had rubber-stamped every benefit request the CEO had made. Nonetheless, the hospital had a contractual obligation to pay the SERP, and it paid the CEO the full $9 million. Combined with the pension plan and the CEO's Social Security benefit, the SERP was equivalent to a retirement annuity of 120 percent of final average total cash compensation.

LAWS, RULES, PRINCIPLES, AND BEST PRACTICES

Boards and their compensation committees should consider four sets of rules or principles to guide their work in overseeing executive compensation:

1. Federal and state laws and regulations
2. The organization's bylaws, committee charters, and policies
3. Principles of governance
4. Best practices in governing executive compensation

Each trustee should know the rules and principles pertaining to executive compensation well enough to be able to question whether the board and committee are complying with the rules and following best practices in governing executive compensation.

Federal and State Laws and Regulations

Three principal sources of federal and state rules establish the basic requirements for governance of executive compensation:

- *Internal Revenue Code (IRC) § 501(c)(3)*, which proscribes private benefit (running a tax-exempt charitable organization for the benefit of private individuals) and private inurement (giving an insider a portion of a charitable organization's revenues, earnings, or assets or paying someone more than the value she provides in return)
- *IRC § 4958*, which authorizes the IRS to penalize participants—both the beneficiary and the individual(s) who knowingly approves it—in an "excess benefit transaction" between a tax-exempt charity and an insider, whether paying too much (more than fair market value) for services delivered or engaging in a bargain sale (paying too much for assets purchased or selling assets for too little)

- *State laws governing not-for-profit corporations,* which define the board's responsibility for acting in good faith, making decisions in the best interests of the corporation, and exercising the care an ordinarily prudent person in a similar position would exercise under similar circumstances

While states' attorneys general have authority to enforce state nonprofit corporation law, some have begun to use state law governing charitable trusts as well to charge a number of organizations with misuse of charitable resources in paying executives too much.[1]

(Another set of federal laws and regulations pertaining to physician compensation prohibits tax-exempt hospitals and health systems from paying physicians for referrals or paying them more than is commercially reasonable. Boards and their compensation committees should also be familiar with these regulations. Physician compensation entails greater legal and regulatory risk than executive compensation does, and many boards are not paying enough attention to these risks.)

Bylaws, Charters, and Policies

The most specific rules a board and its compensation committee must follow are often those found in the organization's own bylaws, committee charter, and policies. They usually charge the board as a whole with determining compensation for the CEO or delegate that responsibility to a standing or ad hoc committee of the board. When the bylaws delegate the responsibility to a committee, they often broaden the charge to overseeing the executive compensation program as a whole or overseeing compensation for some group of executives.

Whereas bylaws state the responsibility for overseeing executive compensation, or the CEO's compensation, in general terms, committee charters typically describe the responsibility in far more detail and even prescribe the process the committee should use in overseeing executive compensation. Committee charters are a relatively new development for hospital and health system boards. Many boards instead choose to articulate these rules in a charge to the committee or a policy statement.

Most boards have a number of policies pertaining to elements of executive compensation, whether the organization's compensation philosophy or other factors address salary administration, incentive compensation, benefits, perquisites, or travel and entertainment expenses. These policies establish rules the committee must follow and may include direction on how the programs are to be governed.

Formal plan documents for incentive plans and executive benefits are, in effect, board policies, too. They set rules the committee must follow and may also prescribe how the plans should be governed.

Principles of Governance

The principles of governance are embedded in corporate law, legal precedent, bylaws, and common practices, whether as a specific set of rules or a set of abstract principles. The most important principle underlying the board's responsibility for governing executive compensation is that the board needs to determine the shape and limits of the executive compensation program so that management is not determining its own compensation, and it must monitor and audit the compensation practice to see that any decisions management makes in administering executive compensation are consistent with the policies and limits the board has set.

A related principle is that boards set policy while management determines how to manage the organization within constraints set by the board. The distinction between governing and managing is critically important in defining the purview of the board in overseeing executive compensation. Many boards and their compensation committees were once content to determine pay for the CEO and allow the CEO to determine compensation for other executives, as long as it was generally consistent with board or committee policy. Recent efforts to strengthen board oversight of executive compensation have clarified the boundary between the board's responsibility for governing and the CEO's responsibility for managing. Boards now generally accept responsibility for overseeing the executive compensation program as a whole, whether just by periodically reviewing compensation for the executive team as a whole, by approving annual salary increases and incentive awards for senior executives, or at least by approving employment agreements, contractual commitments to executives, any new incentive or benefit plan for executives, and significant modifications to executive compensation plans.

Best Practices in Governing Executive Compensation

Best practices in governing executive compensation represent the collective wisdom of governance authorities on the ideal way to handle this responsibility. While different authorities have their own lists of best practices, which do not entirely agree with one another, enough consensus has been reached that boards can generally be sure that any practice prescribed as a best practice is at least a good one.

Sources of best practices include governance organizations, consultants, and attorneys, but the ultimate sources are rules set by stock exchanges or by Congress and the IRS, recommendations from governance organizations and the IRS, and the experience governance authorities have gained from watching boards and their committees deal with executive compensation.

In the not-for-profit sector, the most respected sources for best practices in governing executive compensation are The Governance Institute, the Center for Healthcare Governance, the American Governance & Leadership Group, BoardSource, and the IRS.

The process defined in IRC § 4958 for establishing the presumption of reasonableness is widely recognized as the principal set of best practices for governing executive compensation in the tax-exempt sector.

THE BOARD'S RESPONSIBILITY FOR GOVERNING EXECUTIVE COMPENSATION

The board can delegate responsibility for overseeing executive compensation to a committee, but it is accountable for decisions and actions of its committees. Delegation does not relieve the board of responsibility for defining policies pertaining to executive compensation or monitoring the committee's decisions and actions to ensure that they are consistent with board policies.

Historically, many boards have allowed compensation committees to oversee executive compensation without requiring that they report any details of their work to the board. In turn, committees have been reluctant to share information about executive compensation with the board because boards of hospitals and health systems typically include members of the medical staff. Their concern has been that any disclosure of executive compensation to the board will be soon disclosed to members of the medical staff and eventually to the workforce as a whole.

Now that the disclosures of executive compensation on IRS Form 990 are readily accessible to anyone who wants to see them, now that boards must disclose whether they have reviewed the form before filing it, and now that transparency and full disclosure are recognized as best practices in governance, boards expect to receive detailed information about the compensation committee's actions and decisions related to executive compensation, and committees have begun to comply.

Unless the board insists on approving compensation philosophy, the structure of the executive compensation program, and any contractual obligations with senior executives, and unless it insists on receiving regular reports from the committee on its decisions and actions, the board is not fulfilling its fiduciary duty to oversee executive compensation.

Delegation to a Committee

Most boards delegate oversight responsibility to a compensation committee rather than attempt to handle it on their own. The following are five good reasons for doing so:

1. Governing executive compensation is a highly technical task, so boards delegate this responsibility to those most able and willing to handle it.
2. Governing executive compensation well requires so much time that it cannot easily be accommodated at full board meetings.
3. Where pay levels for executives are significantly higher than those of most trustees, boards prefer that this responsibility be handled by trustees who are comfortable addressing income at this level.
4. Executive pay is controversial enough that boards may want to limit the decision making to a small number of trustees.
5. Some trustees, notably those who are physicians, have a conflict of interest with regard to executive compensation, so they should not be involved in making decisions about it.

Boards that try to govern executive compensation in regular meetings generally do not fare well unless the program is simple and does not involve incentive compensation or supplemental benefits. Just overseeing an incentive compensation plan could take two full meetings of the board, one to set goals and one to determine awards. Even small committees need plenty of time to debate, and the greater the number of trustees involved in determining executives compensation, the longer it takes to reach agreement. The requirements for establishing a rebuttable presumption of reasonableness are burdensome, too, and it is difficult for an entire board to meet them unless it is willing to devote significant meeting time to governing executive compensation.

Holding the Committee Accountable

Boards that delegate responsibility for governing executive compensation to a committee should provide enough guidance that the committee knows how to act on the board's behalf. It should then hold the committee accountable for doing a good job by requiring the committee to report its actions and decisions in summary form or in as much detail as the board wants and by specifying the decisions the committee should bring to the board for approval or ratification.

Composition of the Compensation Committee

The board should establish, either in its bylaws or in the committee's charter, specifications for the composition and leadership of the committee and the process by which members and the chair are chosen. Bylaws often specify the number of committee members and prescribe the process by which members and the chair are appointed. They often name the chair of the board as the chair of the compensation committee. Some bylaws name the board's officers as the members of the compensation committee. This rule occasionally poses a problem because officers may have conflicts of interest that might disqualify them from serving on the compensation committee.

Bylaws rarely specify qualifications for committee membership, but charters often do. Just as finance and audit committees expect their members to be financially literate, compensation committees should expect their members to be able to understand the metrics used in incentive compensation, the financial projections used to estimate retirement benefits and liabilities, and the complex regulations pertaining to supplemental benefit plans. Without these skills, members will not be in a position to question or challenge analyses and recommendations presented by management or consultants.

Scope of the Committee's Governance Role

The board should determine the scope of the compensation committee's role in governing executive compensation because it reflects the scope of the board's role in overseeing compensation. In practice, the decision is usually made by the committee, but it should be ratified by the board, as the committee is operating under a charge from the board as a whole. The days when the compensation committee alone would decide what elements of executive compensation it should oversee and what it should allow management to govern are over.

The most fundamental issues in determining the scope of the committee's responsibility are deciding which positions are within the committee's purview, which ones should be included in the committee's annual review of compensation, whose compensation should be approved by the board or its compensation committee, whose incentive awards need to be approved by the board or committee, how physician compensation should be overseen by the board to ensure compliance with regulation, and how CEO performance appraisal should be conducted. These decisions should not be made to suit the preferences of the current chair or the CEO, but to give the board the ability to defend its governance process to regulators and other external stakeholders.

The board should use a disciplined process to determine the committee's scope of responsibility and document the decision in board minutes or the committee's charter for two reasons:

- The risk of intermediate sanctions for any executive whose compensation is not approved by the committee
- The risk of adverse publicity from public disclosure of executive compensation on IRS Form 990

In the past, some committees limited their purview to the CEO or a handful of senior executives. Others have historically determined compensation for all executives, even a large group of 30 or 40 positions. The introduction of intermediate sanctions regulations encouraged committees to approve compensation for all executives who might be subject to the regulations, and the revised IRS Form 990 encouraged committees to expand their purview even further to cover all executives and physicians whose compensation must be publicly disclosed. As boards have discovered, though, it is not always clear which positions are subject to intermediate sanctions regulations, and it is only those positions whose compensation needs committee approval to be protected from risk of penalties. As a result, many committees are still debating which executives should be included in the annual review.

Special Executive Programs

The scope of the board's or committee's role in overseeing executive compensation must also be defined to cover all special compensation and benefit programs for executives (and perhaps for physicians, unless theirs are handled in some other fashion). Boards generally do not govern pay and benefits for the workforce as a whole, except through the budgeting process, but they should oversee any special programs for executives, especially those in which the CEO participates, so that executives are not managing their own compensation. The norm is for the board or the compensation committee to oversee executive incentive plans, executive benefits, executive perquisites, severance arrangements for executives, and any employment contracts with executives. The governance of these programs is discussed in more detail later in the chapter.

Executives' travel and entertainment expenses should also be reviewed by a committee—the audit committee or the compensation committee—to ensure that none slide across the boundary from expenses to additional compensation.

Bylaws and Charters

Bylaws and charters are the sets of rules boards use to govern themselves and the process they use to govern the hospital or health system. Bylaws explain how a board is supposed to operate across all of its responsibilities. The sections of bylaws defining the roles of committees are usually too short to clearly enumerate a committee's responsibilities or explain how it is supposed to operate.

Charters are the equivalent of bylaws for a committee. They set the rules by which a committee operates; define the responsibilities of the committee; prescribe the process the committee is expected to follow, including the responsibility to report to the board; and sometimes define the process by which the committee is to govern itself.

Formal committee charters are a relatively new development in governance. Their function is to formalize the process that the board used in the past to delegate responsibilities to committees. Often this process was little more than a brief charge documented, if at all, in meeting minutes or in a sentence in the bylaws describing the role of the committee.

In the absence of formal charters or clear charges, committees operate on the basis of precedent. Operating by precedent can work pretty well as long as committee membership is fairly stable. It poses challenges, however, as committee membership and leadership change, especially if committees meet only once a year with nothing but oral tradition to explain the process to new members. Even when membership is fairly stable, members often have difficulty remembering exactly what they are expected to report to the board or bring to the board for approval.

Trustees generally prefer informality to formality, and they usually regard their responsibility for governing themselves as far less important than taking care of the hospital's business. Boards seldom take time to adequately orient new members to the board's rules and processes or to evaluate and strengthen those rules and processes. As a result, committees sometimes develop charters or charges that do not agree with the bylaws or operate in ways that conflict with the charter or bylaws. Unless committees have formal charters requiring them to periodically evaluate the process by which they operate, they are probably not fulfilling all their responsibilities, following the rules the board has set for them, or meeting best practices in governing executive compensation.

Purpose of a Charter

The purpose of a charter is to set the rules the board wants the committee to follow in handling the board's responsibilities, to communicate the rules to all committee members so they understand their role, and to make it easy for the committee chair to lead the committee and see that it meets all its responsibilities. To serve this purpose, a charter needs to be fairly detailed.

Content of a Charter

The charter for a compensation committee generally covers six types of material: (1) the role of the committee or its purpose; (2) its membership and leadership, the duration of members' terms, and the process for selecting members and the chair; (3) the committee's responsibilities; (4) the process the committee is to follow in meeting its responsibilities; (5) requirements for reporting to the board; and (6) the committee's process for governing itself. Sometimes the charter duplicates some of the rules in the bylaws about meetings, quorums, and voting.

A charter for the compensation committee should cover this material in sufficient detail that members understand their responsibilities and the chair knows how to lead the committee.

Purpose statement. A brief statement of the committee's role in carrying out the responsibilities delegated to it by the board.

Makeup of the committee. Statements that identify (1) the number of members the committee should or may have and the process for appointing them, or a list of the officers who are ex-officio members of the committee, and (2) the chair of the committee, or the process for appointing the chair.

List of responsibilities. A list of each committee responsibility, including most or all of the following:

- Recommend to the board a compensation philosophy.
- Recommend to the board the general structure of the executive compensation program.
- Recommend to the board any major change to the executive compensation program, including any new program or benefit.

- Determine compensation for the CEO, including salary, incentive compensation, benefits, perquisites, severance, and any contractual terms.
- Approve compensation for other senior executives potentially subject to intermediate sanctions.
- Administer executive incentive programs.
- Appraise the performance of the CEO (or determine and coordinate the process for doing so).
- Periodically review total compensation for all executives.
- Select, hire, and supervise any consultant, attorney, or other adviser who provides data and advice to the committee.
- Review the disclosure of executive compensation in IRS Form 990 before filing it.
- Periodically review the compensation philosophy and any major policies pertaining to executive compensation.
- Periodically review the structure of the executive compensation program, including incentive plans, executive benefits, and perquisites.
- Periodically review contractual arrangements with executives (e.g., employment agreements, severance agreements or policy, supplemental retirement plans).
- Periodically review the process for approving reimbursement of executives' expenses.
- Determine whether, when, and how to communicate with stakeholders, the press, and the public about executive compensation.

Process requirements. A list of any performance expectations for the committee, including most or all of the following:

- Meet several times a year.
- Distribute the agenda and materials for the meeting well in advance.
- Follow a process that establishes and maintains a rebuttable presumption of reasonableness.[2]
- Document the process and decisions in timely minutes.

- Report decisions to the board, either after each meeting or once a year.
- Bring to the board for approval recommendations on matters the board retains for itself.
- Evaluate the committee's charter and performance annually.

Requirements for reporting to the board. Specifications for what the committee must bring to the board for approval, what the committee must bring to the board for information, and how and how often the committee should report its decisions to the board.

Committee's process for governing itself. A charge to periodically review the committee's charter and evaluate its performance.

The contents of the charter vary according to the board's and the committee's agreement on responsibilities and process; the amount of prescriptive detail specified; the breadth of the committee's responsibilities; and the board's decisions to assign certain responsibilities, such as performance appraisal or review of expense reimbursement, to committees other than the compensation committee.

Considering the time-consuming nature of these responsibilities, a committee needs more than one or two meetings a year, unless the compensation program is simple and the committee's responsibilities are limited to compensation. Any board that allows its committee to meet just once a year ought to be worried about what issues are not getting enough attention.

RELATIONSHIPS AFFECTING EXECUTIVE COMPENSATION GOVERNANCE

Relationship Between the CEO, Board, and Consultant

In most areas of governance, the board tends to follow the CEO's lead. Executive compensation is one area, along with choosing or terminating a CEO, in which the trustees are expected to make decisions independent of the wishes of management. But the boundary between governance and management in this area has shifted recently. While many boards once limited their oversight of executive compensation to determining pay for the CEO (and approving goals for the incentive plan, insofar as those goals are used to determine an award for the CEO), they are now expected to control compensation for any executive who may be subject to intermediate sanctions—and not just salary increases but also incentive awards, supplemental benefits, perquisites, severance, and any other contractual terms. Some boards have been doing this for years, but others are still learning how far they want to go.

Friction over this boundary is not uncommon. CEOs want to be able to decide how other executives are paid. But the regulatory efforts to strengthen governance over the past decade have encouraged boards to be more involved in overseeing pay for the executive team as a whole and emboldened them to challenge, reject, or even change CEOs' decisions. Having boards exercise tighter control of executive compensation has exacerbated friction over turf and changed the dynamic in compensation committee meetings.

The boundary separating board and management turf varies from one organization to another and, to a lesser degree, from one committee chair to another and from one CEO to another. New committee chairs with experience leading compensation committees in publicly traded firms tend to impose a more rigorous process on the committee than previous chairs did. Committees that have generally followed the CEO's lead on executive compensation often begin to exert more control when the CEO retires and a new one takes over.

With this shift in the boundary between governance and management has come a shift of the consultant's obligation from the CEO to the compensation committee, further exacerbating the friction. In the past, the consultant was often chosen by, supervised by, and obligated to the CEO to retain the client relationship. The consultant could only retain the relationship by attending to the CEO's wishes and representing them when working with the committee. In the new paradigm, the consultant is chosen by the committee and is supposed to promote and facilitate the committee's efforts to exercise appropriate control of executive compensation. Some committees even ask the consultant not to show reports to the CEO before the committee sees them.

The pendulum may have swung too far in this direction, as the CEO should exercise considerable influence over executive compensation. The ideal situation is a collaborative working relationship between the compensation committee and the CEO and between the consultant and the CEO in which the committee and the consultant both maintain enough independence to be completely objective.

Role of the CEO
Despite the shift to more board control, the CEO still plays a significant role in shaping the executive compensation program and determining pay for other members of the executive team. It consists of presenting recommendations to the committee based on the CEO's perspective of what it takes to attract, retain, and motivate executives. The recommendations can pertain to compensation philosophy and policy; the peer group used to determine competitive pay levels; the shape of the executive compensation program; the goals used for incentive plans; and salaries, incentive awards, titles, promotions, and promotional increases for other executives.

When it comes to his own compensation, the CEO's role changes. The board or compensation committee determines the CEO's pay. It is totally appropriate, however, for the CEO to communicate any expectations or requests to the committee or committee chair, and even to negotiate with the committee to obtain what he wants, whether an increase in pay, a supplemental benefit or perquisite, a retention incentive, or an employment agreement.

Role of the Committee
Unless the board chooses to exercise control of the program, the compensation committee has the bulk of the responsibility for determining the shape of the executive compensation program;

determining compensation for the CEO; seeing that compensation for other executives conforms to board policy; evaluating the effectiveness of the compensation program; seeing that incentive compensation plans work well; and ensuring that total compensation, including retirement benefits and severance, is reasonable and represents an appropriate use of the organization's resources.

This responsibility entails governing the compensation program well and avoiding problems that arise if the committee does not govern it well. Good governance in this area includes following best practices; promoting compliance; seeing that the program is properly documented and that the committee's process and decisions are appropriately documented in timely minutes; exercising enough diligence that the committee's decisions will not embarrass the organization; working with the board in a spirit of transparency and full disclosure; and developing a plan for addressing any adverse publicity about executive compensation.

To meet its responsibilities, the compensation committee must make sure the data it uses are appropriate and any advice it relies on is unbiased. It should decide how to obtain the data it uses—whether to engage a consultant or get survey data from the state hospital association or from management; see that the data represent pay practices of appropriate peers; and select, hire, and directly supervise any consultant or other adviser it uses to make sure the adviser operates independently of management and understands that it is working for the committee.

Role of the Consultant

The consultant's role is to help the compensation committee do its job well by giving it appropriate comparability data, presenting the data in such a way that the committee understands them, providing information about trends and issues pertaining to executive compensation, alerting the committee to any regulatory issues requiring attention, advising the committee on changes it may consider making to the program, and answering questions committee members may raise. If the committee requests it, the consultant should help the committee strengthen its governance process. The consultant's goal should be to keep the committee well informed and help it make decisions it will not regret.

Specifically, the committee expects the consultant to provide help with or advice on the following:

- Defining the peer group and selecting organizations that fit the group's definition
- Collecting and analyzing the data from the peer group
- Comparing pay, benefits, and total compensation at the committee's institution with those at organizations in the peer group
- Organizing the data and the analysis so they are easy to understand
- Determining competitive salaries and increases
- Deciding whether the incentive plan, benefits, or perquisites should be maintained or changed
- Making the committee's governance process more effective
- Documenting its process and decision making in a way that clearly demonstrates the committee's diligence in governing executive compensation and—to the degree that it does— meeting the requirements for the rebuttable presumption of reasonableness

Compensation committees may also seek assistance from a consultant in modifying elements of the executive compensation program; providing formal, written assurance that compensation for highly paid executives is reasonable; and providing education to the committee and the board. Such education may cover regulations, new developments, best practices in governing executive compensation, or new member orientation. The committee may also ask its consultant to deliver an annual overview of the executive compensation program to the board. This service may be the most valuable one the consultant can provide, as no committee member or executive can field trustees' questions as effectively as the consultant can, put the details of the compensation program into context, or assure trustees that the committee is governing executive compensation well.

Collaboration Versus Independence
Both the committee and any consultant it uses are supposed to be independent of management, so that they can be objective in dealing with executive compensation. The committee cannot meet the requirements for a presumption of reasonableness unless each member of the committee is independent[3] or if it relies on comparability data from a consultant who is not independent. While the IRS has provided no standard definition of *independence* for a consultant, it has indicated that a consultant is independent as long as (1) she does not have prior social or business relationships with the executives whose compensation is being evaluated and (2) the executives whose compensation is being evaluated do not play a role in selecting the consultant or in supervising her work. Some boards worry that a firm that does more work for the organization's management than for the committee or that has worked closely with the management for a long time is not likely to be independent or totally objective. Maintaining independence, however, does not preclude collaboration, and collaboration is essential to the relationships among the committee, the consultant, and the CEO.

A consultant to the compensation committee is caught in the divide between governance and management, even though the consultant works directly for the committee, not for management. The committee expects the consultant to be totally objective and not unduly influenced by management. Like trustees, however, the consultant depends on management to provide critical information about the organization's executive positions, compensation and benefit programs, recruitment and retention issues, competitive challenges, business plans and objectives, and performance relative to the goals of incentive plans.

The only way a consultant can avoid being influenced by management's views is to rely exclusively on written documents rather than interviewing management to obtain information. But this approach does not work because documents never tell the whole story. The solution to this problem is for the board to take a practical approach to information gathering and encourage collaboration while insisting on objectivity. Most committees understand that the relationship among the consultant, the committee, and the CEO can be effective if they make it clear that the consultant works for the committee, the committee expects the consultant to be objective, and the committee expects management to respect the consultant's need to maintain independence and objectivity.

Relationship Between the Board and the Committee

Just as the trustees' expanding role in governing executive compensation can cause friction between the board and management, it can also cause friction between the board and its compensation committee. In the past, committees often told the board little more than that it had completed its duties—determined a salary increase and incentive award for the CEO or reviewed and approved salaries and incentive awards for a group of senior executives. Many boards did not expect more detail because they had never received more and they understood executive compensation to be a confidential personnel matter.

The efforts to strengthen governance and increase transparency have spurred boards to request more information from the committee about executive compensation. Some boards now insist on ratifying all the decisions the compensation committee makes.

The committee should not assume that it has the latitude to decide what to disclose to the committee. That decision should be made by the board. However, most boards allow the committee to decide what it should report to the board, and most committees make those decisions on their own. Some committees even decline

> ### Blunder Deprives Compensation Committee of Authority to Act
>
> A well-respected academic medical center terminated its CEO and paid severance. The board had never seen the CEO's contract and was surprised at the amount of severance payable—three years' compensation in this case—on involuntary termination without cause. It was so upset at having to pay the severance that it relieved the compensation committee of its authority to make decisions without gaining board approval. This change dramatically altered the dynamic between the board and the compensation committee. The board does not have trust in the committee's ability to perform its governance function and now requires full disclosure. Furthermore, the board's decision to limit the committee's ability to act provides committee members with little reason to invest time in committee work.

to honor trustees' requests for more disclosure. Needless to say, boards have good reason to want more information than committees are inclined to disclose, and this sometimes leads to friction between the committee and the board.

Committee Proposes, Board Approves

Boards should delegate administrative control, rather than policy-setting activity, of the executive compensation program to the compensation committee. The committee should not be authorized to approve major elements of the program or contractual obligations such as employment agreements, severance policies, or supplemental retirement plans without the board's approval, if only because a contractual obligation can long outlive members' terms on the committee and board. Instead, the committee should propose to the board the executive compensation philosophy and any related policies, all major elements of the executive compensation program, all contractual agreements with executives, and any major changes to the board-approved program.

Once the board has approved the executive compensation philosophy and the shape of the program, it should generally be content with asking the committee to keep it informed, in as much detail as the board wants, and to bring any significant changes to the program and any new contractual commitments to the board for approval. Administrative decisions should not require board approval.

Special Deals Impede Transparency

One of the largest and most respected health systems in the United States has a representative board made up of trustees from each of its hospitals. Like other representative boards, trustees tend to have as much loyalty to the institution they represent as to the system. The system has had to negotiate special deals with certain executives to bring them on board to avoid distorting internal pay relationships. For example, it agreed to offer long-term incentive opportunity to two newly hired executives rather than pay higher salaries, so now these CEOs have a special deal that the CEOs of the system's other hospitals do not have.

While the compensation committee believes in transparency and full disclosure, it is reluctant to fully disclose this arrangement to the board for fear that the information will cause friction and the committee will be pressured to offer the plan to the other hospital CEOs. So the committee showed the board total compensation for the executives without indicating that the two hospital CEOs had special deals, judging this to be sufficiently transparent.

Overseeing Incentive Compensation

The board is more involved in overseeing incentive compensation than other elements of executive compensation. At the very least, it controls some or most of the goals used in the incentive plan insofar as it approves the budget and operating plan and whatever goals they include. Some boards even reserve the right to approve the goals for the incentive plan, once they have been chosen by the committee. Most boards have received a year-end report on performance before the compensation committee has determined awards and have had ample opportunity to let members of the compensation committee know their assessment of that performance.

The committee's role in overseeing incentive compensation is to select performance measures and goals from an operating plan and set of goals that have already been approved by the board. Goal-setting and, to a lesser degree, evaluation of performance are often handled collaboratively with other committees. For example, the finance committee takes the lead in establishing the budget for the year, including any financial goals it entails, and then helps the compensation committee determine awards related to those goals, and the quality committee sets quality-improvement goals for the year and may help the compensation committee determine awards related to these goals.

Multi-institutional systems sometimes use a collaborative approach whereby the boards of each operating unit set the goals for that unit and evaluate its performance at the end of the year. The compensation committee selects goals from the set approved by the entity boards, weights them, and notifies the entity board of these decisions. At the end of the year, the entity boards evaluate performance and the committee relies on these evaluations to determine incentive awards, then shares its decisions with the entity boards.

Approving and Monitoring Supplemental Executive Benefits, Perquisites, and Employment Agreements

Supplemental benefits and employment agreements entail ongoing obligations and liabilities that stay in place for years, often undergoing little scrutiny, until the liability comes due. For this reason, supplemental benefits and employment agreements should be approved by the board, not just by the compensation committee, and perquisites should be approved by the board, due to the ongoing risk they pose of attracting adverse publicity.

But getting board approval for benefits or perquisites that entail ongoing liabilities is hardly sufficient without ongoing disclosures about the size of the liabilities and the risks to the organization's reputation.

The board should be reminded regularly of each element of the executive compensation program, so newer members can never claim not to know about them—especially those that entail significant liabilities, such as SERPs and severance and retention incentives, and those that are most likely to be criticized as an inappropriate use of resources, such as cars and car allowances and country club memberships. As the board is ultimately responsible for the committee's decisions about executive compensation, and as trustees who have never served on the compensation committee are just as exposed to risk of criticism over executive compensation as committee members, they have a right to be reminded regularly of the elements of the program that expose them to that risk. Not reminding them regularly deprives them of the opportunity to terminate, freeze, or change these programs.

Avoiding Intermediate Sanctions

When the board delegates responsibility for overseeing executive compensation to the compensation committee, it should insist that the committee follow the process for establishing a rebuttable presumption of reasonableness. The risk of intermediate sanctions may be low, as long as compensation is clearly reasonable, but the risk of criticism for laxity in governing executive compensation is high, regardless of how reasonable executive compensation is, and questions in IRS Form 990 require tax-exempt organizations to disclose whether they are following this best practice.

Charging the committee with establishing the presumption forces the board and the committee to specify the committee's authority and any limits on that authority, and it forces the committee to determine which executives are "disqualified persons" covered by the regulation. It sets an expectation for diligence that helps protect the board and an expectation that the committee will report to the board whether it is indeed meeting the requirements for the presumption. To protect itself, the board should insist that the committee report its process, not just its decisions, to the board, in a way that demonstrates that all the requirements have been met. One easy way to do this is to give the board minutes documenting the committee's process every time it approves compensation for an executive covered by intermediate sanctions regulations. After all, documentation of good process is just as important as the process itself, as any IRS audit of executive compensation will focus primarily on documents.[4]

Compliance with Regulation

A key committee responsibility that should be clearly identified in the committee's charter or charge is ensuring that the organization complies with all laws and regulations pertaining to executive compensation. Of course, the committee cannot by itself ensure complete compliance, but it can take the following steps toward achieving it:

- Set an expectation for management to comply with regulations.
- Require a periodic audit by internal or external counsel, the chief compliance officer, or internal or external auditors.
- Require management to provide an annual report on its efforts to ensure compliance.
- Ask its consultant to identify any compensation issue, policy, or practice that may be a compliance risk and inform management and the committee of new regulations requiring a change in the executive compensation program.

The laws and regulations pertaining to executive compensation are too numerous and complicated to expect committee members to know them all, but the committee should also expect management and any advisers it uses to provide enough education that members are aware, at least, of the range of regulations affecting the executive compensation program.

Transparency and Full Disclosure

Boards of many tax-exempt hospitals and health systems have adopted standards calling for transparency and full disclosure when and where appropriate. The IRS requires full disclosure of executive compensation in Form 990; requires that the forms be made available to anyone who asks to see them; and posts the forms on the Internet, where they are readily available to the public. While some compensation committees treat executive compensation as confidential, both to the public and to the entire board, and prefer not to disclose any information sooner than required and in no more detail than required (even knowing that the information will be available to the public about 10 months after the end of the fiscal year), more and more committees are making a commitment to transparency and publish Form 990 on their website. Some publish articles on executive compensation in their employee newsletter when their Form 990 is released to the public.

Because questions about executive compensation arise unexpectedly from a variety of stakeholders and are directed to trustees and executives, not just to members of the compensation committee, the committee should establish a protocol for dealing with questions and requests for information. Each compensation committee must determine the protocol most appropriate for its organization.

Defending Decisions to Stakeholders and Regulators

With accountability for governing executive compensation comes accountability for explaining the program to stakeholders.

If the committee believes the compensation philosophy is appropriate, the structure of the compensation program is appropriate, executive pay is reasonable, and the committee's process is diligent, it is in a good position to defend the program from any criticism it attracts. If the committee is not comfortable defending the program or some aspect of the program, committee members should change it.

The committee should find it easy to defend its decisions if it can assert that it is following best practices in governing executive compensation in the following way:

- The committee is made up entirely of independent trustees who are leaders in the community, respectful of community values, dedicated to the institution's mission, and careful to make decisions that are in the institution's best interests.
- The committee is following the board's policy, making sure that compensation is consistent with a policy developed to allow the organization to attract and retain the caliber of leadership talent it requires to meet the community's needs for high-quality, patient-focused care.
- The policy calls for setting compensation on par with similar leading healthcare organizations so that it is competitive, appropriate, and reasonable.
- The committee follows best practices in governing executive compensation, makes sure it gathers reliable data on compensation from similar organizations, and obtains advice from an independent consultant or adviser with expert knowledge of the field.
- The committee is confident that the compensation of all the institution's executives is reasonable and appropriate.

If a more detailed explanation of the organization's compensation program is requested, it can be based on the fact that the hospital is one of the biggest employers in the community and operates in a highly complex business, requiring extraordinary leadership skills to deal with all the challenges facing healthcare providers today—inadequate reimbursement, narrow margins, community demand for expert services in a broad range of specialties, the extraordinary cost of the technical equipment required to meet that demand, and the challenges of running a complex business 24 hours a day, 365 days a year.

Compensation committees should view these queries and criticisms as opportunities to talk about the caliber of the institution they govern, the talent of its leaders, and the success of the institution in meeting the needs of the community. In that context, they can explain executive compensation as a means to provide a valuable and critical community service.

BEST PRACTICES IN GOVERNING EXECUTIVE COMPENSATION

Following is a list of best practices in governing executive compensation:

- The board should establish a separate compensation committee charged with overseeing executive compensation.
- The committee should be given a charter that spells out the process it should follow, including its obligation to report to the board.
- The board should require that all members of the committee be independent directors with no conflict of interest related to executive compensation.
- The board should see that all members of the committee are able to understand the kinds of data and issues they need to consider in overseeing executive compensation, either by appointing trustees who have experience with the process or by providing ample education in the subject.
- The committee's charter should set an expectation that it follow the process for establishing a rebuttable presumption of reasonableness to minimize the risk of intermediate sanctions.
- The committee should approve compensation for any executive (and for any physician leader, unless another committee

handles physician compensation) who is or may be a disqualified person potentially subject to intermediate sanctions.

- The board should guide the committee's decisions by establishing a compensation philosophy or policy that defines how competitive executive compensation should be, relative to a peer group of comparable organizations.

- The board should make it clear that any major new compensation or benefit program, or any significant change to its structure, especially if it is a significant departure from past practice, needs approval by the full board.

- If the committee uses a compensation consultant to gather comparability data, it should select the consultant and guide the consultant's work. If it decides to collect data on its own, it should make sure that it has several sources of data, understands the data, and makes sure the data are appropriate. It should avoid using data gathered, interpreted, or presented by management.

- The committee should insist that the comparability data it uses represent total compensation (salary plus bonus or incentive compensation plus benefits plus perquisites), not cash compensation alone.

- The committee should insist that the compensation data it uses come from organizations similar to theirs and represent pay for jobs like those at their organization.

- The committee should make its decisions in executive session on any matter that concerns the CEO and any other executive who serves as staff to the committee. These executives may be present while the comparability data is being presented, offer suggestions and even recommendations, and answer questions asked by committee members, but they should then be excused during the committee's deliberations and decision making.

- The committee should allocate plenty of time to deliberations. It usually takes two or three meetings a year to adequately fulfill the committee's responsibilities, especially if it has responsibility for evaluating the CEO's performance or reviewing physician compensation as well as executive compensation.

- The committee should insist on having the opportunity to consider any major change to the executive compensation program in two separate, consecutive meetings.

- The committee should insist on getting reports, recommendations, and other information it needs to make well-informed decisions far enough in advance of a meeting to have ample time to review them.

- The committee should document its decisions in a way that meets the requirements for a rebuttable presumption of reasonableness and demonstrates the committee's diligence in carrying out its responsibilities.

- The committee should review the annual disclosure of executive compensation on the hospital's Form 990 and see that it is also reviewed by the board as a whole before it is filed.

- The committee should exercise control of any incentive plan in which the CEO participates by reauthorizing the plan each year; establishing the performance measures, goals, and weights for the plan at the beginning of the year; reapproving participation in the plan; evaluating performance and determining awards at the end of the year; and authorizing payment of any awards earned.

- The committee should periodically review any executive incentive plan in its entirety to evaluate its effectiveness in supporting the organization's tax-exempt mission, to monitor participation in it, and to understand how goals and awards for executives relate to goals and awards for other participants.

- The committee should exercise control of any other special compensation program or benefit for executives by deciding who is allowed to participate and monitoring the way the plan is used.

- The committee should periodically review standing liabilities related to executive compensation, such as retirement obligations and severance, to make sure it is familiar with them and understands how increases in compensation affect them. It should also periodically remind the board of these obligations and liabilities.

- The committee should annually review its charter, the process it has followed, and the committee's performance in achieving its accountabilities for the year.
- The committee should provide an annual report to the board, reminding the board of its compensation policy, disclosing the CEO's compensation in full, providing a general overview of the competitiveness of compensation for other executives, explaining the process the committee follows, and summarizing the decisions it has made over the year.

NOTES

1. The most notable recent example is the effort of Minnesota Attorney General Michael Hatch to force Allina Health System and its board of directors to restructure (Catlin 2001; Scheck 2001).

2. There are three requirements. (1) The compensation arrangement and the total value of the resulting compensation (cash + benefits + perquisites) must be approved in advance by an authorized body (e.g., a committee) made up entirely of individuals with no conflict of interest with respect to the compensation under consideration. (2) The authorized body must obtain and rely upon appropriate comparability data on total compensation for functionally comparable positions in approving the terms of the compensation arrangement or increase in salary or total compensation. (3) The authorized body must document in timely minutes its decisions and the bases for the determination that compensation is reasonable. The minutes must identify the terms approved and the date of approval, the members present during debate and how they voted, the comparability data relied upon and the way it was obtained, and any action taken by a member who had a conflict of interest with regard to the transaction. If the compensation approved is higher than the comparability data obtained, the minutes must also record the rationale for determining that the compensation approved represents fair market value.

3. Four criteria are listed for determining whether a director (or another individual participating in approving compensation to establish the presumption of reasonableness) has a conflict of interest with regard to executive compensation, all of which must be satisfied: not a "disqualified

person" participating in or economically benefiting from the compensation arrangement under consideration or a family member of the disqualified person; not in an employment arrangement subject to the direction or control of a participating disqualified person; not receiving compensation or other payments subject to the approval of a participating disqualified person; and not having a material financial interest affected by the compensation arrangement. A disqualified person is an individual in a position to exercise substantial influence over the affairs of the organization at any time during the five years before the date of the transaction.

4. The IRS has a checklist of the information it expects to find in minutes. To make sure the minutes provide the evidence an IRS auditor may look for in determining whether the committee has met the requirements for the presumption, the minutes should include all the information listed below.

- The board or committee should explicitly document its *intent to establish a rebuttable presumption of reasonableness.*
- The minutes should indicate that *no member has any conflict of interest* with regard to the executive compensation arrangement being approved, unless that fact is clearly documented somewhere else.
- The minutes should explicitly identify *who is present during debate, deliberation, and decision making*; they should make it clear that any executive whose compensation is being considered was excused from debate, deliberation, and decision making.
- The minutes should explicitly identify *the source of the comparability data* used and explain *how the comparability data were collected.*
- The minutes should explicitly state the *terms* of the compensation arrangement being approved, in detail (even if stated in an appendix to the minutes), identifying the value of total compensation and each element of compensation and benefits.
- The minutes should explicitly state that the board or committee believes that the *comparability data are appropriate in representing like organizations, like positions, and like circumstances.*
- The minutes should explicitly state the *date* on which *the minutes are prepared* and the *date* on which *they are approved.*

Instead of documenting all the terms approved in the minutes themselves, many organizations append to the minutes a spreadsheet with proposed salary increases and incentive awards; indicate that the salary increases and incentive awards were approved as recommended, and as shown on the attached spreadsheets; and record in detail only what was changed by the committee. Likewise, many organizations append a consultant's report to the minutes to show the data the committee relied on in making its decisions and to identify the source of the data and explain how the data were collected.

CHAPTER 10

Addressing Public Perceptions About Executive Compensation

INTRODUCTION

Executive pay is lower in public and tax-exempt hospitals than in for-profit firms with publicly traded stock, if only because executives of for-profits often receive stock options. No CEO of a tax-exempt hospital or health system is paid as much as a CEO of a publicly traded firm of the same size. That does not impress the public, however, because it believes that executives of tax-exempt charities should be willing to work for less than executives of for-profit firms.

This expectation is based on a misunderstanding of the role of hospitals in our society. They are not charities in the usual sense of the word. They are big, complicated businesses that do not rely on donations for much of their revenue and do not exist primarily to provide free services to the poor. They are tax exempt because they are organized to serve the public. In a sense, they are "owned" by the public—by the communities they serve—not by private shareholders, even when they are sponsored by a church or a religious order.

Executive jobs in hospitals and health systems are more difficult than comparable jobs in for-profit businesses, for several reasons. First, hospitals are far more labor intensive than other businesses, and hospital executives manage far more people than do their counterparts in other businesses with the same revenue. Second, each patient needs to be treated differently, so work processes are not as standardized and repetitive as they are in other businesses. Third, hospitals deal with life-threatening illness, pain and suffering, and death, where the consequences of even minor errors are greater than in most businesses. Fourth, hospitals are heavily regulated and must comply with far more rules than most other businesses do. Fifth, outsiders dictate much of what a hospital does, with enough variation that hospitals have difficulty establishing standardized practices for most activities. Every payer sets different policies on what they will pay for and what they will not cover; every payer sets different requirements for submitting bills and documenting services; and different physicians, even those in the same specialty, treat patients with the same symptoms differently and order different tests, procedures, and supplies.

Few hospital administrators join the profession because of a calling to a charitable vocation for which they would willingly work for less than the appropriate rate of pay for a leadership position with significant responsibility. Boards want the best executives they can find, people who are expert leaders and managers. Having a calling to serve is not even considered an important attribute for an executive—at least not outside of Catholic health systems.

PUBLIC PERCEPTION

Comparisons with Public Sector Administrators

The public often compares pay for hospital executives with pay for administrators of public agencies. Why should a hospital CEO, they wonder, be paid more than the mayor or the governor? These comparisons are irrelevant because the jobs, the labor markets, and the processes for determining pay are different for each.

The city or the state may have a bigger budget and more employees than the hospital, but elective positions require political acumen rather than management skills. The pay for the mayor and the governor are set in a political and legislative process, not subject to market forces of supply and demand. The salary for an elected official is not set high enough to attract and retain the best available leader, and it is not adjusted to acknowledge the competencies of the incumbent or the incumbent's ability to earn more in another position. Pay is not the reason people want the job of mayor or governor.

Concern About Tax Exemption and Charitable Care

Legislators and regulators often focus on the relationship between executive pay and tax exemption. They expect executives of tax-exempt organizations to be paid less than their counterparts in tax-paying organizations. They also have an interest in making sure executives are not enriched by misallocation of charitable resources that could be put to better use.

They tend to be concerned as much with the way executives are paid as with how much they are paid. Legislators and regulators are particularly skeptical of bonuses or incentive awards because they associate these with profit sharing in the for-profit sector. They are skeptical of supplemental benefits and perquisites, whether retirement plans, country club memberships, or automobile allowances.

Tax exemption represents a significant subsidy by taxpayers and a competitive advantage that tax-paying hospitals do not get. Legislators and regulators want to see that the public receives something in exchange for the subsidy and make sure that the hospital is not skimping on charitable care in order to pay bigger bonuses. This concern gets translated into an expectation that executive pay should be lower in tax-exempt hospitals than in tax-paying hospitals, and that incentive awards should not be tied to financial performance.

Concern About Rising Cost of Care

The press, legislators, and regulators often seem to link executive compensation to the rising cost of care. If nothing else, both are rising, and it is easy to reach the conclusion that escalating executive pay contributes to increases in the cost of care.

What this viewpoint misses is that executives take every available measure to control cost increases—short of cutting their own pay. But executive compensation is a tiny fraction of operating costs, in the vicinity of 1 percent. While increases in executive compensation have virtually no impact on the cost of care, increases in pay for the workforce as a whole do, and even that adjustment is driven largely by market forces of supply and demand or determined through contract negotiations with unions.

Link to Efforts to Control Pay and Benefits for Employees

Employees and unions view executive compensation through the prism of employee pay and benefits. Efforts to control the cost of healthcare over the past decade have inevitably focused on payroll costs, as payroll accounts for half of all costs and three-quarters of all controllable costs. Hospitals have reduced headcount, reduced retirement benefits, shifted a good portion of the cost of medical premiums to employees, and expected the remaining employees to produce better results while taking care of sicker patients. Most employees become cynical about executive pay, as pay rises faster for executives than for other employees and as executives receive bonuses for reducing costs, increasing productivity, and improving quality.

Unions have used executive pay as leverage for organizing, negotiating, and conducting corporate campaigns because it works. Employees and the public are willing to be manipulated because they, too, believe that executives are overpaid.

Biggest and Most Complex Organization in Most Communities

In most communities, the local hospital is the biggest employer in town. Even in bigger cities with corporate headquarters or in state capitals with lots of government employees, hospitals are among the biggest employers. However, the public has little understanding or appreciation of the size and complexity of a hospital or health system and thus compares pay for hospital executives with pay for managers or administrators of much smaller organizations.

Even trustees who own their own businesses or lead one have difficulty grasping the size and complexity of a healthcare organization. Trustees often focus on the number of high-paid executives in a hospital and wonder why a hospital needs so many more executives than they have in their own businesses. They have a hard time understanding the intensity of the management challenges in a hospital.

THE PRESS

The press tends to keep executive compensation in the news, and that keeps the public attuned to it. The public could find the data on its own, as data on executive compensation are readily available, yet the data are not very interesting. Only when the information is put into context by the press does it become a story.

Adverse publicity about executive compensation is typically limited—at the local level, at least—to a once-a-year story after Internal Revenue Service (IRS) Form 990 statements are released. In most communities, the story fades within a day or two. On the other hand, the reappearance of the story every year reminds people regularly that executive compensation is an issue.

In the main, local newspapers' stories on executive compensation cover local or regional organizations because those are the institutions their readers are most interested in. The stories cover organizations of different sizes and types but often do not point out that pay varies in fairly predictable ways: big organizations pay more than small ones, independent organizations pay more than subsidiaries of the same size, and so on. Furthermore, the stories do not compare executive pay at local organizations with national norms, which would help demonstrate that, in general, local organizations pay on par with their counterparts of similar size across the country.

Newspapers need a good headline and a good first paragraph to draw readers into the story. Reporters tend to focus on four aspects of executive compensation: who is paid most, how much pay has increased since the previous year, any large increases since the previous year, and pay at any organization that has experienced newsworthy trouble over the past year.

Small and mid-size organizations generally end up in the middle or at the bottom of the list. The largest organizations almost always get the most attention because their CEO's pay is usually among the highest on the list.

The anomalies are always highlighted in such stories, especially if the numbers are unusually high. Severance always makes a good story because it is essentially pay for not working and pay for someone who was fired. Also making news are payments of lump-sum retirement benefits earned over a long career, as the numbers distort the picture of what is otherwise annual compensation.

CEOs and trustees often view the press as hostile in its approach to executive compensation. On the whole, however, the press is just doing its job, trying to create an interesting story from the facts it uncovers. Criticizing the press for publishing these stories is tantamount to saying that executive pay should be kept secret, which in turn implies there is something to hide.

STAKEHOLDERS' PERCEPTIONS

Dealing effectively with criticism of executive pay is far more complicated in not-for-profit healthcare than it is in the for-profit sector because of the range of stakeholders to be considered. Hospitals and health systems depend for their success on the goodwill of not only their employees, physicians, and patients but also local employers, local tax authorities, community leaders, state legislators, and the public.

Hospitals need to maintain high morale on their workforce and a good relationship with their medical staff to deliver good patient care—at the same time they are trying to improve productivity, control costs, and stretch resources. Any sign that executives are treated unusually well could undermine that balance.

And they need to maintain good relationships with local business and community leaders, as local employers pay for much of the hospital's operating expenses; with local and state authorities, to maintain tax exemption and government funding for public healthcare benefits; and with the community at large, to burnish their image as a good place to go for care, to raise funds, to recruit and retain volunteers, and to ensure the public's continuing support for Medicare, Medicaid, and other publicly funded healthcare programs.

POLITICAL CRITICISM

Some criticism of executive pay is politically motivated. As one of the largest employers in the community, one of the richest organizations in the community, and one of the largest recipients of public funding, hospitals are an easy target for politicians seeking to enhance their position of influence by acting tough.

Attorneys General

Some of the most damaging attacks against hospitals and health systems have come from states' attorneys general, who have targeted executive compensation as a means to advance their own careers.

In at least one case, a tax-exempt system's use of incentive compensation was used as evidence that it was no different from a for-profit corporation and therefore did not deserve its property-tax exemption. In another case, a board's failure to follow its own rules in governing executive compensation led to a dismissal of the board (Sullivan 2002; Catlin 2001).

One attorney general began an investigation of executive pay while running for governor and announced that the attorney general's office would henceforth exercise more oversight of tax-exempt healthcare organizations because, she noted, federal efforts had been ineffective (Office of Massachusetts Attorney General 2009). One announced an investigation of executive compensation while opposing a merger of two systems (Bakhtiari 2010).

Connection to Tax Exemption

Political criticism of executive compensation in the tax-exempt sector is often related to tax exemption. Critics attack executive compensation practices in ways that make it difficult to tell whether they are targeting tax exemption or excessive pay.

As cities' need for tax revenue grows, hospitals and health systems are likely to be asked to pay property taxes or make payments in lieu of taxes. If the request comes in the form of litigation, the claims are likely to cite executive compensation as evidence that hospitals are operating like for-profit organizations by diverting a portion of their profits to executives in the form of bonuses.

Connection to Taxpayer Funding for Services

Political criticism of executive compensation in healthcare is also related to taxpayer funding of services. Both federal and state legislators and officials look at examples of unusually high executive compensation at publicly funded service providers as evidence of inappropriate use of resources.[1]

REGULATORY RISKS

Widespread concern that executive compensation in tax-exempt hospitals is excessive poses a number of regulatory risks. Criticism of executive pay as excessive is only two, albeit giant, steps removed from calling it private inurement, and the penalty for private inurement is loss of tax exemption. The more likely penalties, however, are an end to the rebuttable presumption and initial contract safe harbors, limits on executive compensation, and erosion of popular support for public health programs and the consequent tightening of reimbursement.

As the United States struggles to find ways to pay for expanding access to healthcare, executive compensation will be part of the debate. Congress and state legislatures have already entertained limits on executive compensation for tax-exempt healthcare providers and even for tax-paying healthcare insurers. For example, the Senate Finance Committee has considered proposals to eliminate the presumption of reasonableness and the initial contract exemption. Some legislators, including Senator Chuck Grassley (R-Iowa), view their widespread use as an indication of abusive practices—even though the IRS promotes the process for establishing the presumption as a best practice in governing executive compensation.

Given hospitals' dependence on the goodwill of taxpayers, legislators, and regulators, they would be wise to shape their decisions about executive compensation with appropriate concern for their impact on public relations. In particular, they should consider abandoning practices that attract unnecessary criticism and are especially hard to defend, such as providing car allowances, tax gross-ups, and generous severance benefits.

SHAPING PERCEPTIONS

Until recently, compensation committees made decisions about executive compensation without much regard for public perception, as executive compensation was regarded as confidential information that did not need to be disclosed to the public or even to the hospital's board. The typical approach to dealing with media reports on executive compensation was to wait until a reporter called, then quickly put together some explanation and wait for any reaction to the story to fade away.

The ready availability of Form 990 on the Internet, with its mandatory disclosure of executive compensation, means that everyone now has access to this information. Hospitals are accordingly beginning to shape public perception of their executive compensation programs in a number of ways.

First, they are framing all descriptions and documentation of the executive compensation program in terms that go beyond the usual explanations of recruitment and retention and motivation and reward. These characterizations may seem persuasive to consultants, executives, and trustees, but they do not impress other stakeholders.

Second, they are beginning to shape their decisions in terms of what they are willing to disclose to the public and the impression the decisions will make when they become public. In the early years of Form 990, hospitals sought to pay executives in ways that were not required to be reported on the form. Now they talk about transparency and full disclosure, recognizing that any action they take related to executive compensation must be reported on Form 990.

Third, many hospitals and health systems are developing comprehensive strategies to shape public perception of their executive compensation programs. Some now use Form 990 to explain their compensation philosophy, their governance process, and their compensation programs. Some explain anomalies and answer questions before they arise. Some post their policies on executive compensation, and even their Form 990s, on their websites. Others publish articles on their executive compensation programs in employee newsletters.

Supply and Demand

The traditional justification for executive compensation is that it is set in a free market through the interaction of supply and demand.

In other words, "we're just paying what we have to pay to get and keep our executives." The fact that it often costs more to replace an executive than to keep one gives credence to this argument. Organizations commonly find it costs more to hire the next executive than what the last one was paid, unless they promote from within.

This argument is most persuasive for organizations that position pay at median or average, and less persuasive for those that intentionally position pay at the 75th percentile. The 75th percentile position is higher than the going rate—higher than what three-quarters of comparable organizations pay—and therefore higher than necessary.

Organizations often express the supply and demand argument in terms of a shortage of talent capable of doing the job. While no shortage of talent exists for executive jobs generally—almost 6,000 hospitals and several hundred multihospital systems operate in the United States, so the total size of the labor market is enormous—institutions do face a shortage of executives who have ample experience in jobs just like the one to be filled.

One hears this argument most often at large health systems, as there are relatively few of them. Because, presumably, the only executives qualified to lead the largest organizations are those who have already done so, there are not enough executives to go around. This argument implies that second-level candidates are not qualified to be promoted to the top job in their own organizations, or at others the same size. It also seems to suggest that an executive who has successfully led a five-hospital system with $1 billion in net revenues is not qualified to lead an eight-hospital system with $3 billion in net revenues, as if the jobs were fundamentally different due to size.

Given that executive pay levels have been rising only 3 to 5 percent per year for the past decade or two, at about the same rate as inflation in workforce pay levels generally, little evidence exists that a shortage of talent is driving executive pay inexorably upward.

A justification based on supply and demand is not persuasive to anyone who does not understand the challenges involved in leading a healthcare institution. Countless doctors, for example, assume that they could lead a hospital just as well as someone with a master's degree in healthcare administration. The justification, then, needs to be expressed in terms of the competency requirements for leading a hospital or health system. Perhaps the most important competencies for a healthcare CEO are the following:

- Lead change successfully
- Inspire and engage people across the organization to support and achieve the changes needed
- Build and maintain effective relationships with a wide variety of constituencies
- Shape and implement strategy in a highly competitive environment
- Manage operating costs in a volatile, low-margin business
- Shape and develop a management team that can keep operations running smoothly 365 days a year, 24 hours a day

The challenges of managing such an organization make the job of a healthcare CEO more difficult than a job leading most other businesses. The same is true for many other leadership positions in healthcare—chief financial officers, chief information officers, chief human resources officers, and so on.

When trustees conduct an external search for a new CEO, they set their expectations high. They want a seasoned executive with ample experience performing the job who is impressive enough to quickly win the support of the medical staff and the board, fits like a glove into the culture of the organization, and seems like the right person to lead the organization over the next decade.

Search consultants know how difficult it is to find candidates who meet high expectations like these. Even if they can identify 100 people who could do the job and 50 who could meet the expectations, finding 5 or 10 who are willing to consider the job is a challenge because it generally entails giving up a good job elsewhere, moving across the country, and proving oneself all over again in new circumstances to an unknown board and medical staff.

Now go back to the argument about supply and demand. Any executive who can meet high expectations is presumably already well ensconced in a secure job, well paid, and successful enough to have no reason to move unless the recruiting organization is willing to overcome all the reasons not to move.

The going rate for an external recruit is not average pay for the job. It may be the average of what the ideal candidates are already paid. More likely, it is whatever it takes to persuade the best candidate to leave her current post—at a hefty premium, no doubt, over what she is currently paid.

The going rate for current executives is whatever it takes to keep them from considering offers from other hospitals or systems. It might be median or average pay, but it might be more. If an executive is well known and recognized as a successful leader, he typically gets a lot of calls from recruiters. If other positions pay more, those higher compensation levels become the threshold required to keep the executive in his current job. If an organization really wants to retain its executives, it tends to position pay well above average, often at the 75th percentile, so that executives will be less likely to consider other job offers.

Defending Executive Compensation

The healthcare field ought to do a better job defending its executive compensation practices than it currently does. Community hospitals are especially vulnerable to criticism of their executive pay because it hurts their relationships with physicians, employees, and business and community leaders and undermines legislative support for the hospitals.

The corollary, of course, is that hospitals and health systems should avoid pay practices that cannot be defended or that attract needless attention. They do not necessarily need to pay executives less but they must make sure that pay programs and pay decisions can be defended as reasonable and appropriate.

Hospitals and health systems have several vehicles available for communicating effectively about executive compensation, including the following:

1. The internal documents that are used to define executive compensation programs and policies
2. Any material that goes to the compensation committee or board to help it understand the program and make good decisions about it
3. Form 990 Schedule O, which has room to explain the program, its goals, and the process by which the board governs executive compensation
4. The organization's website and employee newsletter

A persuasive message about executive compensation addresses four themes—the need for effective leaders, so that the hospital can achieve its mission and meet community needs; the importance of the institution to the community and all the benefits it provides; the diligence with which executive compensation is governed by community leaders who have the best interests of the community and the institution in mind; and the reasonableness of the compensation philosophy.

Need for Effective Leaders

One key is to focus on the real reason for paying leaders well: to meet the community's needs to the extent possible; ensure that the hospital delivers safe, high-quality clinical care; and achieve the hospital's other goals. The public wants the community to have a good local hospital that is big enough to meet the community's needs for a variety of services and good enough to provide safe, effective clinical care. If the community understands that the hospital cannot survive or thrive without strong, effective leaders, the issue changes from how much to pay to what kind of talent we need to keep the hospital strong.

Value of Institution to Community

Organizations should emphasize the value of the institution to the community. Most communities can get along fine with one less motel or one less restaurant but would suffer with one less hospital. The hospital is one of the community's most important institutions. Its employees keep the economy and the community going by supporting other business and community services. It attracts doctors to town who might otherwise be reluctant to practice there. And it provides opportunities for other businesses that sell products and services to the hospital, its employees, and the medical staff. The hospital cannot fulfill that role in the community without effective leaders capable of managing the biggest and most complex business in town.

Strong Governance Process

Another essential part of the message is explaining how executive compensation is set. If the community understands that executive compensation is determined by the board—that is, by community leaders, with proper consideration for community values and with the best interests of the institution and the community in mind—it is more likely to believe that the decisions are well intentioned and well considered. The public is also more likely to accept the decisions if it knows they are made by people it respects. An explanation of the board's role in governing executive compensation, and the process it uses, can take people beyond thinking that executives determine their own pay and that "the hospital" pays too much.

Reasonable Compensation Philosophy

Compensation philosophy needs to be part of the explanation of why pay levels are set where they are. If the philosophy is to pay at median or average, actual pay levels seem more appropriate, as no one wants to be paid less than median or average. If the philosophy is to pay above median or average, it is important to explain why the board thinks pay should be set there, and the most persuasive reason is to make it proportional to performance. If the board expects the hospital to perform well above average, a reasonable approach to achieving that performance is to give executives the opportunity to earn more than average as a reward. If the reason for paying above average is to attract and retain the best possible leaders, that, too, helps make pay seem appropriate.

Value of Stability

One nuance worth remembering is that stability is valuable in itself. Stability of the executive team is likely to improve performance and strengthen the hospital, whereas high turnover is likely to hurt performance and weaken the hospital.

Research shows that organizations with stable leadership tend to perform better than organizations with high turnover.[2] Good performance requires sustained effort and continuous attention to detail.

Research also shows that turnover is expensive (Waldman et al. 2004). A hospital may save money while a position is vacant, but it typically ends up spending more to fill a vacancy than what was paid to the previous incumbent. Additional cost factors may include the fee for a recruiter, a hiring bonus, a special bonus to buy an executive out of benefits forfeited on leaving the previous employer, or a higher salary than the last incumbent earned. External hires tend to be paid more competitively than internally promoted executives and therefore tend to drive up pay levels for other executives over time.

Turnover is also risky. New executives often fail and need to be replaced. That process can lead to extended periods without strong leadership, which can slow down the implementation of new programs or strategies and even lead to deterioration in performance for want of attention to important issues.

Any institution that performs well and has a stable management team would be wise to explain that its good performance is due in significant part to its success in holding onto its leadership team, and that it does so in part by paying executives enough to keep them from being recruited away by an organization willing to pay more.

Public Benefit from Effective Leadership

Another theme worth developing is the benefit the community gains from the hospital's success in recruiting and retaining effective leaders, beyond the success of the institution itself. Perhaps the most important of these is preservation of healthcare services in the local community, or preservation of competition if more than one hospital is operating in town. Corollaries are preservation of good jobs in the community; a large base of well-educated citizens who are likely to support public education; a stable property tax base; and the benefit of a healthy community with a highly skilled workforce—good volunteers, dependable donors, and good board members for local churches and community service organizations.

The benefits a hospital delivers to its community are more varied and important than the few that are typically tallied in a report on community benefits. This broader set of benefits is well worth mentioning in explaining why it is important to bring to the community talented leaders who would not otherwise come if the hospital were not willing to pay them competitively.

BEST PRACTICES IN ADDRESSING PUBLIC PERCEPTIONS ABOUT EXECUTIVE COMPENSATION

Following is a list of best practices in working with public perceptions:

- Make sure all trustees know enough about the executive compensation program that adverse publicity does not generate divisiveness on the board.

- Appoint the chair of the compensation committee or the chair of the board as the principal spokesperson for the institution in defending executive compensation.
- Tell trustees to refer press inquiries to that spokesperson and give simple, brief answers in response to other inquiries.
- Prepare a set of general responses to help the spokesperson respond to questions that may arise.
- Publish brief descriptions of the institution's compensation philosophy and process for governing executive compensation on Form 990.

NOTES

1. One example is Governor Andrew M. Cuomo's 2012 executive order 38 limiting reimbursement for executive pay at agencies contracting with the State of New York to $199,000.

2. Not all studies reach this conclusion, but some do. See the citations in Cao, Maruping, and Takeuchi (2006).

References

Bakhtiari, E. 2010. "New Hampshire AG Reviews CEO Salaries at Nonprofit Hospitals." *HealthLeaders Media*. Published June 15. www.healthleadersmedia.com/content/LED-252517/New-Hampshire-AG-Reviews-CEO-Salaries-at-Nonprofit-Hospitals.

Bebchuk, L., and J. M. Fried. 2004. *Pay Without Performance: The Unfulfilled Promise of Executive Compensation*. Cambridge, MA: Harvard University Press.

Bivens, J. 2011. "CEOs Distance Themselves from the Average Worker." *Economic Policy Institute*. Published November 9. www.epi.org/publication/ceo-ratio-average-worker/.

Brauer, L. M., and C. F. Kaiser III. 2000. "C. Physician Incentive Compensation." *Update on Healthcare*. Accessed February 1, 2012. www.irs.gov/pub/irs-tege/eotopicc00.pdf.

Cao, Q., L. M. Maruping, and R. Takeuchi. 2006. "Disentangling the Effects of CEO Turnover and Succession on Organizational Capabilities: A Social Network Perspective." *Organization Science* 17 (5): 563–76.

Catlin, B. 2001. "A Break-up for Allina." *Minnesota Public Radio*. Published July 20. http://news.minnesota.publicradio.org/features/200107/20_catlinb_allina/.

Conference Board, The. 2009. "The Conference Board Taskforce on Executive Compensation." *The Conference Board*. Accessed January 31. www.conference-board.org/pdf_free/ExecCompensation2009.pdf.

Council of Institutional Investors. 2011. "Executive Compensation," 10–18. In *Corporate Governance Policies*. Washington, DC: Council of Institutional Investors.

Cuomo, A. M. 2012. "No: 38—Limits on State-Funded Administrative Costs & Executive Compensation." *State of New York Executive Chamber*. Published January 18. www.governor.ny.gov/executiveorder/38.

Drucker Institute. 2011. "Turning Up the Heat on CEO Pay." *The Drucker Exchange.* Published February 17. http://thedx.druckerinstitute.com/2011/02/turning-up-the-heat-on-ceo-pay/.

Heritage Institute. 2007. "Examples of Large Executive Compensation in the US." *Corporate Governance News.* Updated February 8. http://heritageinstitute.com/governance/compensation.htm.

Institute for Policy Studies. 2010. *CEO Pay and the Great Recession.* Washington, DC: Institute for Policy Studies.

Institute for Policy Studies and United for a Fair Economy. 2008. *Executive Excess 2008.* Washington, DC: Institute for Policy Studies.

Integrated Healthcare Strategies. 2010. *2010 National Healthcare Leadership Compensation Survey.* Kansas City, MO: Integrated Healthcare Strategies.

Internal Revenue Service. 2006. IRS letter boilerplate. *Internal Revenue Service.* Published January 6.

———. 1990. "Overview of Inurement/Private Benefit Issues in IRC 501(c)(3)." *1990 EO CPE Text.* Accessed January 31, 2012. www.irs.gov/pub/irs-tege/eotopicc90.pdf.

———.1987a. General Counsel Memorandum GCM 39674. *Legalbitstream.* Published October 23. www.legalbitstream.com/scripts/isyswebext.dll?op=get&uri=/isysquery/irlc227/1/doc.

———. 1987b. General Counsel Memorandum GCM 39670. *Legalbitstream.* Published June 17. www.legalbitstream.com/scripts/isyswebext.dll?op=get&uri=/isysquery/irlc22b/2/doc.

———. 1969. Revenue Ruling 69-383. *Internal Revenue Service.* Accessed October 17, 2011. www.irs.gov/pub/irs-tege/rr69-383.pdf.

Kaplan, R. S., and D. P. Norton. 1996. *The Balanced Scorecard: Translating Strategy into Action.* Boston: Harvard Business Review Press.

Kay, I. T., and S. Van Putten. 2007. *Myths and Realities of Executive Pay.* New York: Cambridge University Press.

McDowell, S. R. 2007. "Nonprofit Compensation: Tax and Corporate Governance Issues." Presentation to 2008 Washington NonProfit Legal & Tax Conference, Steptoe & Johnson, Washington, DC, February 28–29. www.steptoe.com/assets/attachments/3447.pdf.

Office of Massachusetts Attorney General. 2009. Memorandum addressed to the Massachusetts Hospital Association, Blue Cross Blue Shield of Massachusetts,

Harvard Pilgrim Health Plan, Tufts Health Plan, and Fallon Health Plan. Published September 2. www.mass.gov/ago/docs/nonprofit/bcbs-memo-090209.pdf.

Scheck, T. 2001. "Assessing the Impact of Allina's Break-up." *Minnesota Public Radio*. Published July 20. http://news.minnesota.publicradio.org/features/200107/20_catlinb_allina/scheck.shtml.

Sullivan, K. 2002. "Minnesota Fat Cats." *In These Times*. Published July 8. http://images.indymedia.org/imc/twincities/text/minnesota_yqo6gn.txt.

Waldman, J. D., F. Kelly, S. Arora, and H. L. Smith. 2004. "The Shocking Cost of Turnover in Health Care." *Health Care Management Review* 39 (1): 2–7.

Additional Resources

Abramowitz, R. L., and B. J. Brown II. 2002. "Deferred Compensation for Hospital Executives." The Health Lawyer [article index]. Published in August. www.abanet .org/health/03_publications/HealthLawyer/vol_14.html.

Ackerman, F. K. 2008. "The Compensation Committee." In *Governance for Healthcare Providers*, edited by D. B. Nash, W. J. Oetgen, and V. P. Pracilio, 204–26. Boca Raton, FL: CRC Press.

American College of Healthcare Executives. 2009. *Employment Contracts for Healthcare Executives: Rationale, Trends, and Samples*, 5th ed. Chicago: Health Administration Press.

————. 2003. *Evaluating the Performance of the Hospital CEO*, 3d ed. Chicago: Health Administration Press.

American Hospital Association and American College of Healthcare Executives. 2009. "Executive Compensation Resources for Non-profit Hospitals." *American Hospital Association*. Accessed February 1, 2012. www.aha.org/aha/issues/ Tax-Exempt-Status/execcomp.html.

Bainbridge, S. M. 2005. "Executive Compensation: Who Decides?" *Texas Law Review* [book review]. Accessed October 3, 2011. http://fedsoc.server326.com/ FacultyDocuments/Shareholder%20Voting/Bainbridge.pdf.

Barragato, C. A. 2002. "Linking For-Profit and Nonprofit Executive Compensation: Salary Composition and Incentive Structures in the U.S. Hospital Industry." *Voluntas: International Journal of Voluntary and Nonprofit Organizations* 13 (3): 301–11.

Bebchuk, L., and J. M. Fried. 2003. "Executive Compensation as an Agency Problem." *Journal of Economic Perspectives* 17 (3): 71–92.

Bebchuk, L. A., J. M. Fried, and D. I. Walker. 2002. "Managerial Power and Rent Extraction in the Design of Executive Compensation." *University of Chicago Law Review* 69: 751–846.

Bebchuk, L. A., and R. J. Jackson Jr. 2005. "Executive Pensions." *Journal of Corporation Law* 30: 823–55.

Becker, I. S., and W. M. Gerek (eds.). 2009. *Understanding Executive Compensation: A Practical Guide for Decision Makers.* Scottsdale, AZ: WorldatWork.

Bjork, D. A. 2010a. "Regulation of Executive Compensation at Nonprofit Health Care Organizations: Coming Changes?" *Inquiry, the Journal of Health Care Organization, Provision, and Financing* 47 (1): 7–16.

———. 2010b. "Rethinking Executive Pay in Community-Based Organizations." In *Executive Compensation: A Collection of Articles from WorldatWork,* 209–17. Scottsdale, AZ: WorldatWork Press.

———. 1989a. "Compensation Patterns in HMOs, Clinics, and Other Health Care Organizations." In *The Hay Group Guide to Executive Compensation: How to Meet the Complicated and Sensitive Challenge of Rewarding Key Executives in the Health Care Field,* edited by T. P. Flannery, 150–72. Chicago: Pluribus.

———. 1989b. "Incentive Compensation in For-Profit and Not-for-Profit Organizations: A Comparison." In *The Hay Group Guide to Executive Compensation: How to Meet the Complicated and Sensitive Challenge of Rewarding Key Executives in the Health Care Field,* edited by T. P. Flannery, 85–107. Chicago: Pluribus.

Bjork, D. A., and D. J. Fairley. 2004. *Strengthening Governance in Hospitals and Health Systems: What Boards Are Doing Well, and What They Could Do Better. A Survey of Governance Reform Initiatives in Not-for-Profit Hospitals and Health Systems.* Bozeman, MT: American Governance and Leadership Group.

Bjork, D. A., D. J. Fairley, and K. McManus. 2004. *Health Care Governance in an Era of Reform.* Bozeman, MT: American Governance and Leadership Group.

Brancato, C. K., C. Peck, and D. Hervig. 2001. *Compensation Committee of The Board: Best Practices for Establishing Executive Compensation.* New York: The Conference Board.

Brancato, C. K., and A. A. Rudnick. 2006. *The Evolving Relationship Between Compensation Committees and Consultants.* New York: The Conference Board.

Chingos, P. T. (ed.). 2004. *Responsible Executive Compensation for a New Era of Accountability.* Hoboken, NJ: Wiley & Sons.

———. 2002. *Paying for Performance: A Guide to Compensation Management,* 2nd ed. Hoboken, NJ: Wiley & Sons.

Cotter, T. J. 2009. "Navigating in a Shifting Executive Compensation Environment." *Executive Action Series*. Accessed February 1, 2012. http://nchl.org/ Documents/Ctrl_Hyperlink/NCHL_Executive_Action_Series_-_Executive_ Compensation_uid1302012524222.pdf.

Cotter, T., M. Peregrine, L. Woods, and J. Zybach (moderator). 2004. "Compensating Directors and Trustees of Nonprofits: What the Federal Tax Law Allows." Presentation to meeting of American Bar Association, Committee on Nonprofit Corporations and Committee on Health Law. April 2. www.abanet.org/buslaw/ newsletter/0028/materials/pub/39.pdf.

Crystal, G. S. 1991. *In Search of Excess: The Overcompensation of American Executives*. New York: W.W. Norton.

Davidson, G. A., and D. K. Feller. 2002. "What Every Director of a Nonprofit Organization Needs to Know to Avoid Intermediate Sanctions." In *Nonprofit Governance and Management,* edited by V. Futter, J. A. Cion, and G. W. Overton, 669–78. New York: American Society of Corporate Secretaries.

DiPrete, T. A., G. Eirich, and M. Pittinsky. 2010. "Compensation Benchmarking, Leapfrogs, and the Surge in Executive Pay." *American Journal of Sociology* 115 (6): 1671–712.

Doubleday, D., and B. Greenblatt. 2010. "How to Create Minimum Standards for Assessing Executive Pay." In *Executive Compensation: A Collection of Articles from WorldatWork,* 7–12. Scottsdale, AZ: WorldatWork Press.

Ellig, B. R. 2007. *The Complete Guide to Executive Compensation*, rev. ed. New York: McGraw Hill.

Ericson, R. N. 2004. *Pay to Prosper: Using Value Rules to Reinvent Executive Incentives*. Scottsdale, AZ: WorldatWork Press.

Feldstein, M. S. 2003. "Why Is Productivity Growing Faster?" *Journal of Policy Modeling* 25 (5): 445–51.

Flannery, T. P. 2002. *Executive Compensation: Guidelines for Healthcare Leaders and Trustees*. Chicago: Health Administration Press.

———. (ed.). 1989. *The Hay Group Guide to Executive Compensation: How to Meet the Complicated and Sensitive Challenge of Rewarding Key Executives in the Health Care Field*. Chicago: Pluribus.

Frydman, C., and R. E. Saks. 2008. "Executive Compensation: A New View from a Long-Term Perspective, 1936–2005." *Massachusetts Institute of Technology*. Published August 8. http://web.mit.edu/frydman/www/trends_frydmansaks_0808.pdf.

Fulmer, I. S. 2009. "The Elephant in the Room: Labor Market Influences on CEO Compensation." *Personnel Psychology* 62 (4): 659–95.

Gabaix, X., and A. Landier. 2006. "Why Has CEO Pay Increased So Much?" MIT Department of Economics Working Paper No. 06-13 (May 2006).

Graham, M. D., T. A. Roth, and D. Dugan. 2008. *Effective Executive Compensation: Creating a Total Rewards Strategy for Executives.* New York: AMACOM.

Harvard Business School. 2009. "Executive Compensation: A Broader View." *Summary of the Proceedings of the Conference on Executive Compensation.* Conference held September 14–15. Accessed February 1, 2012. www.hbs.edu/news/pdf/HBS%20Executive%20Comp%20Conference%202009%20-%20Exec%20Summary.pdf.

Healthcare Association of New York State and Healthcare Trustees of New York State. 2004. "Compensation and Interested Party Transactions. In *Nonprofit Corporate Accountability: A Guidebook,* 131–33. Rensselaer, NY: Healthcare Association of New York State.

Herzberg, F. 1987. "One More Time: How Do You Motivate Employees?" *Harvard Business Review.* Published September-October. www.sph.ukma.kiev.ua/images/Seminar_4_One_More_Time_How_Do_You_Motivate_Employees%20(Herzberg).pdf.

Hogan & Hartson LLP. 2009a. "Compensation Compliance Checklist: What Steps Should a CEO Take to Assure Compliance with Legal Standards and Reporting Obligations?" *American Hospital Association and American College of Healthcare Executives.* Accessed February 1, 2012. www.aha.org/aha/content/2008/pdf/08CompChecklist.pdf.

————. 2009b. "Excess Benefit and Reasonable Compensation: An Analysis of the Intermediate Sanctions Rules." *American Hospital Association and American College of Healthcare Executives.* Accessed February 1, 2012. www.aha.org/aha/content/2008/pdf/08ExcessBenefitAnalysis.pdf.

————. 2009c. "Executive Compensation: A Primer for Establishing Reasonable Compensation." *American Hospital Association and American College of Healthcare Executives.* Accessed February 1, 2012. www.aha.org/aha/content/2008/pdf/08ExecCompPrimer.pdf.

————. 2009d. "Sample Compensation Committee Charter." American Hospital Association and American College of Healthcare Executives. Accessed February 1, 2012. ww.aha.org/aha/content/2008/pdf/08SampleCompCommCharter.pdf.

Internal Revenue Service. 2009. *IRS Exempt Organizations (TE/GE) Hospital Compliance Project Final Report.* Published February 12. www.irs.gov/pub/irs-tege/frepthospproj.pdf.

————. 2007. *Report on Exempt Organizations Executive Compensation Compliance Project—Parts I and II.* Published in March. www.irs.gov/pub/irs-tege/exec._comp._final.pdf.

———. 1998. "Section 457 Deferred Compensation." *EO CPE Text*. Published in August. www.irs.gov/charities/article/0,,id=96421,00.html.

Joyce, J. W. 2010. "Revisiting Executive Compensation Philosophy." In *Executive Compensation: A Collection of Articles from WorldatWork*, 173–80. Scottsdale, AZ: WorldatWork Press.

Karp, D. C., J. L. Goldstein, and J. Unger. 2007. *Compensation Committee Guide and Best Practices*. Wachtell, Lipton, Rosen & Katz. Published January 20. www.corpgov.deloitte.com/binary/com.epicentric.contentmanagement.servlet .ContentDeliveryServlet/USEng/Documents/Compensation%20Committee/ Compensation%20Committee%20Guide%20Best%20Practices_Wachtell _012007.pdf.

Kohn, A. 1993a. *Punished by Rewards: The Trouble with Gold Stars, Incentive Plans, A's, Praise, and Other Bribes*. Boston: Houghton Mifflin.

———. 1993b. "Why Incentive Plans Cannot Work." *Harvard Business Review*. Published September-October. www.fbe.hku.hk/doc/courses/ug/2010-2011/ BUSI0029A/R7-Why%20Incentive%20Plans%20Cannot%20Work.pdf.

Kramer, J., and R. E. Santerre. 2010. "Not-for-Profit Hospital CEO Performance and Pay: Some Evidence from Connecticut." *Inquiry* 47 (3): 242–51.

Levinson, H. 1973. *The Great Jackass Fallacy*. Boston: Harvard University Press.

Lipman, F. D., and S. E. Hall. 2008. *Executive Compensation Best Practices*. Hoboken, NJ: Wiley & Sons.

Lorsch, J., and R. Khurana. 2010a. "The Pay Problem." *Harvard Magazine* (May-June): 30–35.

———. 2010b. "Towards a New Paradigm for Executive Compensation." *Harvard Law School Forum on Corporate Governance and Financial Regulation*. Published May 12. http://blogs.law.harvard.edu/corpgov/2010/05/12/towards-a-new-paradigm-for-executive-compensation/#more-9227.

Main, B. G. M., and C. A. O'Reilly III. 2007. "Setting the CEO's Pay: It's More than Simple Economics." *Organizational Dynamics* 36 (1): 1–12.

McGuire Woods. 2009. "Executive Compensation Limits Under the ARRA: A Sign of Things to Come for Not-for-Profit Healthcare Organizations?" *Legal Updates*. Published March 12. http://mcguirewoods.com/news-resources/ item.asp?item=3795.

Mercer. 2009. *Pay for Results: Aligning Executive Compensation with Business Performance*. Hoboken, NJ: Wiley & Sons.

Mercer Human Resource Consulting. 2006. "The Board's Role in Enhancing Stakeholders' Understanding of Executive Compensation." *Compensation*

Committee Leadership Network ViewPoints. Accessed February 1, 2012. www.tapestrynetwork.net/documents/Tapestry_Mercer_CCLN_Oct06_View.pdf.

Murphy, K. J. 2002. "Explaining Executive Compensation: Managerial Power Versus the Perceived Cost of Stock Options." *University of Chicago Law Review* 69 (3): 847–69.

Nelson, J., D. A. Bjork, and K. McManus. 2009. "Rethinking Executive Pay: Responsible Governance in an Era of Healthcare Reform." *E-Briefings.* Published in November. www.governanceinstitute.com/ResearchPublications/Resource Library/tabid/185/CategoryID/63/List/1/Level/a/ProductID/984/Default.aspx?Sort Field=DateCreated+DESC%2cDateCreated+DESC.

O'Reilly, C. A., and B. G. M. Main. 2010. "Economic and Psychological Perspectives on CEO Compensation: A Review and Synthesis." *Industrial and Corporate Change* 19 (3): 675–712.

O'Reilly, C. A., III, B. G. M. Main, and G. S. Crystal. 1988. "CEO Salaries as Tournaments and Social Comparison: A Tale of Two Theories." *Administrative Science Quarterly* 33 (2): 257–74.

Panel on the Nonprofit Sector. 2005. *Strengthening Transparency, Governance, and Accountability of Charitable Organizations: A Final Report to Congress and the Nonprofit Sector.* [Log-in required to access report.] www.nonprofitpanel.org/ Report/index.html.

Peregrine, M. W., and T. J. Cotter. 2010. "Dodd-Frank: The Spillover Impact on Nonprofit Healthcare." *Health Lawyers Weekly.* Published July 30. www.sullivan cotter.com/sites/default/files/Article_Dodd-Frank_July2010_Cotter_0.pdf.

Peregrine, M. W., R. E. DeJong, and T. J. Cotter. 2010. "The 2011 Agenda for the Executive Compensation Committee." *E-Briefings.* Published November 20. www.sullivancotter.com/2011-agenda-executive-compensation-committee.

———. 2004. "New EO Focus—the Board Compensation Committee." *The Exempt Organization Tax Review* 43 (3): 265–71.

Peregrine, M. W., R. E. DeJong, T. J. Cotter, and K. Hastings. 2006. "Updated Guidance for the Board's Executive Compensation Committee. A Governance Institute White Paper." San Diego: The Governance Institute.

———. 2005. "The Board's Role in Approving Executive Compensation. A Governance Institute White Paper." San Diego: The Governance Institute.

Porter, E. 2011. *The Price of Everything: Solving the Mystery of Why We Pay What We Do.* Virginia Beach, VA: Portfolio.

———. 2010. "How Superstars' Pay Stifles Everyone Else." *New York Times,* December 26, 1–4.

Rich, J., and C. Peck. 2005. *Executive Compensation Consulting: A Research Working Group Report on Best Practices*. New York: The Conference Board.

Snyder, F. G. 2003. "More Pieces of the CEO Compensation Puzzle." *Delaware Journal of Corporate Law* 28 (1): 129–211.

Swinford, D., and M. Vnuk. 2008. "The Compensation Committee: From Competence to Excellence." *Directors Monthly* (October): 16–18.

Tosi, H. L., S. Werner, J. P. Katz, and L. R. Gomez-Mejia. 2000. "How Much Does Performance Matter? A Meta-analysis of CEO Pay Studies." *Journal of Management* 26 (2): 301–39.

Van Dalsem, S. A. 2007. "CEO Separation Bonuses: Shareholder Wealth Enhancing or Rent Extraction?" Published online September 11. http://69.175.2.130/ ~finman/Orlando/Papers/SeparationBonus.pdf.

Index

224, 225, 275–276; confusion about, 269; customized service for, 274; documentation of, 270–271, 307, 315–316, 331; employment agreement provisions for, 310, 336; flexible, 229, 252, 261–262, 264–265, 269; formal plan documents of, 345; health and welfare benefits, 234–243; implication for employers, 227–228; as incentive compensation component, 63; incentive compensation *versus,* 47–48, 71; increase in, 224; influence on organizational culture, 67; as market value component, 78–79; overview of, 226–227; paternalism of, 208, 226, 271; as percentage of payroll, 229; as percentage of salary, 47, 111n., 227; as percentage of total compensation, 78–79; perquisites as, 278; perquisites differentiated from, 231–232, 279–280; perquisites *versus,* 231–232; personal responsibility for, 271–272; prevalence of, 266–269; principles for, 275; provisions and structure of, 233–264; purposes of, 227–231; qualified *versus* nonqualified, 232–233; rationale for, 228–231; record-keeping for, 274; regulatory compliance regarding, 274; relationship to community values, 44; review of, 354; role in recruitment, 39, 223, 228–229, 230; role in retention, 39–40, 223, 228–229, 230; salary *versus,* 47–48, 229; special, 307, 351; standard packages of, 226–227; taxation on, 232–233, 275, 276; tax gross-ups on, 224–225, 231, 281, 297–298, 301; terms, complexities, and provisions of, 269–271; timeliness of, 274; value of, 269–270

Best practices, in executive compensation, 55–56, xxviii; in benefits, 275–276; in compensation philosophy, 70–72; in employment agreements, 336–337; in goal setting, 219; in governance, 8, 9, 343, 346–347, 368, 369–372; in incentive compensation design, 218–220; in market value determination, 109–110; in perquisites, 302; in public perception of executive compensation, 391–392; in salary administration, 151–152

Bias, in executive compensation, 48–49

Boards. *See also* Trustees: adoption of compensation philosophy by, 35–36; attitudes toward incentive compensation, 46–47; as community leaders, 389; executive compensation responsibility of, 347–355; incentive compensation governance role of, 209, 220, 364; membership turnover of, 304, 325; peer group selection by, 54–57; relationship with CEOs, 339, 355–357; relationship with compensation committees, 361–366

BoardSource, 346

Bonuses, 8; for acquisitions or projects, 18–20; as executive compensation measure, 11; hiring, 64, 211, 213, 390; incentive compensation *versus,* 47–48, 71, 155; for performance, 145–146; as reward *versus* incentive, 15; rolling stay, 214; stay, 24, 210–211, 215–216

Broadbanding, in salary administration, 131

Budgets, for salaries, 60–61, 118, 127–128, 136–137, 152

Business expenses, differentiated from perquisites, 280–281

Bylaws, 349, 351–352; affecting executive compensation, 344–345;

Children's hospitals, executive pay levels in, 55

CIOs. *See* Chief information officers

"Circuit breakers," for incentive plans, 183, 188

Claims, release from, 331, 333

Clawbacks, 172

Cleveland Clinic, 94

Cliff vesting, 194, 233, 248

Clinical quality, 135; *versus* financial performance, 67

Clinical quality performance measures/goals, 196, 197, 199, 205

Club memberships, as perquisites, 231, 302; country club memberships, 278, 281, 282, 283–284, 286–287, 300, 301, 365; luncheon club memberships, 278, 279, 281, 283–284, 286, 287–288, 300

"Club" (custom) surveys, 83, 92–93, 95

CNOs. *See* Chief nursing officers

Collaboration: with consultants, 357, 360–361; effect of pay mix on, 69; in governance, 357; obstacles to, 163, 164

Communication: about benefits, 269–270, 275; about executive compensation, 148–151, 388; about flexible benefit plans, 265; with the media, 354; with the public, 354; with stakeholders, 354

Communities, justification of executive compensation to, 387–391

Community health status performance measures, 199

Community hospitals, 387; closure of, 50; justification of executive compensation by, 387–391

Community values, 43–44

Commuting expenses, reimbursement for, 296–297

Comparability data. *See also* Peer groups

Compensation committees: accountability of, 349; boards' relationship with, 361–366; bylaws of, 353; charters of, 340, 344–345, 349, 350, 353–355, 369, 372; compliance with compensation philosophy, 32–33; composition of, 349; conflicts of interest of, 369; consultants' relationship with, 8–9, 356–357, 358–361, 370; decision making by, 27, 370–371; defense of compensation programs by, 367–369; disclosure compliance by, 347, 361–362; executive sessions of, 370; goal approval by, 202–203; goal-setting role of, 364; governance role of, 220, 350–351; incentive compensation governance role of, 168–173, 209, 220, 364; leadership of, 50–51, 353; limitations on ability to act, 362; meetings of, 7–8, 355, 370–371; membership of, 50–51, 349, 353; oversight responsibility of, 348–351; performance expectations for, 354; presumption of reasonableness and, 365–366; proposals offered by, 362–363; regulatory compliance responsibility of, 366–367; reports provided by, 355, 372; responsibilities of, 353–354, 357–358, 366–367, 369–372; salary administration role of, 119, 128; salary review by, 119; self-governance of, 355

Compensation levels: benchmark levels of, 36; consultants' effects on, 6, 8–11; exceptions from, 32–33; factors affecting, 5–8; reasonable, xxiv; regional differences in, 10, 55; relationship to cost control, 21–22; relationship to executive talent, 45; relationship to performance, 46–47. *See also* Above-average compensation; Median compensation;

Overpayment; Percentiles; Under-payment

Compensation opportunity, definition of, xxix

Compensation philosophy, 21, 29–72; affordability issue of, 42–43; as basis for compensation levels, xviii; best practices in, 70–72; board approval of, 340, 363; challenges to, 50–51; communication to stakeholders, 44–45, 52–54; compensation level issue of, 39–40; of competitive compensation determination, 57–60; competitive labor market issue of, 40–42; consistency of, 50–51; definition of, 30–33, 34; development of, 38–49; differenti-ated from compensation policy, 34; of external recruitment, 42; fairness issue of, 48–49; of fixed *versus* vari-able pay balance, 63–65; formal, 31, 35, 36; functions of, 29–30; of incentive compensation, 60–63; influence on compensation pro-grams, 52; informal, 31, 51; multi-ple, 33; of peer group choice, 54–57; proposals of, 362–363; rationale for, 31–32, 35–36, 38–39; reasonable, 389–390; regional impact on, 74; relationship to goals, 207; relationship to incentive opportunity, 181; review of, 72, 354; specificity of, 29, 36, 52; trade-offs in, 47–48; unintended consequences of, 36–38; values issue of, 43–44

Compensation policy, 25; definition of, 34; formal, 38–39; informal, 38; rationale for, 49–50

Compensation strategy, definition of, 34

Competence: as basis for salary increase, 145–146, 151; definition of, 145; seniority *versus*, 152

Competencies: as basis for salary increases, 146–147; of CEOs, 386; comparison with performance, 147; definition of, 145; performance measures for, 199; seniority *versus*, 152; undervaluation of, 144–145

Competition: employment agreement prohibition of, 310; for leadership talent, 40; separation agreement prohibition of, 331

Competitiveness, of executive compen-sation, 7; compensation philosophy of, 31, 57–60; consultants' effects on, 9; determination of, 57–60; of median compensation, 38; patterns of, 59; relationship to cost control, 21–22

Compliance, regulatory, 274, 366–367

Compounding effect, of above-average incentives/benefits, 59, 60

Compound (combined) jobs, 98

Conference Board, 27n., 224–225

Conferences: continuing education programs offered at, 291; employer-paid attendance at, 279, 281, 300–301, 302

Confidentiality, of executive compen-sation, 44, 367, 383–384

Conflicts of interest, 348, 369, 372–373n.

Consistency, of compensation policies, 50–51

Consultants: board's relationship with, xxi; CEO's relationship with, 9, 356–357; collaboration with, 357, 360–361; compensation committee's relationship with, 8–9, 356–357, 358–361, 370; data-gathering tech-niques of, 10–11; independence of, 360–361; influence on compensa-tion levels, 6, 8–11; responsibilities of, 358–360; selection and supervi-sion of, 354, 370

Consulting firms: as peer group data source, 95, 96; surveys by, 83–84

Continuing education: employer-paid, 278, 288–289, 300–301, 302; provided by professional societies, 290–291

Continuity, as organizational goal, 69

Contracts, employment. *See* Employment agreements

Contractual obligations: for benefits, 226; for deferred compensation payment, 263–264; duration of, 362

Conventions, employer-paid attendance at, 279, 281

Cost control, xix, 53, 378; exemptions from, 42–43; in the for-profit sector, xx–xxi; organizational focus on, 67; perquisites as exceptions to, 281–282; relationship to compensation level, 21–22; as salary administration goal, 115

Cost-effectiveness performance measures, 199

Cost of living, inflation in, 135

Council of Institutional Investors, 27n.

Country club memberships, as perquisites, 278, 281, 282, 283–284, 286–287, 300, 301, 365

Criminal activities, as cause for termination, 322

Criticism, of executive compensation, 1, 375–392; from the media, 378, 379–380; from politicians, 381–382; from the public, 376–379; regulatory risks of, 383; response to, 383–391; from stakeholders, 380–381

Cuomo, Andrew M., 392

Custom ("club") surveys, 83, 92–93, 95

Customization, of compensation packages, 316

Death, implication for severance payments, 328

Decision making, regarding executive compensation, 1, 4–5, 7–8; by compensation committees, 27, 370–371; compensation philosophy and, 29; by directors, 7–8; influence of values on, 43; influence on organizational culture, 67

Deferred compensation, 64. *See also* Supplemental executive retirement plans (SERPs): buyouts of, 213; due on termination, 308; as liability, 257; life insurance–funded, 262–263; as offset to supplemental executive retirement benefits, 255; rationale for, 252; recordkeeping for, 274; reported on Internal Revenue Service Form 990, 87; as retention incentive, 211; severance benefits as, 319; taxation on, 232–233

Dental benefits, 234

Department heads: incentive compensation for, 175; incentive plan goals of, 186

Directors: decision making by, 7–8; incentive compensation for, 175; incentive plan goals of, 185, 187

Disability: implication for severance payments, 328; job termination for, 308

Disability benefits/insurance, 24, 227, 292–293, 321–322; compensation strategy for, 34; long-term, 228, 238, 239, 267, 328; purpose of, 228; short-term, 226, 238–239; supplemental, 238–239

Disability salary continuation, 239, 241, 243, 267

Disabled persons, discrimination toward, 336

Disclosure, of executive compensation, 44; accessibility of, 347; by

206–208; levels in, 203–205; in long-term incentive plans, 192; for maximum-award levels, 176–178, 179, 190–191, 201–202, 206, 207; for multihospital systems, 364; negotiations over, 153–154; for on-plan performance awards, 200, 201; operating plan–based, 195; organization-wide *versus* departmental goals in, 162–164; pass/fail goals in, 189, 190–191, 205, 206; range of outcomes in, 189; for target-award levels, 177, 178, 179, 180, 190–191, 200, 206; team (institutional) and individual (job-related) goals in, 162–164, 184–188; three-point scale for, 178, 189, 190–191, 200, 201; for threshold-award levels, 190–191, 200, 201–202, 206; two-point scale for, 189, 191–192, 200

"Going rates," for jobs, 81, 387

Golf club memberships. *See* Country club memberships

Governance, 339–373. *See also* Salary administration

Governance Institute, The, 346

Grants, retention incentives as, 214

Grassley, Charles E. "Chuck," 339, 383

Growth, of healthcare organizations, 12–13

Growth/market share performance measures, 199

GuideStar, xxii, 88

Hatch, Michael, 372n.

Hay Group, 276n.

Healthcare benefits, 24–25, 223–224, 226–227, 234–235; costs of, 229; employers' responsibility for, 229, 231; post-retirement, 234, 235, 266–267, 276; prevalence of, 266; purpose of, 228; shared costs of, 234; supplemental, 234–235

Healthcare costs, relationship to executive compensation, 378

Healthcare executive positions: compound (combined), 98; unique or unusual, 97

Healthcare executives. *See also* Chief executive officers (CEOs); Chief financial officers (CFOs); Chief information officers (CIOs); Chief nursing officers (CNOs); Chief operating officers (COOs): attitudes toward incentive compensation, 15–16; challenges faced by, 6–7, 375–376; comparison with public-sector administrators, 376–377

Healthcare industry, executive positions within, 40–41

Healthcare insurance. *See* Healthcare benefits

Health club memberships, 278, 283–284

Health insurance industry, incentive compensation in, 63

Heritage Institute, 27n.

Hiring: cost of, xix, 75–76, 81, 114; retention incentives in, 213

Hiring bonuses, 64, 211, 213, 390

Holidays, as paid time off, 226, 228, 229, 240–241

Home computer allowances, 231, 283–284

HCAHPS (Hospital Consumer Assessment of Healthcare Providers and Systems), 197

Hospitals: community benefits provided by, 391; as executive work environment, xxv–xxvi, 386; 375–376; management challenges in, xxv–xxvi, 375–376, 386, 389; number of, 385; public role of, 375; size and complexity of, 379; tax-exempt status of, 375

Housing allowances/subsidies, 213, 278, 295, 296

Housing loans, as retention incentive, 211

Hurdles, for incentive plans, 183, 188

Incentive compensation, 153–221; above-average, 59, 62, 68; administrative guidelines for, 172–173; advantages and disadvantages of, 157, 158–159; all-employee, 176, 216–217; annual, 62, 65, 154, 155, 156, 173–174, 175–176, 177, 182, 184–187, 218, 219–220; award amount determination in, 61–62, 188–192, 208–210; below-average, 62; benefits *versus,* 47–48, 71; best practices in, 218–220; boards' attitudes toward, 46–47; bonuses *versus,* 155; CEOs' administration of, 168; compensation committees' administration of, 354, 371; decentralized, 186; deferral of awards in, 193–194; definition of, 60; design of, 160–161, 218–220; discretionary, 178–179, 192–193; documentation of, 173; effectiveness of, 160–161; eligibility for, 175–176, 218; elimination of, 71; emphasis on, 60–63; equity-based, 217; executives' attitudes toward, 15–16; fixed *versus* variable components of, 63; formal plan documents of, 170–172, 345; "free-rider problem" of, 163; funding for, 182–184; goal-setting scales for, 178, 188–192, 200, 201–202, 206; governance of, 220, 351; hybrid short-term/long-term, 174–175; importance of, 153; internal champions of, 161; limits to, 166; long-term, 62, 65, 68, 154, 156, 174–175, 176, 177, 182, 184, 188, 213, 218, 220; management of, 62; as market value component, 78–79; maximum-award levels of, 176–178, 179, 190–191, 200, 201–202, 206; at median

or average levels, 64–65; outcomes of, 71; with overlapping long-term cycles, 182, 183; oversight of, 168–173, 348, 364; overview of, 154–157; as percentage of salary, 47, 61; as percentage of total compensation, 14, 78–79; performance effects of, 67; performance measures of, 188, 194–199; performance period duration of, 182; performance scales of, 219; plans , 6, 25, 67, 153–221; prevalence of, 14–15, 61, 173–175; as private inurement, 158, 159; as profit-sharing mechanism, 165; pro rata payment of, 308; purpose of, 157–159; for recent performance, 145–146; regulations pertaining to, 164–168; relationship to tax status, 158, 159; review of, 169–170, 171, 220, 371; salary increase *versus,* 126, 152; special-purpose, 174; structure of, 181–194, 219; target-award levels of, 177, 178, 179, 180, 190–191, 200; three-point scales for, 177, 178, 180–181, 200, 201; threshold-award levels of, 177, 178, 180–181, 200, 201–202; trustees' administration of, 168–169; trustees' attitudes toward, 16; two-point scales for, 200; unintended consequences of, 61; utility of, 156–157

Incentive opportunity, 176–181; annual, 177, 178–179, 180–181; best practices for, 218; definition of, xxix, 176–177; long-term, 177, 180–181; relationship to compensation philosophy, 181; total, 181

Income, of physicians, 53

Industry meetings attendance, employer-paid, 300–301, 302

Inflation, 5, 11, 36; compensation data adjustment for, 107, 110; competitive compensation–related, 36; in cost of living, 135; in costs and revenues, 11; drivers of, 135; effect of surveys on, 11; market value effects of, 10; merit pay effects of, 137, 138–139, 141–142; as salary increase determinant, 133–135, 143, 385

Information, impact on compensation levels, xxii

Information gathering, 361

Information technology executives, pay levels of, 135

Insiders, xxiii, 165

Institute for Policy Studies, 27n.

Insubordination, as basis for termination, 309

Insurance policies: life insurance premium reimbursement for, 273. *See also* Healthcare benefits

Integrated Healthcare Strategies, 276n.

Intellectual capacity, of workers, 20

Intermediate sanctions, 3, 55–56, 79, 119, 164–165, 210, 354. *See also* Reasonableness, rebuttable presumption of, 3; avoidance of, 365–366, 369–370; compensation committees' response to, 350–351; definition of, xxiii; effects of, xxiv; implication for board's oversight responsibility, 355–356; as private inurement, 165–166; relationship to presumption of reasonableness, 79, 119; retention incentives–related, 18; severance benefits–related, 323

Internal equity, 113, 130

Internal equity analysis, 105–106

Internal Revenue Code (IRC): excess benefit transaction regulation of, 343; private inurement and private benefit regulations of, 164–165, 166–167, 169–170, 171, 343; Section 457, 248; Section 457(b), 233, 248; Section 457(f), 233; Section 501(c)(3), 343; Section 4958, xxiii, 152n., 167, 343, 347. *See also* Intermediate sanctions

Internal Revenue Service (IRS): audits by, 366, 373n.; comparability data regulation of, 56; fair market value definition of, 79, 80–81; as governance best practices source, 346–347; governance ruling of, 340; incentive compensation rulings of, 158; taxation on benefits regulations of, 232–233

Internal Revenue Service Form 990, xxiv, 44, 96, 365. *See also* Disclosure: availability of, 347, 367, 384; disclosure requirements of, 126; effect on compensation levels, xxii; effect on public perception of executive compensation, 380, 384; as market data source, 85–88; as peer group data source, 93, 110; perquisite disclosure requirement of, 301; recency of data on, 107; Schedule J of, 278; Schedule O of, 388; supplemental benefits disclosure on, 273, 274; weaknesses of, 86–88; wrong or misleading data on, 104

Internal Revenue Service Form W-2, 64

Japan, salary disparity in, 20

Job analysis, 89

Job candidates, personal value determination of, 113, 114

Job changes, costs of, 75

Job descriptions, 306, 315

Job evaluation, 21, 77

Job responsibilities. *See* Responsibilities

Jobs: economic value of, 3; "going rates" for, 81, 387

Job size, comparison with benchmark jobs, 108–109, 110

Job titles: changes in, 120; as incentive plan eligibility criterion, 175; on Internal Revenue Service Form 990, 86–87; as job value indicator, 89; as perquisites, 278, 299; relationship to job responsibilities, 49, 89, 90

Job value determination, of executive compensation. *See* Market value determination, of executive positions
Johns Hopkins Medicine, 94
Joint ventures, 324–325, 326

Kaiser Permanente, 91

Labor markets, for healthcare executives, 40–42, 73–74; effect on compensation levels, xix, 3; regional, 73–74, 75; size of, 75, 385
Large healthcare organizations. *See also* Multihospital systems
Laws, compliance with, 366–367
Leaders: competencies of, 146–147; public benefits provided by, 391
Leadership: of compensation committees, 50–51, 353; need for effective, 388; recruitment and retention of, 39; stability of, 390–391; transitions in, 212
Leadership development programs, 42, 146–147
Legal services allowances, 283–284
Legislators: concern about executive compensation levels, 377; concern about healthcare cost increase, 378; explanation of compensation philosophy to, 52–53
Liabilities, executive compensation-related, 364–365, 371–372; retirement benefits as, 255–256, 257, 261
Life insurance, 23, 24, 25, 227, 235–237, 252, 292–293, 321–322, 328; compensation strategy for, 34; as deferred compensation funding source, 262–263; group policies, 236, 237, 268; permanent policies, 236–237, 268; post-retirement, 276; prevalence of, 268; purposes of, 236; as retention incentive, 211; split-dollar, 236, 262, 263, 268,

274; supplemental, 235–237; term policies, 237, 268
Long-term care/disability benefits, 238, 239–240, 267, 292–293; post-retirement, 276
Loyalty, effect of benefits on, 228
Luncheon club memberships, 278, 279, 281, 283–284, 286, 287–288, 300

Management, differentiated from governance, 209, 345–346, 355–357, 360–361
Market adjustments, of salary increases, 135–136
Market data: selection of, 88–89; sources of, 83–88
Market movement, 107, 134–135; relationship with salary increase, 137–138
Market pricing, 77
Market value: communication about, 148; definition of, 75–83; differentiated from fair market value, 79–80; as executive compensation measure, 11; rates of change of, 132; relationship to labor market size, 75
Market value determination, of executive positions, 73–111, 77; benchmarks for, 96–98; best practices in, 109–110; data adjustment in, 107–109; data samples for, 98–103; data validation for, 104–106; degree of dispersion in, 106–107; dispersion of pay component of, 76–78; inflation factor in, 10; job analysis in, 89–90; organization analysis in, 90–91; organization size as determinant in, 98–103; peer group comparability data sources for, 95–96; peer group selection for, 91–94; prestige as determinant in, 98–103; as salary administration component, 114; for setting of base salary, 113; value of person *versus* value of job in, 82–83

Mayo Clinic, 91, 94

Media: communication with, 354; executive compensation coverage by, 379–380, 384

Median compensation, 5, 7; competitiveness of, 38; effect of inflation on, 36; explanation to stakeholders, 53; fair market value of, 80–81; implication for executive recruitment, 42; influence on organizational culture, 67–68; less than, 5, 7; as market value basis, 77–78; prevalence of, 58, 77–78; regionally based, 43

Median salary, 16, 64–65; capping of, 123; positioning of, xxx

Medicare, 267; retrospective settlements in, 209

Membership dues, as executive perquisite, 231–232. *See also* Country club memberships; Luncheon club memberships

Mercer, 276n.

Mergers, 13, 212; as change-of-control cause, 324–325, 326; retention incentives and, 215

Merit increase guidelines, 137–39

Merit pay, 60–61. *See also* Incentive compensation plans: comparison with incentive compensation, 161–162; definition of, 137; goals of, 133; guidelines for determination of, 138, 139; inflationary component of, 137, 138–139, 141–142; integration with performance appraisal, 137–138; performance-based component of, 137–139, 140–142

Middle managers, incentive compensation for, 176

Midpoint salaries: adjustments for achievement of, 142–143; capping of, 142; market adjustments for, 136; merit-pay-based, 133

Minority groups, salary discrimination toward, 126–127

Misconduct, as cause for termination, 322

Mission, 70

Morale, 7, 228, 381

Multihospital systems: benefits offered by, 224; centralized, 198; compensation philosophies of, 21, 33; goal setting for, 364; incentive compensation eligibility in, 176; incentive compensation plans of, 176, 185–186; incentive compensation plans of, 61, 62, 63, 175; increase in, 13; internal promotions in, 42; number of, 385; organization-wide performance goals of, 164; pay mix in, 66; travel perquisites of, 294

Negotiations: arms'-length, xxii, 80; discretionary, 334–336; over goal setting, 153–154; of special deals, 363

Net operating income, 196

Net operating margin, 196

New positions, salary ranges for, 118

90th percentile compensation, 12, 37, 58–59, 60, 207; "aspirational" peer group-based, 94; without incentive compensation plans, 91

Not-for-profit organizations, state laws governing, 344

Not-for-profit status, impact on compensation levels, xix–xxi

Offer letters, 307, 336

Offices and office furnishings, as perquisites, 231, 281, 298–299

Operating expenses: as organization size measure, 10–11; reductions in, 21–22

Operating plans, 194, 195, 200

Operating profit margins, xxv, 42

Opportunity, definition of, xxix

Organizational culture, effect of pay mix on, 65–70

Organization analysis, 90–91

Organization size: as compensation level determinant, xviii, 10, 12–13; as market value determinant, 90, 98–103; measures of, 10–11; as salary level determinant, 6, 20–21

Outsourcing, 4, 20, 21, 224

Overpayment, 2–8. *See also* Intermediate sanctions

Paid time off (PTO), 226, 228, 229, 240–243; prevalence of, 268; relationship to flexible benefit plans, 265; supplemental, 241–243; unused, conversion to compensation, 242–243

Part-time workers, 231

Patient satisfaction performance measures/goals, 196–197, 199, 205, 208

Pay at risk. *See* Incentive compensation

Pay for performance. *See* Incentive compensation: definition of

Pay mix: effect on organizational culture, 65–70; performance-oriented, 68–69; standard, 67–68

Payroll cost control. *See* Cost control

Pay Without Performance: The Unfilled Promise of Executive Compensation (Bebchuk and Fried), 7–8

Peer groups: appropriateness of, 10; "aspirational," 94; CEOs' selection of, 71; choice of, 54–57, 70, 71, 91–94; as compensation policy focus, 38; custom-tailored, 93, 95–96, 96, 110; disclosure of, 54; inappropriate, 70; for market value determination, 91–94, 95–96, 109–110; national (broadly defined), 54, 55, 56–57, 71, 92, 96, 110; performance relative to, 205; of physician-led systems, 92; redefini-

tion of, 74; regional (narrowly defined), 43, 55, 56–57, 93; selection of, 88; specialized, 74; survey data about, 92–93

Pension Benefit Guarantee Corporation (PBGC), 245

Pension restoration plans, 252, 253

Percentage, definition of, xxix

Percentiles, of executive compensation: definition of, xxix; 10th percentile, 12; 25th percentile, 12, 129; 50th percentile, xxix; 60th percentile, 16, 59, 64–65, 136; 65th percentile, 16, 59, 64–65; 75th percentile, xxix, 12, 16, 36, 37, 42, 58–59, 64–65, 106–107, 123, 129–130, 385, 387; 90th percentile, xxix, 12, 37, 58–59, 60, 94, 207

Perceptions, of executive compensation, 1, 375–392; best practices for addressing, 391–392; of executive compensation governance, 389; media perceptions, 378, 379–380; politicians' perceptions, 381–382; public perceptions, 376–379; regulatory risks of, 383; response to, 383–391; shaping of, 383–391; stakeholders' perceptions, 380–381

Performance and incentive compensation: above-average compensation relationship, 57–58; best-in-class, 206; breakthrough, 206; comparison with competencies, 147; compensation level relationship of, xviii, 13–16, 46–47; components of, 145; departmental, 162, 163, 164; fixed pay relationship of, 63; ideal, 205–206; implications for involuntary termination, 323; long-term, 68–69; peer group selection based on, 93, 94; retirement benefits relationship, 63–64; salary increase based on, 115, 125–216, 133–134, 140–142, 151, 152

Performance appraisals: of CEOs, 350, 354; comparison with incentive compensation, 161–162; differences in, 140, 141; integration with merit pay, 137–138; metrical scales for, 204–205; pass/fail approach in, 205; relationship to salary increases, 147–148

Performance evaluations: differentiated from performance measurement, 210; for incentive awards determination, 208–210

Performance management, incentive plans as basis for, 161–164

Performance measurement, differentiated from performance evaluation, 210

Performance measures, of incentive plans, 194–199, 208; for annual incentive plans, 195–196; best practices in, 219–220; for long-term plans, 198–199; number of, 197; weighted, 197, 220

Perquisite allowances, 301

Perquisites, 22–25, 277–302; approval and monitoring of, 364–365; as benefits, 278; benefits *versus,* 231–232; best practices in use of, 302; changing patterns in use of, 301–302; compensatory, 232; definition of, 277; differentiated from business expenses, 280–281; differentiated from supplemental executive benefits, 279–280; disclosure of, 277, 301; documentation of, 315–316; economic value of, 278; effect on productivity, 282; employment agreement provisions for, 310, 336; governance of, 351; as incentive compensation component, 63; noncompensatory, 231–232; overview of, 278–281; as percentage of salary, 47; as percentage of total compensation, 78–79; prevalence of, 283–284;

public relations risks of, 299–300; purpose of, 281–282; reduced emphasis on, 72; relationship to community values, 44; review of, 354; special, documentation of, 307; taxation of, 300–301; tax gross-ups on, 224–225, 231, 281, 297–298, 301

Personal days, 240

Personal value: as basis for salaries, 151; determination of, 113, 114; relationship to salary range, 122–123

Phantom equity, 166

Philosophy, of compensation. *See* Compensation philosophy

Physicians: as CEOs, 135; compensation for, legal and regulatory risks of, 344; as hospital administrators, 386; income of, 53

Planning, influence of incentive compensation on, 16

Politicians, criticism of executive compensation by, 381–382

Positioning, of salaries, xxx

Precedent, as basis for compensation committee operation, 352

Prestige. *See* Privileges

Private benefit, 164–166, 209–210; definition of, 221n.; differentiated from private inurement, 221n.

Private inurement, 164–167, 209–210; definition of, xxiii, 221n.; differentiated from private benefit, 221n.; effects of, xxiii; profit pools and, 183–184

Privileges, as job value determinant, 98; perquisites as, 231, 277, 279, 281

Productivity, effect of perquisites on, 282

Professional societies: continuing education provided by, 290–291; employer-paid memberships in, 279, 281, 288–289, 300–301

Professional society meetings, employer-paid attendance at, 300–301, 302
Profit margins: operating, xxv, 42; of tax-exempt hospitals, 3
Profit pools, for incentive plans, 183–184, 188
Profit-sharing plans, 14; avoidance of, 219; defined-contribution retirement plans as, 247
Profit-sharing pools, 166
Projects: bonuses for, 18–20; retention incentives and, 212
Promotion: external, 67–68; incentive compensation *versus,* 152; internal, 39, 67–68; salary increases associated with, 120; salary ranges associated with, xix; of second-level executives, 41
Proxies, as market data source, 86
Public, communication with, 354
Public perceptions, of executive compensation, 375–392
Public relations aspect, of employment agreements, 337

Quality control, in data validation, 104–106
Quality dashboards, 196
Quality improvement plans, 196

Rabbi trusts, 264, 276n.
Racial discrimination, in executive compensation, 48, 336
Raises. *See* Salary increase
Reasonableness, rebuttable presumption of, 55–56, 79, 119, 167, 168; as abusive practice, 383; based on salary ranges, 152n.; as best practice, 383; compensation committees' responsibility for, 365–366, 371; "disqualified persons" issue in, xxiii, 366, 372–373n.; establishment of, 347, 348–349, 383; evidence of, 373n.; of incentive

awards, 209–210; regional differences in, 56; of retention incentives, 216
Recruitment, 22; at above-average compensation levels, 45; compensation levels required for, xx; competitive labor market for, 41–42; difficulties in, 386–387; employment agreements used for, 336; external, xx, 40, 42, 76, 386; external, *versus* internal, 5; hiring costs in internal, xx, 39, 40, 42, 76; regional factors in, 54, 73–74; role of benefits in, 39, 223, 228–229, 230; role of executive compensation in, xix; severance policies used for, 336; use of employment agreements in, 307
Referrals, payment for, 344
Regional differences/factors: in compensation levels, 10, 55; in compensation philosophy, 74; in executive job choices, 41; in executive recruitment, 54, 73–74; in reasonableness of compensation, 56
Regional labor markets, 73–74, 75
Regression analysis: definition of, 111n.; in market value determination, 95, 99
Regression formulas: definition of, 111n.; or data validation, 104–105
Regulations, executive compensation–related, 2–3; compliance with, 274, 366–367; impact on compensation levels, xxii–xxv
Religious discrimination, 336
Relocation expenses, 295–296, 335
Reorganization, 212
Resignation, notice of, 305
Resource allocation, 42, 53, 70
Responsibilities: as basis for executive compensation, xviii, 21; of benchmark jobs, 108; clarification of, 306; of composite jobs, 98; employ-

ment agreement descriptions of, 314–315; for executive compensation, 347–355; failure to perform, 322; increase in, 120; relationship to job titles, 49, 89, 90; for salary administration, 117; as salary level determinant, 6; shared, 90; for understanding benefits, 271–272

Restructured positions, salary ranges for, 118

Retention: compensation levels required for, xx, 115, 387, 390–391; competitive labor market for, 41–42; cost of, 75, 76, 114; effect of high salaries on, 143–144; role of benefits in, 39–40, 223, 228–229, 230; role of executive compensation in, xix; salary adjustments and, 115; salary ranges required for, 126

Retention agreements, 307; documentation of, 330

Retention incentives, 17–18, 210–216; definition of, 210–211; effectiveness of, 215; prevalence of, 211; retirement benefits as, 256; special bonuses as, 19–20; types of, 213–215; uses for, 211–213; value of, 215–216

Retirement: early, 327–328; implication for severance benefits, 327–328

Retirement age, 327–328, 329; cliff vesting at, 248; implication for retirement benefits, 335; retention incentives related to, 212–213, 214

Retirement benefits and plans, 23, 243–264. See also Supplemental executive retirement plans (SERPs)

Retirement planning, 292–293

Retirement savings plans, 223, 226–227, 243, 245

Revenues, as organization size measure, 10–11

Risk, retention benefits as response to, 211–212

Risk taking: entrepreneurial, 68; unnecessary, 69

Roth plans, 247

Rural hospitals, executive compensation levels of, 10, 55

Sabbaticals, 283–284

Safe harbors, for intermediate sanction risk minimization, 167, 168

Salary: appropriate, 113; benefits as percentage of, 47; benefits versus, 47–48, 229; capping of, 122–123, 142; communication about, 148–151; definition of, 116; disparities in, 20–21, 27n., 225; documentation of, 315; effect on executive retention, 143–144; fairness of, 126–127; as foundation of executive compensation, 113; freezing of, 142; hierarchy of, 6; inappropriate, 113; incentive compensation as percentage of, 47; as market value basis, 78–79; median, 16; for new executives, 151; perquisites as percentage of, 47; positioning of, xxx; relationship with total cash compensation, 16; role in recruitment, 39; role in retention, 39; as total compensation determining factor, 59

Salary administration, 6, 114–116; best practices in, 8, 151–152, 343, 346–347, 368, 369–372; broadbanding in, 131; bylaws, charters, and policies for, 343, 344–345; communication in, 148–151; by community leaders, 389; compensation committee's role in, 220, 350–351; definition of, 114, 117; differentiated from management, 209, 345–346, 355–357, 360–361; fairness of, 126–127; goal of, 120–121; impact on compensation levels, xxi–xxii; impediment to, 7; of incentive plans, 220, 351; lack of, 340–342;

cause–based, 322–323; lump sum payments of, 319; media reports on, 380; purpose of, 317–318; relationship with years of service, 319–320; release from claims requirement for, 316, 320–321; retention incentives and, 211, 215; at retirement, 327–329, 337; *versus* retirement benefits, 321–322; separation agreement provisions for, 331; tenure-based, 320, 333; voluntary termination–based, 305, 322, 325

Severance packages, 24

Severance policies, 332–333; boards' objections to, 335; as income security, 307; for recruitment, 336

Severance practices, 334

Sex discrimination, 336

Sick-leave benefits, 226, 228, 229, 238–239, 240, 241; unlimited, 241, 243

Silo orientation, 163

Small healthcare organizations/hospitals: above-average compensation policies of, 57–58; closure of, 13; executive pay levels in, 55; executive recruitment from, 40, 41–42, 45; incentive compensation plans of, 61, 62, 175; incentive opportunity in, 179; organization-wide performance goals of, 164

Smart phones, as perquisites, 231–232, 278–279, 300, 302

Social contract, 244

Social justice, 20

Social Security, 243–244, 245–246, 257–258, 261, 264

Solicitation: employment agreement prohibition of, 310; separation agreement prohibition of, 331

Spouse travel perquisites, 284–285, 295, 301

Stability, of healthcare executive leadership, 390–391

Stakeholders: communication with, 354; explanation of compensation philosophy to, 44–45, 52–54; influence on tax-exempt status, 66; justification of executive compensation to, 44–45, 367–369; perception of organizational values by, 66; perceptions of executive compensation by, 380–381

State hospital associations: as market data source, 84; surveys sponsored by, 95

Stay bonuses, 24, 210–211. *See also* Retention incentives

Stock options, xxi

Strategic initiatives performance measures, 199

Subsidiary hospitals, employment agreements with, 304

Succession planning, 328

Sullivan Cotter, 276n.

Sunset clauses, 329, 337

Supplemental executive retirement plans (SERPs), 64, 247–264, 307; account-balance plans, 263; after-tax basis for, 248, 249; amendments to, 330; cash-balance, 244, 246; choices among, 226–227; cliff vesting of, 248, 249–250; compensation strategy for, 34; Conference Board recommendations regarding, 224; defined-benefit, 87, 111n., 214–215, 223, 229, 244–246, 252, 253–257, 259, 260–261, 264, 268; defined-contribution, 229, 244, 246–247, 252, 257–261; definition of, 247; documentation of, 330; employment agreement provisions for, 330; excessive, 340–342; expansion of, 224; as fixed compensation, 63–64; funding for, 263–264; implication for severance benefits, 329; as liability, 257; life insurance as, 236–237; life insurance–funded, 262–263;

lump sum value of, 256; non-executive retirement benefits *versus,* 225; for non-executive workforce, 24–25; nonqualified, 247–264; payment in lieu of, 335; pension restoration plans, 252, 253; prevalence of, 268; qualified, 64, 243–244, 258; rabbi trusts for, 264; rationale for, 24, 252; recordkeeping for, 274; as retention incentive, 39–40, 211, 214–215, 249, 256; risks of, 256; severance benefits *versus,* 321–322; Social Security, 243–244, 245–246, 257–258, 261, 264; substantial risk of forfeiture (SRF) of, 248, 250, 251; target-benefit, 23, 252, 259–261, 268; taxation on, 232–233; as unfunded benefit, 263; vesting requirements for, 8; voluntary savings plans, 243, 245

Supply and demand, 134, 135, 384–387

Surveys, of executive compensation, 27n., 276n.; adjustment of data from, 107; "all systems"/"all hospitals" data sets of, 99, 100–103; data comparability tables of, 99, 100–103; data validation in, 104–105; influence on compensation levels, 12; limitations to, 85; as market value data source, 83–85; national (general-purpose), 83–84, 85, 99; regional, 84, 99; specialized, 84; wrong or misleading data in, 104

Taxable benefit allowances, 273, 301

Taxation: on benefits, 232–233, 275, 276; as deferred compensation, 232–233; on executive compensation, xxii, xxiv; on perquisites, 300–301; on severance benefits, 319

Tax-exempt organizations, incentive compensation regulations affecting, 164–168

Tax-exempt status: implication for compensation levels, 377; political criticism of, 382; stakeholders' influence on, 66

Tax gross-ups, 224–225, 231, 281, 297–298, 301

Tax obligations, of executives, 8

Taxpayer Bill of Rights 2, 167

Taxpayer funding, for hospital services, 382

Taxpayers, explanation of compensation philosophy to, 52–53

Tax planning, 293–294

Tenure, 24; as basis for severance benefits, 320, 333; as salary disparity cause, 124

Termination: for cause, 321, 322–323, 331; change of control–related, 324–326; constructive, 324, 325, 326, 334; death-related, 321–322, 328; disability-related, 321–322, 328; double-trigger, 325, 326; employment agreement provisions for, 308, 309, 310, 316, 322–326; higher-than-average incidence of, 69; involuntary, 308, 309, 310, 313, 319–320, 321, 325; involuntary with cause, 323; involuntary without cause, 322–323, 328, 329, 333–334; nonrenewal-related, 326–327; reasons for, 317; retirement-related, 321–322, 327–328; single-trigger, 325, 326; voluntary, 321, 322, 325, 334; without severance benefits, 321–322; wrongful, 320

Top-hat plans. *See* 457(b) plans

Total compensation: annual review of, 152n.; benefits as component of, 270; comparability data for, 370; expected, xxix; as market value basis, 78–79; regulatory requirements regarding, 79

Towers Watson, 276n.

Trade associations: continuing education provided by, 291; employer-paid memberships in, 289
Trade-offs, in compensation philosophy, 47–48
Training programs, 290–291
Transparency: as best practice, 347; in board–compensation committee relations, 361; in communication about executive compensation, 148–151; in salary administration, 127; special deals–related impediment to, 363; standards and protocols for, 367; in tax-exempt charities, 54
Travel, paid time off during, 241–242
Travel accident and life insurance policies, 235
Travel expenses: for attendance at conferences and meetings, 290; employer-paid, as perquisite, 231–232, 278, 281, 283–284, 294–295; review of, 351
Trustees: attitudes toward growth, 13; attitudes toward incentive compensation, 16; attitudes toward retention incentives, 17; executive compensation governance responsibility of, 1, 25, 26–27, 117; goal-negotiation role of, 153–154; incentive plan control by, 168–169; influence on compensation levels, xxi; intermediate sanctions on, 3; perception of executive compensation, 379; salary administration responsibility of, 119
Tuition reimbursement, as perquisite, 290
Turnover: in board membership, 304, 325; cost and risk of, 390; effect on compensation levels, xx; effect on performance, 390; in peer group

organizations, 56–57; reasonable amount of, 68; relationship to lack of incentive compensation, 155; relationship to salary level, 144; voluntary, 22

Uncompensated work, bonuses for, 19
Underpayment: compensation philosophy–based, 30; market adjustments in, 136; retention incentives–related, 18
Unemployment benefits, 317
Unions, 378
University of California–Los Angeles Medical Center, 94
Urban areas, labor markets in, 74
Urban hospitals, executive compensation levels of, 10, 55

Vacation benefits, 24, 226, 227, 228, 229, 240, 283–284; length of, 243; prevalence of, 268; use-it-or-lose-it policy for, 241
Values: of the community, 43–44; of executive job candidates, 41; represented in compensation philosophy, 30, 43–44, 70; stakeholders' perception of, 66
Variable pay, 47, 48; balance with fixed pay, 63–65
Vice presidents, incentive plan goals for, 185, 187
Vision care benefits, 234
Voluntary Hospital Association, 70

Welch, Jack, 224
Welfare benefits, 226
Windfalls, incentive awards as, 209–210
Women, discrimination toward, 48, 49, 126–127

About the Author

David A. Bjork, PhD, is senior vice president and senior advisor of the Executive Compensation and Governance practice at Integrated Healthcare Strategies in Minneapolis. He joined the firm as a partner in 1994 to start a division focused on executive compensation. Over the next decade, as practice leader, he helped develop the largest and one of the most respected executive compensation consulting practices serving the healthcare industry. He developed the standards the firm now uses for governance of executive compensation, compliance with intermediate sanctions regulations, CEO performance appraisal, and surveys of executive compensation.

Dr. Bjork has 30 years' experience consulting with healthcare organizations and helping their boards of directors with executive compensation issues. He has worked with major clients, for-profit and not-for-profit, in every segment of the healthcare industry. In addition to advising boards on executive compensation and governance of executive compensation, he has helped health systems reorganize to become more effective, work through post-merger integration, and maintain management continuity through major transitions.

One of the country's authorities on executive compensation in the healthcare industry, he frequently presents seminars on the topic to industry and professional associations and client organizations. He has published a number of articles, monographs, and book chapters on governance and on executive compensation in the healthcare industry.

Dr. Bjork earned an AB degree at Harvard University, an MBA in finance at the University of Chicago, and a PhD from the University of California at Berkeley. Before joining Integrated Healthcare Strategies, he was a consultant with the Hay Group for 12 years and, before that, taught at the University of California and the University of Chicago.

Dr. Bjork can be contacted at david.bjork@ihstrategies.com or davidabjork@comcast.net.